GL
AF443219

# ANIMAL LAPAROSCOPY

# ANIMAL LAPAROSCOPY

---

*Edited by*

## Richard M. Harrison, Ph.D.

Delta Regional Primate Research Center,
Tulane University
Covington, Louisiana

*and*

## David E. Wildt, Ph.D.

Institute of Comparative Medicine,
Baylor College of Medicine,
Houston, Texas


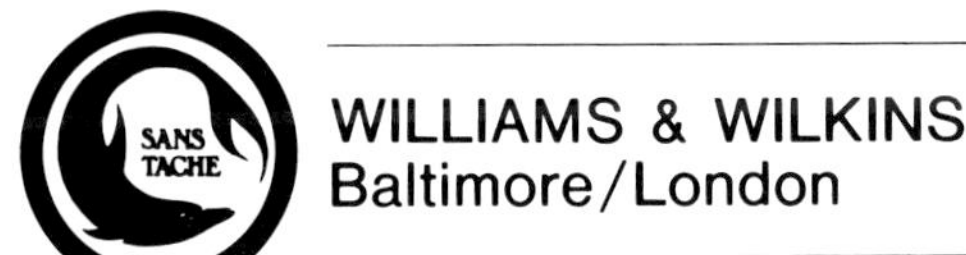


**WILLIAMS & WILKINS**
Baltimore/London

Copyright ©, 1980
The Williams & Wilkins Company
428 E. Preston Street
Baltimore, Md. 21202, U.S.A.



*Made in the United States of America*

Library of Congress Cataloging in Publication Data

Main entry under title:
Animal laparoscopy.

   Includes index.
   1. Abdomen—Diseases—Diagnosis. 2. Laparoscopy. 3. Veterinary gastroenterology. I. Harrison, Richard M. II. Wildt, David E.
SF851.A54      636.089'63'0754      79-9305
ISBN 0-683-03881-8

Composed and printed at the
Waverly Press, Inc.
Mt. Royal and Guilford Aves.
Baltimore, Md. 21202, U.S.A.

# FOREWORD

In recent years the science of laparoscopy has made noticeable strides in advancing our knowledge of physiology and anatomy. Initial advances were made in clinical medicine, particularly with advances in reproductive physiology. In the early 1970s, however, attention turned to research application of the laparoscope. Early studies were descriptive in nature, but soon procedures and techniques were developed which allowed a wide variety of research projects to be performed. Subsequent work allowed reapplication of new research techniques back to clinical practice and veterinary medical use.

Considerable contributions to the field of laparoscopy came from the Endocrine Research Unit of Michigan State University. Beginning in 1969 and continuing to the present, a small group of investigators first developed ancillary research techniques and then applied them to a wide variety of experimental animals ranging from wild to domestic species and including most common laboratory animals. The editors of the present volume were active participating members of that research group.

Dr. R. M. Harrison was instrumental in the application of laparoscopy to the squirrel monkey (*Saimiri sciureus*) and, particularly, the use of this instrument for testing contraceptive effectiveness in this nonhuman primate. Dr. Harrison's subsequent research at the Delta Regional Primate Research Center has further contributed to the knowledge concerning the reproductive physiology in a variety of nonhuman primates.

Dr. D. E. Wildt first developed laparoscopic techniques and procedures for the observation of ovaries in domestic swine. Working with Dr. Harrison, both in Michigan and in Louisiana, he gained experience with the laparoscopy of nonhuman primates and subsequently, at the Institute of Comparative Medicine in Houston, extended his laparoscopic studies to include other domestic animals and many wild species.

Drs. Harrison and Wildt are eminently qualified to edit this book. Their contributions, as individual chapters, are also welcome additions to the libraries of those who use laparoscopy in their research or clinical practice.

W. RICHARD DUKELOW, PH.D.

# PREFACE

Laparoscopy (observation through an endoscope inserted into the peritoneal cavity) allows direct viewing of the abdominal and pelvic organs with minor surgical interference and negligible animal trauma. Consequently, for the clinical veterinarian and veterinary or biomedical researcher this procedure has developed into a valuable and positive alternative to laparotomy. The book *Animal Laparoscopy* has been prepared as a guide and source of reference to these professions. The editors' goal has been to provide a definitive text on laparoscopic techniques in animals. To achieve this purpose, information has been presented for the novice or student as well as the experienced laparoscopist. Written and illustrative details have been included to introduce the beginner to various types of laparoscopy equipment and provide step-by-step procedures for performing anesthesia, animal restraint, and various diagnostic and surgical procedures. The experienced laparoscopist will discover that this text provides previously unpublished information, including a detailed explanation on the optical mechanisms of the laparoscope, methods for improving laparoscopic photography, and a description of the most recent laparoscopy equipment suitable for most animal species. Both the beginning and experienced operator should benefit from the discussions for resolving procedural complications and performing the latest clinical and research techniques.

The authors of the various chapters are undoubtedly some of the most experienced in the field and we, the editors, are fortunate to have contributions by some of the pioneers in animal laparoscopy. The experience of the authors varies over a wide range of species, providing the reader with the opportunity to study laparoscopic methods not only in common domestic and laboratory animals but in monkeys, zoo mammals, birds, and reptiles. This information has not been previously available in this detail.

The editors realize that laparoscopy is only one specialized procedure under the general terminology of endoscopy. We have resisted the temptation to dilute the text through descriptive detail of other endoscopic procedures. However, those interested in these other specialized areas of endoscopy (i.e., arthroscopy, cystoscopy, hysteroscopy) will find valuable information in sections on optical principles and instrumentation.

Finally, we acknowledge that, comparatively, animal laparoscopy is a relatively new field, particularly with respect to clinical veterinary medicine. Where applicable, the authors have been encouraged to emphasize their experiences on the use of laparoscopy for performing various clinical procedures, both diagnostic and surgical. In addition, the reader will discover that the authors have discussed the future implications of this technique, often suggesting exciting areas which to date have been essentially untouched. Consequently, it is hoped that this text will not only serve as a valuable teaching and reference source, but also provide impetus for further studies designed to eventually determine the ultimate applicability of laparoscopy in animals.

R. M. H.
D. E. W.

# ACKNOWLEDGMENTS

The editors wish to acknowledge the support of their respective institutions, colleagues, and staffs for assisting in the compilation of material for this text. Special thanks are due to Richard S. Hall, for providing the illustrations associated with the color plate figures, Carol Shull, Marie Schlenker, and Brenda Wildt for typing the manuscripts, and Sylvia Guthrie and Pat Schmidt for assistance and proofreading.

R. M. H.
D. E. W.

**Mitchell Bush, D.V.M.**
Office of Animal Health,
National Zoological Park,
Smithsonian Institution,
Washington, D.C.

**W. Richard Dukelow, Ph.D.**
Endocrine Research Unit,
Michigan State University,
East Lansing, Michigan

**Richard M. Harrison, Ph.D.**
Delta Regional Primate Research
Center,
Tulane University,
Covington, Louisiana

**Peter R. Klatt, Dr. Med. Vet.**
Department of Veterinary Medical
Research,
Hoechst AG,
Frankfurt, West Germany

**Duane C. Kraemer, D.V.M., Ph.D.**
Department of Veterinary Physiology
and Pharmacology,
Texas A&M University,
College Station, Texas

**Duane P. Maxwell, M.S.**
Department of Veterinary Physiology
and Pharmacology,
Texas A&M University,
College Station, Texas

**Rochelle Prescott, B.S. Ch.**
Dyonics, Incorporated,
Woburn, Massachusetts

**Stephen W. J. Seager, M.R.C.V.S.**
Institute of Comparative Medicine,
Texas A&M University/
Baylor College of Medicine,
Houston, Texas

**Karl H. Seeger, Dr. Med. Vet.**
Bacteriological Laboratory,
Hoechst AG, Frankfurt,
West Germany

**David E. Wildt, Ph.D.**
Veterinary Resources Branch
Division of Research Services
National Institutes of Health
Bethesda, Maryland

**Don M. Witherspoon, D.V.M.,
Ph.D.**
Division of Veterinary Services,
Spendthrift Farms,
Lexington, Kentucky

# CONTENTS

# CHAPTER 1

# Historical Development of Laparoscopy in Animals

## Richard M. Harrison, Ph.D.

---

### INTRODUCTION

The development of laparoscopic techniques in animals is historically unique. Unlike other biomedical techniques, which were first perfected in animal subjects and later applied to humans, laparoscopy had its origin in human application. Only in the last decade have these techniques been intensively applied to a wide variety of animal species for research and diagnostic evaluations.

### EARLY HISTORY

#### Bozzini's Light Transmitter

The broad field of endoscopy, of which laparoscopy is a specialized component, had its earliest beginnings with the "light transmitter" developed by Philipp Bozzini in 1804 (Rathert *et al.*, 1974). Bozzini's device was a vase shaped, leather covered tin lantern using a wax candle light source (Fig. 1.1). He indicated that it was possible to view into the mouth, nose, ears, vagina, dilated cervix, urethra, female urinary bladder, and rectum with this device. Bozzini claimed that script on a piece of paper, placed in the fundus of a human uterus immediately postpartum, could be seen as clearly using the device inserted through the vagina as if the paper was the same distance from a candle on a table (Bozzini, 1806). In spite of his success, some contemporaries considered his device a mere toy. Bozzini died 5 years later and the ridicule he had received apparently stifled other public reports of such devices for approximately 50 years, although efforts to improve viewing into body cavities continued.

#### Latter 19th Century

By the mid-1850s, Desormeaux had developed an "endoscope" for examining the urinary bladder (Benedict, 1951). This instrument employed an alcohol lamp flame for light, directing the light by a series of lenses and mirrors to the desired area (Figs. 1.2 and 1.3). In 1868, Kussmaul used a professional sword swallower as a subject to attempt viewing the inside of the stomach through a rigid tube (Balin *et al.*, 1966). Because of the inherent problem of transmitting light down a long viewing tube, this effort was unsuccessful. Bruck, a dentist, used a platinum wire loop, heated by an electrical current

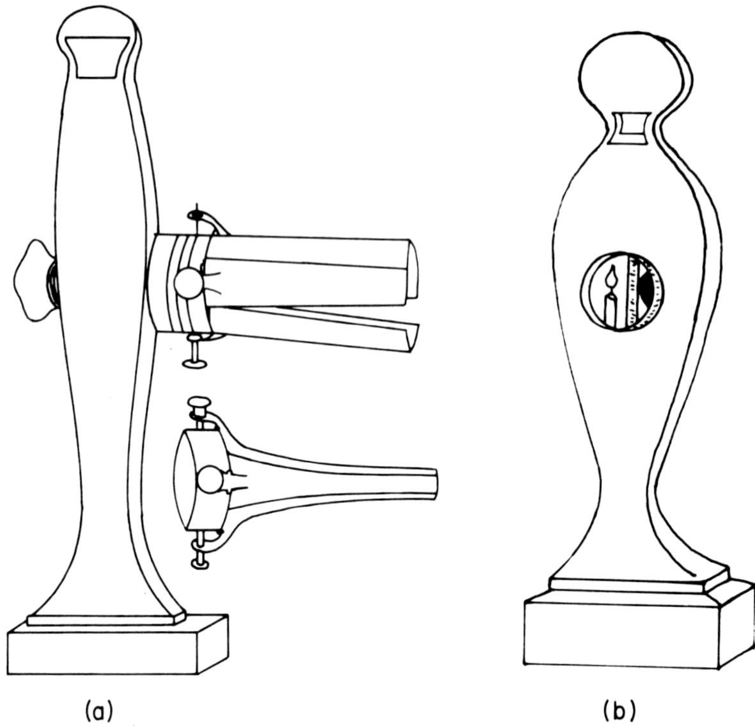

(a)                                                    (b)

**Figure 1.1**  Bozzini's light transmitter, circa 1806. **(a)** Device with eyepiece on the left and an expandable cannula attached on the right for viewing cavities such as the vagina or rectum. The cannula in its insertion mode appears below. (Reproduced with permission from *Journal of Medical Primatology* 5:73–81, 1976.) **(b)** Device as viewed from cannula side with cannula removed. Viewing passage is to the right of the central partition, the candle for light is to the left.

to provide greater illumination for inspection of the oral cavity. His "lamp" was the first internal light source (Fig. 1.4) and was later adapted for use in cystoscopy (i.e., examination of the urinary bladder cavity through the uretha). At about this same time, Pantaleoni used a device in women, similar to that developed by Desormeaux, to examine the uterine cavity transcervically (Silander, 1963), a procedure currently termed hysteroscopy.

These early endoscopists encountered two technical problems. First, when viewed through a cylindrical tube without the aid of lenses, the field of vision decreases as the length of the tube increases. This was the circumstance in these early investigations and, consequently, only those structures directly in line of sight could be observed. Second, these attempts were stifled by the lack of an adequate light source. The use of flames was often insufficient and necessitated reflection of the light into the cavity to be examined. Although the incandescent platinum wire loop did provide the additional light required for endoscopy, it had a short life expectancy and was also capable of traumatizing tissue due to heat generation. By the late 1870s, significant technological advancements in instrumentation had partially solved these problems. To broaden the visual field, Nitze, in cooperation with Leiter, incorporated optical lenses into the cystoscope (Fig. 1.5) so that structures outside the direct line of vision could be observed. The incandescent lamp was invented by Edison in 1880, and by 1883, Newman had miniaturized the electric light bulb. Dittel, in 1887, incorporated a small bulb into the distal end of the cystoscope to provide adequate illumination within the bladder cavity

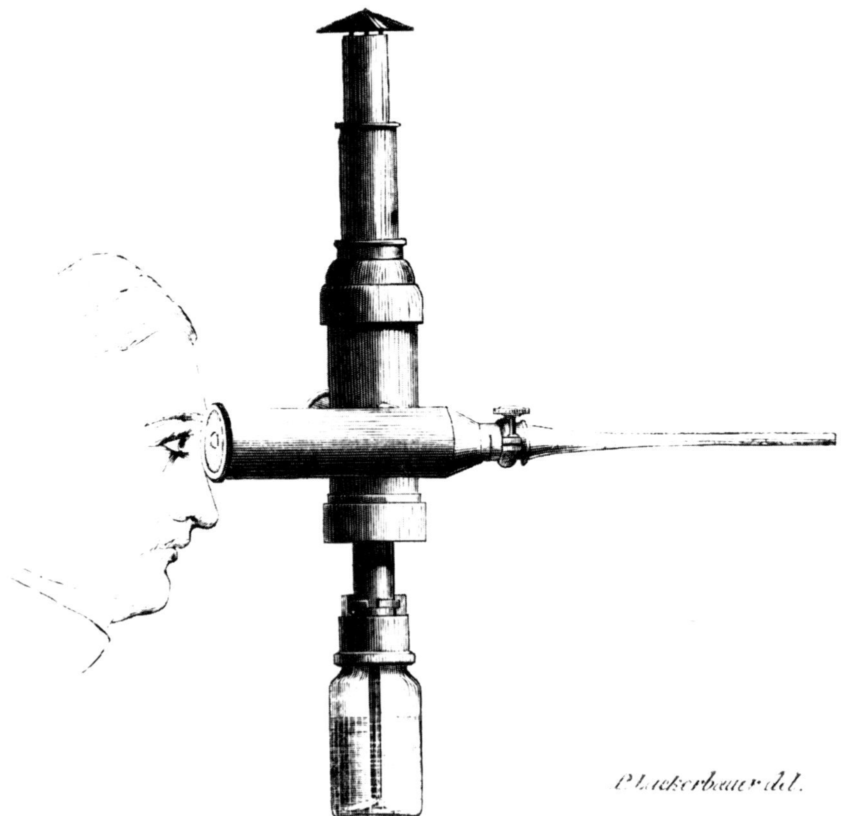


**Figure 1.2**  Desormeaux's endoscope, circa 1853. Device as it appeared in use. (Reproduced with permission, courtesy of National Library of Medicine, Bethesda, Maryland.)

(Fig. 1.6). Although this did solve the illumination problem, new problems developed, including trauma burn, excessive heat generation, and frequent bulb burn-out requiring the withdrawal of the instrument and bulb replacement.

### Early 20th Century

A new approach was described in 1901 by von Ott of Petrograd who placed patients in an extreme Trendelenburg position and then viewed the pelvic organs through an incision in the vaginal cul-de-sac. Illumination was provided by an incandescent lamp reflected by a head mirror through the incision. Although von Ott termed his procedure ventroscopy, it is considered the forerunner of the modern culdoscopy procedure.

The Nitze cystoscope provided the investigator with adequate illumination within a cavity and a wide field of vision. These characteristics allowed for the eventual adaptation of this instrument for viewing into cavities other than the urinary bladder. Kelling (1902) first reported the use of such a device for examining the abdominal organs of a dog and termed the procedure coelioscopy. The technique, as later described by Nadeau and Kampmeier (1925), involved applying a local anesthetic to a small area of the ventral abdominal wall, followed by the intraabdominal insertion of a Fiedler puncture needle. Filtered air was passed through the needle to establish a pneumoperitoneum, and then a trocar-cannula was inserted into the cavity through the anesthetized area and its stylet replaced with the thinnest Nitze cystoscope. Some eight years later Kelling (1910) announced that the procedure had been used on humans. In 1923, he

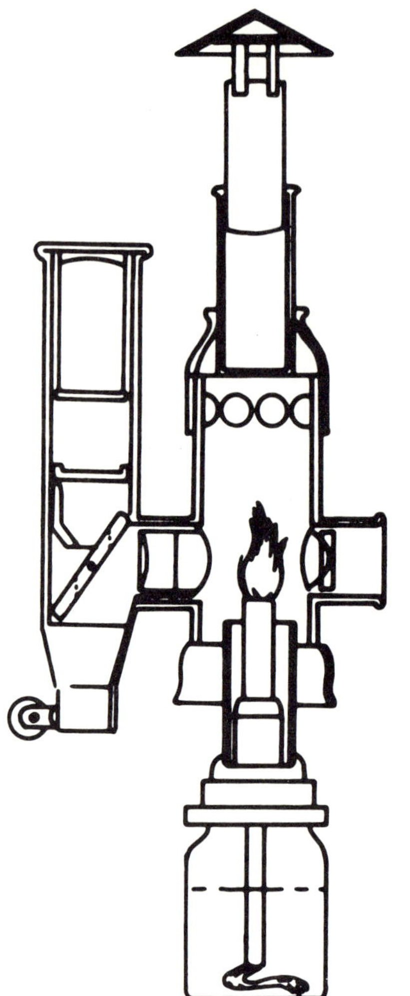

**Figure 1.3** Desormeaux's endoscope. Cut-away view with cannula removed and viewing tube rotated 90°. The mirror and lens to the right and left, respectively, of the alcohol lamp flame concentrated light into the viewing tube. The mirror in the viewing tube reflected the light into the desired area and had a hole in the middle to allow viewing. (Reproduced with permission from *Journal of Medical Primatology* 5:73–81, 1976.)

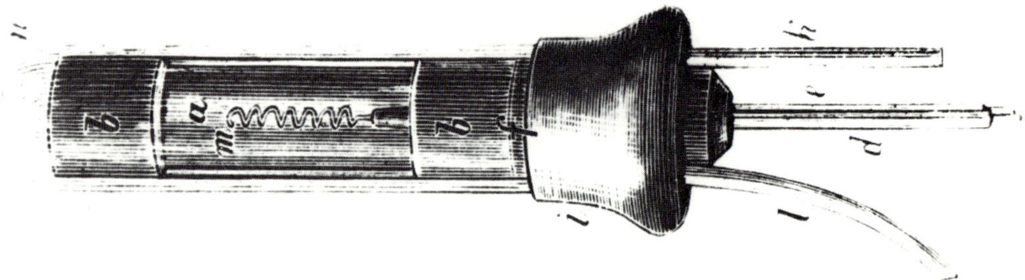

**Figure 1.4** Bruck's platinum wire loop, 1868. This electric lamp required circulating water for cooling but provided the first internal light source for endoscopy. (Reproduced with permission, courtesy of National Library of Medicine, Bethesda, Maryland.)

reported that the postwar economic situation in Germany had made it necessary to reduce hospital costs and that he had reduced the number of surgeries by increasing the diagnostic use of his procedure. By this time, Kelling's methodology had been simplified to a single puncture technique with pneumoperitoneum being established after trocar insertion.

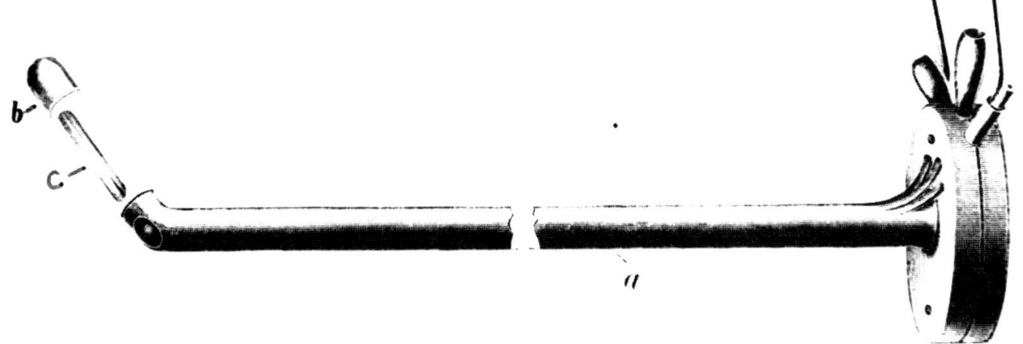

**Figure 1.5**   Nitze's cystoscope—early model with heated wire light source **(c)**. (Reproduced with permission, courtesy of National Library of Medicine, Bethesda, Maryland.)

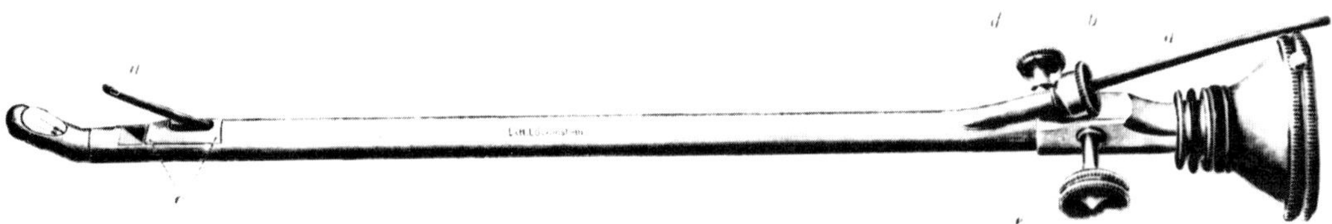

**Figure 1.6**   Nitze's cystoscope—later model with electric bulb illumination shown with ureteral probe inserted through channel. (Reproduced with permission, courtesy of National Library of Medicine, Bethesda, Maryland.)

Much of the honor Kelling should have received was instead accorded to Jacobaeus who independently developed a technique similar to Kelling's and reported the details eight years later (Jacobaeus, 1910). Jacobaeus published a number of reports on the clinical application of "thoraco-laparoscopy," i.e., endoscopy of the pleural, pericardial, and peritoneal cavities. In this latter procedure, initial insufflation was achieved through separate puncture needles and the trocar-cannula contained a trap valve which prevented air from escaping when the stylet was removed.

Jacobaeus is credited with the first use of the term "laparoscopy" to describe the technique of endoscopy of the peritoneal cavity. Although Kelling did not use the term to refer to his own work, this investigator's earlier use of the techniques in dogs would establish Kelling as the "father of veterinary laparoscopy."

The procedure used by Jacobaeus in humans was reported to be useful for the diagnosis of metastatic nodules of the liver, gastric carcinoma, and general carcinosis of the intestines. Using a modified procedure, he performed thoracoscopy and developed techniques for separating pleural lesions by galvanocautery to gain maximum therapeutic value of artificial pneumothorax in the treatment of pulmonary tuberculosis. After 1913, most of Jacobaeus' efforts continued in thoracoscopy, which he believed to be the procedure of most future value.

At about the same time, but unaware of the works of Kelling and Jacobaeus, Bernheim (1911) described a procedure termed "organoscopy" for visually diagnosing the abdominal state. This investigator used a proctoscope and an electric headlight for illumination. Details of his procedure were not reported, but clear viewing of the ventral surfaces of the liver and stomach and all portions of the gallbladder were claimed. This procedure of examining abdominal organs through a lensless tube appeared to be a retrogressive step to the procedure described by von Ott. However, others have continued to use similar techniques for many years and the modern minilaparotomy procedures may be considered the eventual result of these initial efforts.

During the next 30 years, the technique of abdominal endoscopy or laparoscopy was refined and used for the diagnosis of many abnormal conditions in human patients. Nordentoeft (1912) developed and patented an instrument called a "trocar-endoscope." He claimed the instrument could be used for suprapubic cystoscopy, arthroscopy of the knee, and observations within the body cavities of animals. By placing a female cadaver in a Trendelenburg position, Nordentoeft observed the pelvic organs, and reported a striking view when the abdomen was inflated. His clinical use of the technique was not reported, but his paper was the first to focus on the usefulness of endoscopy to view the pelvic organs in contrast to the upper (cranial) abdominal organs. In the same year, Tedesko reported trials with laparoscopy in patients with ascites before the Society of Internal Medicine and Pediatrics in Vienna. The resulting discussion by participants of this meeting indicated that some of those who had tried the procedure were satisfied and continued to use it, whereas others rejected it as too dangerous. Stolkind (1919), a Russian, restricted the use of laparoscopy to those cases where an exploratory laparotomy was contraindicated, an opinion almost diametrically opposed today. Renon (1913) of France, considered laparoscopy an excellent tool for the diagnosis of certain liver and peritoneal diseases but of little value in the diagnosis of intestinal lesions. Laparoscopy, in concert with X-ray and fluoroscopy, was used by Orndoff (1920) to diagnose tubercular peritonitis, hemoperitoneum, hydroperitoneum, ectopic pregnancy, and abnormalities of the ovaries and oviducts. The use of a pneumoperitoneum to facilitate laparoscopic examinations was well-presented by Orndoff (1920), Alvarez (1921), van Zwaluwenburg and Peterson (1921), and Peterson (1922). In 1921, Case reported four deaths resulting from air embolism following pneumoperitoneum. However, six years later, Sante (1927) reported 1000 cases where pneumoperitoneum was used with no side effects. As a result of these and other studies, some form of pneumoperitoneum continues to be used by all modern laparoscopists.

In Italy, Roccavilla (1914, 1920) modified the Kelling and Jacobaeus method by designing an instrument which used an external light source that was reflected into a trocar tube. An ocular placed above the tube and in direct line of view magnified the internal illuminated field. The trocar tube was designed to accommodate a Nitze cystoscope. In an effort to document laparoscopic observations, Korbsch (1921) of Germany, had watercolor sketches made of the views seen by laparoscopy. In some cases, the laparoscope was in place in the patient's abdominal cavity for three hours with no reported postoperative patient discomfort. Korbsch inflated the abdomen through a puncture needle that was closed at the lower end but had a lateral slit, similar to the Verres needle used today. Zollikofer (1924) of Switzerland reported that laparoscopy was the most practical means for the diagnosis of liver diseases. This investigator's efforts were noteworthy since he was the first to use carbon dioxide for insufflation because of its rapid absorptive characteristics. A nasopharyngoscope was used through the abdominal wall in dogs by Stone (1924). The trocar tube was fitted at its outer end with a rubber gasket to prevent insufflatory air loss. His experiences were limited to experimental work on dogs.

An unusual report by Steiner in 1924 described a technique termed "abdominoscopy," endoscopy of the abdominal cavity. Steiner considered this a "new" means of diagnosing abdominal diseases but described a technique quite similar to those of Kelling, Jacobaeus, Orndoff, and others. Steiner's abdominoscope resembled a cystoscope but with a moveable curved end which was used to move organs and thereby facilitate visualization. Insufflation was performed through a canal in the endoscope. Steiner's report is of value in that it emphasized the importance of patient positioning to examine various organs and described techniques for viewing the gallbladder, stomach, spleen, appendix, and other pelvic organs.

# MODERN HISTORY

## Developments in Human Laparoscopy

Many endoscopists consider Kalk the father of modern endoscopy because of his prolific publication in the field and his contributions to instrument development. He published more than 20 papers on laparoscopy between 1929 and 1939 which contributed to its widespread promotion. In addition, Kalk introduced the forward oblique 135° viewing system which was responsible for improving the popularity of laparoscopy in Europe (see Chapter 2 for illustrations of various directions of view). In comparison to the direct forward telescope, the forward oblique instrument provided a larger viewing area by rotating it on its long axis without changing the direction of the axis. Kalk's laparoscope with certain modifications is still used today.

Ectopic pregnancy was successfully diagnosed by Hope (1937) using laparoscopic techniques. Ruddock (1937) reviewed 500 laparoscopic cases and found that the technique was 67 to 100% effective for correctly diagnosing diseases of the abdominal organs. He also reported one death due to excessive biopsy hemorrhage, eight punctures of small bowel, colon, or stomach, and three unsuccessful attempts due to extensive adhesions in the abdominal cavity. By 1949, Ruddock had made laparoscopic examinations for diagnostic purposes in over 2500 cases. The patients ranged in age from six months to 85 years and were about equally distributed as to sex. Over 1000 biopsy samples were obtained. Ruddock (1937) noted that by changing the tilt of the table various organs could be viewed, including the liver, gallbladder, lower tip and edge of the spleen, the omentum, occasionally the appendix, greater curvature and anterior surface of the stomach, small intestine, large intestine, urinary bladder, uterus, oviduct, and ovary, all from a single infraumbilical puncture.

Anderson (1937) began to conduct experiments in living dogs using a right angle cystoscope and the flexible cannula and trocar designed by Nadeau and Kampmeier (1925). Anderson had a special gastrodiaphane (small electric light bulb passed through an esophageal tube to the stomach) made for use in humans that allowed for air dilation of the stomach and transillumination of the anterior wall and greater curvature. Similar techniques allowed study by transillumination of the colon and urinary bladder. Anderson reported that laparoscopy could be used to sever abdominal adhesions, incise ovarian cysts, and sterilize women by endothermic coagulation of the oviducts. This was the first reported use of laparoscopic techniques for sterilization.

Distal illumination with the light source as a component of the telescope itself is still employed in some laparoscopes today. However, the development of proximal light projection systems which eliminated the dangers of thermal tissue injury increased the practicality and usefulness of laparoscopy. Initially, quartz rods were used to transmit light from a proximal light source. The endoscope developed by Fourestier utilized this means of proximal light projection. Light from an external projector was reflected by a prism to the end of a clear rod of fused quartz. The quartz rod and the telescope both passed through a common sheath or cannula (Fig. 1.7, Balin *et al.*, 1966). This removed all danger to the patient and provided sufficient light for photographic documentation, but the quartz rods were costly, fragile, and cumbersome. By the early 1950s, Hopkins and Kapany in England, and van Heel in Holland (Kapany, 1958) had begun development of a system for light transmission through flexible fiber optic glass bundles. The use of a "cold" light transmission from an external projector and the return of a clearer, brighter image from the internal structures viewed was possible with the new laparoscopic telescopes containing the Hopkins lens system and fiber light bundles (Fig. 1.8). These refinements allowed the investigators to obtain true color photographs, motion pictures, and television images of the internal organs as seen by laparoscopy.

Palmer (1947) used laparoscopy to investigate causes of infertility. This investigator

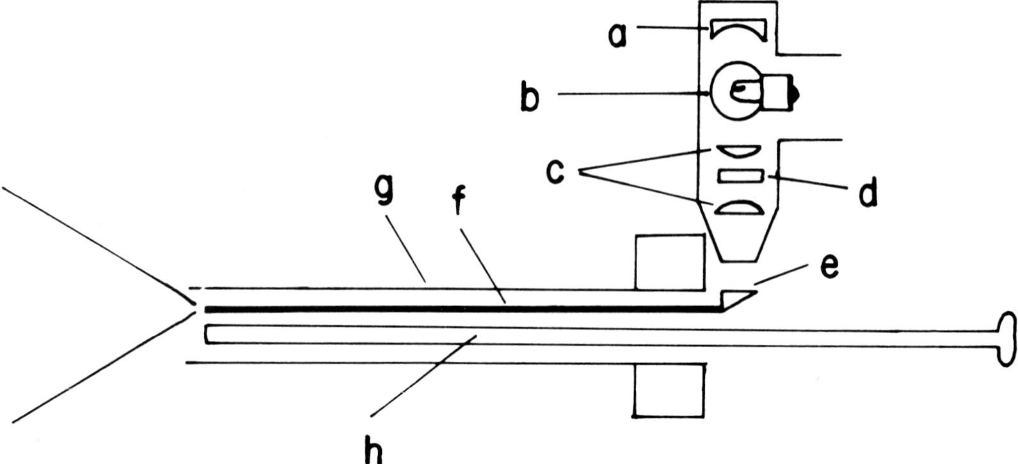


**Figure 1.7**  Diagram showing early light projection system using a quartz rod as a light guide: **(a)** reflecting mirror; **(b)** incandescent bulb; **(c)** condenser lenses; **(d)** catathermic glass; **(e)** prism; **(f)** quartz rod; **(g)** common sheath; and **(h)** telescope.

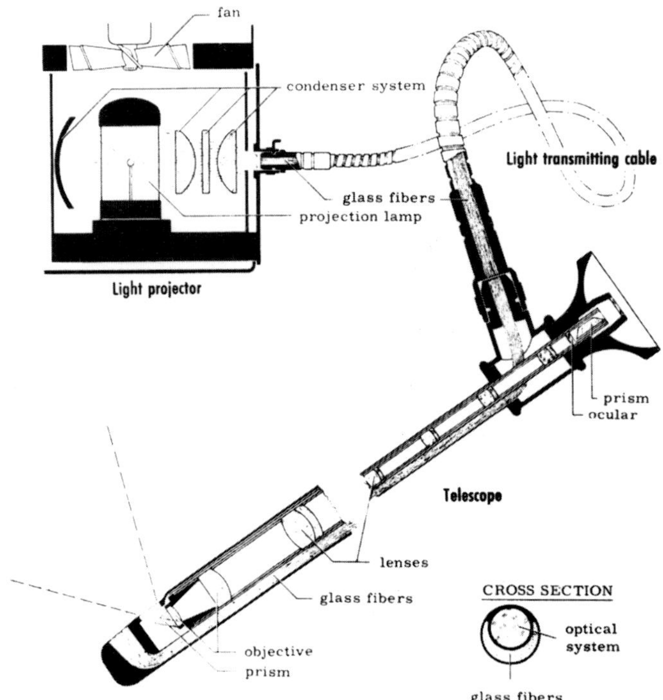


**Figure 1.8**  Diagram of fiber optic light system in a modern laparoscope. Light from the projector is transmitted via a detachable, flexible light cable to the laparoscope and through the instrument by the glass fiber guides. Heat produced by the lamp is mainly eliminated by filters; the rest is absorbed by the glass fibers so that the light leaving the distal end of the laparoscope is cold light. (Reproduced with permission of M. R. Cohen, *Laparoscopy, Culdoscopy and Gynecography*, W. B. Saunders Co., Philadelphia, 1970.)

used insufflation to establish a pneumoperitoneum and cautioned against intraabdominal pressure in excess of 25 mm mercury. Palmer also designed a uterine cannula to assist in the movement of the uterine fundus. Frangenheim (1960, 1965) of Germany described complications associated with laparoscopy, such as emphysema, thermal injury, hemorrhage, and infection. He recommended the avoidance of laparoscopy puncture through any previous laparotomy scars because of adhesions and possible puncture of attached bowel. In England, Steptoe (1967) published the first English language textbook on laparoscopy and promoted the safety and effectiveness of laparoscopic sterilization. He also developed techniques for the laparoscopic recovery of follicular ova. Semm (1969, 1970) described the surgical procedure of laparoscopy in detail and developed ancillary equipment for a number of procedures, including uterine biopsy and tubal sterilization. The value of the laparoscope as a precise and acceptable diagnostic tool for the gynecologist, as well as the indications, contraindications, and complications associated with this technique, were discussed by Smith and Dillon (1970). Ancillary techniques, including biopsy of ovaries, oviducts, and uterus; aspiration of fluid from the cul-de-sac, ovarian cysts, and hydrosalpinges; as well as tubal sterilization and lysis of avascular adhesions, have been described (Siegler and Garret, 1970). The laparoscopic recovery of human oocytes has also been well-discussed (Steptoe and Edwards, 1970; Lopata *et al.*, 1974; Berger *et al.*, 1975) and according to Steptoe (1979) was the method used to obtain an ovum for subsequent *in vitro* fertilization that resulted in the birth of Louise Brown in 1978. The number of laparoscopic sterilizations reported by the American Association of Gynecologic Laparoscopists (AAGL) exceeded 233,000 in the period 1971 to 1975. Large sterilization studies by Edgerton (1974) and Wheeless and Thompson (1973) reported more than 1000 patients each. The number of diagnostic procedures recently reported by members of the AAGL would raise the total number of laparoscopic procedures to more than 500,000 for the 1971 to 1979 period.

## Developments in Animal Laparoscopy

With the background of extensive human clinical studies, it has been relatively easy to adapt laparoscopic techniques for use in animals. As indicated earlier, the first report of laparoscopy in animals was conducted in dogs in the early 1900s (Kelling, 1902). Orndoff (1920) reported on the successful development of endoscopic techniques in animals but did not specify the species used. Anderson (1937) used dogs to perfect his skills prior to human clinical trials, but it was not until much later that laparoscopic techniques were considered for animal research or clinical veterinary medicine.

The increased desire in the 1950s and 1960s for a better understanding of reproductive function in animals stimulated interest in developing a means for directly observing the ovaries. Initially, some investigators implanted metal or plastic viewing ports, "windows," in the abdominal wall of the animal to provide direct visual access to ovaries. Others placed a chronic cannula into the abdominal wall for serial insertion of the laparoscope. These pelvic viewing ports or ovarian chambers were used in the rhesus monkey to observe follicular development and ovulation (Balin *et al.*, 1963). The chronic indwelling cannula placed in the flank of cows (Megale *et al.*, 1956; Dziuk *et al.*, 1958; Lamond and Holmes, 1965), sheep (Dierschke and Hyatt, 1969), or pigs (Betteridge and Raeside, 1962) provided means to repeatedly observe reproductive changes in these animals. In some studies, an open cylinder was inserted through the cannula with a light at the distal end; in other studies, a laparoscope with proximal light projection was used. The primary problem with these indwelling devices was the formation of intraabdominal peritoneal granulomas which obstructed vision and insertion of instruments. Various hormonal and enzymatic preparations were used in attempts to prevent granuloma formation, but these efforts produced concern over the effects of these treatments on ovarian structure and function. By the end of the 1960s, most investigators had abandoned the use of the indwelling cannula and adapted the trocar puncture techniques developed previously by laparoscopists in human patients. In part, the acceptance of the trocar puncture technique was due to the realization that numerous punctures could be made in a relatively small area without noticeable trauma to the animal. Extensive details of the procedures currently used and accepted will be provided in later chapters. However, the pioneering efforts of the numerous investigators responsible for the development of contemporary laparoscopy procedures in animals deserves discussion.

In domestic animals laparoscopy was first utilized in the cow by Goetze (1926) and then by Liess (1936) and Megale *et al.* (1956). These last investigators successfully viewed the ovaries by insertion of the laparoscope through a cannula placed in the vaginal fornix or paralumbar fossa. Megale (1967) later adapted similar techniques to the goat and sheep. Improvements in laparoscopic techniques for cattle, which included rumen displacement, were later reported by Wishart (1972) and Wishart and Snowball (1973). Recently, Seeger (1977) described his laparoscopic procedure using the trocar puncture technique and presented excellent color photographs of bovine ovaries to illustrate a clinical case. Similar work has also been published by Japanese investigators (Mori *et al.*, 1977). Ovulation in mares has been studied using 135° and 180°, 9 mm in diameter laparoscopes inserted in the flank area (Witherspoon and Talbot, 1970a, b). Additional descriptions of laparoscopy techniques for the mare as well as the donkey were reported by Heinze *et al.*, (1972) and by Heinze and Klug (1973). In general, successful laparoscopy in the cow and mare is performed under local anesthesia with the animal restrained in a stanchion or holding chute with the hindquarters elevated.

Hulet and Foote (1968) described a laparotomy restraining device for use in sheep and described a minilaparotomy technique for rapid examination of the reproductive tract. A number of investigators have reported on the procedural techniques for laparoscopy in sheep and goats. Roberts (1968) was the first to use laparoscopy in concert with the ventral trocar-cannula insertion technique. Thimonier and Mauleon (1969) used a similar approach in studies concerned with determining the effects of various hormonal treatments on ovarian function in the ewe. These investigators reported performing as many as 40 laparoscopic examinations per animal over a two year period with no adverse effects. Two years later, laparoscopy was reported as a safe procedure for the diagnosis of pregnancy in the ewe (Phillippo *et al.*, 1971). At this same time, Dukelow *et al.*, (1971), using techniques similar to those described in sheep, characterized ovarian morphology in the cycling African pygmy goat. More recent studies in the sheep have concentrated on the usefulness of various anesthetics (Boyd and Ducker, 1973), descriptive reports (Seeger, 1973), and auxiliary laparoscopic techniques such as ova collection (Snyder and Dukelow, 1974). Studies by Morris *et al.* (1976, 1977) have demonstrated the usefulness of the pregnant ewe as a model for studying fetoplacental circulation using combined laparoscopic-fetoscopic techniques.

Laparoscopy in the pig by the midventral approach was initially described by Wildt *et al.* (1973). Subsequent study established that this technique could be successfully utilized in this species for early pregnancy diagnosis and the serial collection of uterine fluids (Wildt *et al.*, 1975).

Lettow (1972) used laparoscopy in the dog to assist in obtaining liver biopsies but reported no procedural details. More recently, Wildt *et al.* (1977b) have described the specifics of anesthesia and laparoscopy in the dog and cat and have reported the uses of this technique for studying reproductive function and for making clinical diagnostic evaluations. Laparoscopy has also been utilized in the dog for characterization of ovarian morphology and ovulation (Wildt *et al.*, 1977c).

The versatility of a single laparoscopic telescope can be illustrated from the wide range of animals examined at the Endocrine Research Unit of Michigan State University.

All of the laparoscopy studies from this laboratory have been performed using a 5 mm in diameter, 130° laparoscope. The Endocrine Research Unit investigators have been responsible for adapting laparoscopy to more than 23 species ranging from mice to cattle and including rabbits, mink, chickens, sheep, goats, swine, and at least nine species of nonhuman primates.

Laparoscopy in rabbits requires some special techniques because of the flaccid nature of the abdominal organs. A suture threaded through the abdominal wall, around the ovarian ligament, and back through the wall allows the ovaries to be elevated for better viewing. Using this technique, the investigators were able to determine the time sequence of ovulation following mating, human chorionic gonadotropin (HCG) alone, or HCG and pregnant mares' serum gonadotropin (PMSG) administration (Fujimoto *et al.*, 1974).

Numerous studies in nonhuman primates have been conducted using laparoscopic techniques to examine the female reproductive organs. Balin and Wan (1969) detected induced ovulation in rhesus monkeys. With the use of specialized instruments, Dierschke and Clark (1976) were able to detect the ovulatory follicle in rhesus monkeys as early as day 3 of the cycle in 43% of the cases. Natural and hormonally controlled ovulations in cynomolgus monkeys were observed laparoscopically and allowed for short fertile matings (Jewett and Dukelow, 1971a, b; Dukelow *et al.*, 1972). The correlation of hormonal levels, sexual behavior, external physical features, and follicular morphology as detected by laparoscopy has provided better insight into the reproductive physiology of rhesus (Bosu, 1973; Bosu *et al.*, 1973; Bosu and Johansson, 1974; Batta and Brackett, 1974), pigtail (White *et al.*, 1973; Blakley *et al.*, 1977), and Japanese macaques (Nigi, 1977). Similar studies have also been conducted in baboons (Wildt *et al.*, 1977a; Eddy *et al.*, 1976). Ovarian anatomy, endometrial histology, and perineal swelling in chimpanzees have also been interrelated using this technique (Graham *et al.*, 1973).

Laparoscopy was first used to detect ovulation in squirrel monkeys in 1971 (Harrison and Dukelow). These same investigators also used the technique to examine seasonal adaptations (Harrison and Dukelow, 1973), follicular morphology (Harrison and Dukelow, 1974), and effects of a progestogen on ovulation (Harrison and Dukelow, 1971; Harrison *et al.*, 1974). Specialized laparoscopic techniques have also been developed for this species and include laparoscopically assisted recovery of uterine ova and uterine fluids (Ariga and Dukelow, 1977a, b). More recently, studies showing correlation of vaginal cytology and laparoscopically confirmed ovulation have been performed in the squirrel monkey (Jarosz *et al.*, 1977).

Laparoscopy for reproductive and clinical procedures in zoo or "exotic" animals has recently received attention. Standard laparoscopy procedures have been performed in the lion, tiger, jaguar, leopard, cheetah, bear, and numerous other wild species (Wildt *et al.*, 1978; Bush *et al.*, 1978b). The anesthetic procedures vary among species but in all of these animals, the laparoscope was inserted through a midventral incision. Laparoscopy has also proven to be a practical and safe procedure for sexing exotic avian species by direct inspection of the gonads (Bush *et al.*, 1978a).

Details of the above procedures for various species will be presented in subsequent chapters. It should be noted that, with the exception of the dog, cat, and zoo animals, laparoscopy generally has been utilized for only the study of reproductive function (Dukelow, 1978) and largely ignored as a clinical veterinary tool. It should be emphasized that the latter use of this technique is a relatively new field and that only slight modifications are necessary, in most species, to successfully examine the liver, intestines, gallbladder, portions of the stomach, diaphragm, urinary bladder, spleen, and abdominal wall. In addition, most studies have been conducted in female animals, but recent studies indicate the usefulness of laparoscopy in males to observe most abdominal organs as well as the abdominal portion of the vas deferens and reproductive vasculature.

**References**

Alvarez, W. C. (1921) The use of $CO_2$ in pneumoperitoneum. *A.J.R.* 8:71–72.

Anderson, E. T. (1937) Peritoneoscopy. *Am. J. Surg.* 35:136–139.

Ariga, S., and Dukelow, W. R. (1977a) Recovery of preimplantation blastocysts in the squirrel monkey by a laparoscopic technique. *Fertil. Steril.* 28:577–580.

Ariga, S., and Dukelow, W. R. (1977b) Nonsurgical (laparoscopic) uterine flushing and egg recovery techniques in the squirrel monkey (*Saimiri sciureus*). *Primates* 18:453–457.

Balin, H., Halpern, B. D., and Israel, L. (1963) An *in vivo* pelvic "ovarian chamber" for direct visualization procedures. *Am.J. Obstet. Gynecol.* 87:152–159.

Balin, H., and Wan, L. S. (1969) A study of induction of ovulation in *Macaca mulatta*. *J. Reprod. Med.* 2: 273–284.

Balin, H., Wan, L. S., and Israel, S. L. (1966) Recent advances in pelvic endoscopy. *Obstet. Gynecol.* 27: 30–43.

Batta, S. K., and Brackett, B. G. (1974) Ovulation induction in rhesus monkeys by treatment with gonadotropins and prostaglandins. *Prostaglandins* 6:45–54.

Benedict, E. B. (1951) *Endoscopy as Related to Diseases of the Bronchus, Esophagus, Stomach, and Peritoneal Cavity.* Williams and Wilkins, Baltimore.

Berger, M. J., Smith, D. M., Taymor, M. L., and Thompson, R. S. (1975) Laparoscopic recovery of mature human oocytes. *Fertil. Steril.* 26:513–522.

Bernheim, B. M. (1911) Organoscopy. *Ann. Surg.* 53: 764–767.

Betteridge, K. H., and Raeside, J. I. (1962) Observations of the ovaries by peritoneal cannulation in pigs. *Res. Vet. Sci.* 3:390–398.

Blakley, G. A., Blaine, C. R., and Morton, W. R. (1977) Correlation of perineal detumescence and ovulation in the pigtail macaque (*Macaca nemestrina*). *Lab. Anim. Sci.* 27:352–355.

Bosu, W. T. K. (1973) Laparoscopic techniques for the examination of the ovaries in the rhesus monkey. *J. Med. Primatol.* 2:124–129.

Bosu, W. T. K., and Johansson, E. D. B. (1974) Effects of postovulatory norethindrone and estrogens on the plasma levels of estrogen and progesterone in rhesus monkeys. *Contraception* 9:357–367.

Bosu, W. T. K., Johansson, E. D. B., and Gemzell, C. (1973) Ovarian steroid patterns in peripheral plasma during the menstrual cycle in the rhesus monkey. *Folia Primatol.* 19:218–234.

Boyd, J. S., and Ducker, M. J. (1973) A method of examining the cyclic changes occurring in the sheep ovary using endoscopy. *Vet. Rec.* 93:40–43.

Bozzini, P. (1806) Lichtlieter, eine Erfindung zur Anschauung inneren Theile und Krankheiten nebst der Abbildung. *J. Pract. Arzneykunde Wundarzneykunst.* 24:107–124. (English trans.: Bush, R. B., et al., 1974.)

Bush, M., Kennedy, S., Wildt, D. E., and Seager, S. W. J. (1978a) Sexing of birds by laparoscopy. *Int. Zoo. Yearb.* 18:197–198.

Bush, M., Wildt, D. E., Kennedy, S., and Seager, S. W. J. (1978b) Laparoscopy in zoological medicine. *J. Am. Vet. Med. Assoc.* 173: 1081–1087.

Bush, R. B., Leonhardt, H., Bush, I. M., and Landes, R. L. (1974) Dr. Bozzini's Lichtleiter. *Urology* 3:119–123.

Case, J. T. (1921) A review of three years' work and articles on pneumoperitoneum. *A.J.R.* 8:714–721.

Dierschke, D. J., and Clark, J. R. (1976) Laparoscopy in *Macaca mulatta*: specialized equipment employed and initial observations. *J. Med. Primatol.* 5: 100–110.

Dierschke, D. J., and Hyatt, J. L. (1969) Peritoneoscopy via a chronically implanted cannula to observe ovarian activity in ewes. *J. Anim. Sci.* 28:645–649.

Dittel, V. (1887) Neue Apparate zur Elektro-Endoskopie. *Z. Therap. Einbzhng. Elect. Hydrotherap., Wien.* 5:41.

Dukelow, W. R. (1978) Laparoscopic research techniques in mammalian embryology. In: *Methods in Mammalian Reproduction.* J. C. Daniels, ed., Academic Press. New York, pp. 437–460.

Dukelow, W. R., Harrison, R. M., Rawson, J. M. R., and Johnson, M. P. (1972) Natural and artificial control of ovulation in nonhuman primates. In: *Medical Primatology 1972, Part 1*, E. I. Goldsmith and J. Moor-Jankowski, eds., Karger, Basel, pp. 232–236.

Dukelow, W. R., Jarosz, S. J., Jewett, D. A., and Harrison, R. M. (1971) Laparoscopic examination of the ovaries in goats and primates. *Lab. Anim. Sci.* 21:594–597.

Dziuk, P. J., Conker, J. D., Nichols, J. R., and Peterson, W. E. (1958) *In vivo* observation of the internal genital organs in the cow. *Tech. Bull. Univ. Minnesota Agr. Exp. Station* No. 222:65–67.

Eddy, C. A., Turner, T., Kraemer, D. C., and Pauerstein, C. J. (1976) Pattern and duration of ovum transport in the baboon. *Obstet. Gynecol.* 46:658–664.

Edgerton, W. D. (1974) Laparoscopy in the community hospital: set-up, performance, control. In: *Gynecological Laparoscopy: Principles and Technique.* J. M. Phillips and L. Keith, eds., Stratton Intercontinental, New York, pp. 79–90.

Frangenheim, H (1960) Erfahrungen mit der Laparoskopie und der Culdoskopie in der Gynakologie. *Med. Welt.* 41:2153–2154.

Frangenheim, H. (1965) Technical errors in peritoneoscopy. *German Med. Monthly* 10:405–411.

Fujimoto, S., Rawson, J. M. R., and Dukelow, W. R. (1974) Hormonal influences on the time of ovulation in the rabbit as determined by laparoscopy. *J.*

Reprod. Fertil. 38:97–103.

Goetze, R. (1926) Zur Fremdkoerperoperation beim Rind. D.T.W. 34:764–765.

Graham, C. E., Keeling, M., Chapman, C., Cummins, L. B., and Haynie, J. (1973) Method of endoscopy in the chimpanzee: relations of ovarian anatomy, endometrial histology, and sexual swelling. Am. J. Phys. Anthropol. 38:211–216.

Harrison, R. M. (1976) The development of modern endoscopy. J. Med. Primatol. 5:73–81.

Harrison, R. M., and Dukelow, W. R. (1971) Megestrol acetate: its effect on the inhibition of ovulation in the squirrel monkey. J. Reprod. Fertil. 25:99–101.

Harrison, R. M., and Dukelow, W. R. (1973) Seasonal adaptation of laboratory-maintained squirrel monkeys. J. Med. Primatol. 2:277–283.

Harrison, R. M., and Dukelow, W. R. (1974) Morphological changes in the Saimiri sciureus ovarian follicle as detected by laparoscopy. Primates 15:305–309.

Harrison, R. M., Rawson, J. M. R., and Dukelow, W. R. (1974) Megestrol acetate. II. Effects on ovulation in nonhuman primates as determined by laparoscopy. Fertil Steril. 25:51–56.

Heinze, V. H., and Klug, E. (1973) Endoskopische Beobachtungen an der inneren Genitalorganen (Pelviskopie) bei pferd und Esel. Die Blauen Hefte fur den Tierarzt. 50:555–560.

Heinze, V. H., Klug, E., and von Lepel, J. D. (1972) Optische Darstellung der inneren Geschlechtsorgane bei Equiden zur Diagnostik und Therapie. D.T.W. 79:49–51.

Hope, R. B. (1937) The differential diagnosis of ectopic gestation by peritoneoscopy. Surg. Gynecol. Obstet. 64:229–234.

Hulet, C. V., and Foote, W. C. (1968) A rapid technique for observing the reproductive tract of living ewes. J. Anim. Sci. 27:142–145.

Jacobaeus, H. C. (1910) Ueber die Moglichkeit die Zystoskopie bei Untersuchung seroser Hohlungen Anzuwenden. Munch. Med. Wochenschr. 57:2090–2092.

Jarosz, S. J., Kuehl, T. J., and Dukelow, W. R. (1977) Vaginal cytology, induced ovulation, and gestation in the squirrel monkey (Saimiri sciureus). Biol. Reprod. 16:97–103.

Jewett, D. A., and Dukelow, W. R. (1971a) Laparoscopy and precise mating techniques to determine gestation length in Macaca fascicularis. Lab. Prim. Newsl. 10:16–17.

Jewett, D. A., and Dukelow, W. R. (1971b) Follicular morphology in Macaca fascicularis. Folia Primatol. 16:216–220.

Kalk, H. (1929) Erfahrungen mit der Laparoskopie (Zugleich mit Beschreibung eines neuen Instrumentes) Z. Klin. Med. 111:303–348.

Kapany, N. S. (1958) Fiber optics. In: Concepts of Classical Optics. J. Strong, ed., Freeman, San Francisco, pp. 553–596.

Kelling, G. (1902) Ueber Oesophagoskopie, Gastroskopie, und Kolioskopie. Munch. Med. Wochenschr. 49:21–24.

Kelling, G. (1910) Ueber die Moglichkeit, die Zystoskopie bei Untessuchungen seroser Hohlungen anzuwenden. Munch. Med. Wochenschr. 57:2358.

Korbsch, R. (1921) Die Laparoskopie nach Jacobaeus. Berl. Klin. Wochenschr. 58:696–698.

Lamond, D. R., and Holmes, J. H. G. (1965) Suitable endoscopy and laparotomy techniques for ovarian examination in the cow. Aust. Vet. J. 41:324–325.

Lettow, E. (1972) Laparoscopic examinations in liver diseases in dogs. Vet. Med. Rev. 2:159–167.

Liess, J. (1936) Die endoskopic beim Rinde. Schaper, Hannover, Germany.

Lopata, A., Johnston, I. W. H., Leeton, J. F., Muchnicki, D., McTalbot, J., and Wood., C. (1974) Collection of human oocytes at laparoscopy and laparotomy. Fertil. Steril. 25:1030–1037.

Megale, F. (1967) Endoscopic photography of ruminants. Vet Med. Small Anim. Clin. 62:555–557.

Megale, F., Fincher, M. G., and McEntee, K. (1956) Peritoneoscopy in the cow: visualization of the ovaries, oviducts, and uterine horns. Cornell Vet. 46:109–121.

Mori, J., Kariya, T., and Tsujimura, S. (1977) Direct ovarian observation in the cow by means of laparoscopy. Jpn. J. Anim. Reprod. 23:126–127.

Morris, J. A., Davidson, E. C., Jr., Maidman, J. E., Arce, J. J., Brown, J. E., and Frazer, R. (1976) Sampling the fetoplacental circulation. I. The pregnant ovine. Am. J. Obstet. Gynecol. 125:1121–1124.

Morris, J. A., Davidson, E. C., Jr., Maidman, J. E., Arce, J. J., Brown, J. E., and Frazer, R. (1977) Sampling the fetoplacental circulation. II. Combined laparoscopy-fetoscopy in the pregnant ovine. Am. J. Obstet. Gynecol. 128:279–286.

Nadeau, O. E., and Kampmeier, O. F. (1925) Endoscopy of the abdomen: abdominoscopy. Surg. Gynecol. Obstet. 41:259–271.

Nigi, H. (1977) Laparoscopic observation of ovaries before and after ovulation in the Japanese monkey (Macaca fuscata). Primates 18:243–259.

Nordentoeft, S. (1912) Ueber Endoskopie geschlossener Cavitaten mittels meines Trocar-Endoskops. Verh. dt. Ges. Chir. 42:78–81.

Orndoff, B. H. (1920) The peritoneoscope in diagnosis of diseases of the abdomen. J. Radiol. 1:307–325.

Palmer, R. (1947) Coelioscopie par la vois Transvaginale. C. R. Soc. Fr. Gynecol. 17:229–233.

Peterson, R. (1922) Value of pneumoperitoneal roentgenography in obstetrics and gynecology. J.A.M.A. 78:397–400.

Phillippo, M., Swapp, G. H., Robinson, J. J., and Gill, J. C. (1971) The diagnosis of pregnancy and estimation of foetal numbers in sheep by laparoscopy. J. Reprod. Fertil. 27:129–132.

Rathert, P., Lutzeyer, W., and Goddwin, W. E. (1974) Philipp Bozzini and the Lichtleiter. Urology 3:113–

118.

Renon, L. (1913) Technique et indications de la laparoscopie. *Rev. Gen. Clin. Ther.* 27:148–150.

Roberts, E. M. (1968) Endoscopy of the reproductive tract of the ewe. *Proc. Aust. Soc. Anim. Prod.* 7: 192–194.

Roccavilla, A. (1914) L'endoscopie delle grandi cavita siercse mediante un movo apparecchio ad illuminazione diretta. *Rif. Med.* 30:991–995.

Roccavilla, A. (1920) Laparoscopie e pneumoradiologie abdominale. *Radiol. Med. Milano* 7:411–421.

Ruddock, J. C. (1937) Peritoneoscopy. *Surg. Gynecol. Obstet.* 65:623–639.

Ruddock, J. C. (1949) The application and evaluation of peritoneoscopy. *Calif. Med.* 71:110–116.

Sante, L. R. (1927) Present status of pneumoperitoneum as an aid in the radiologic diagnosis of abdominal lesions. *SWest. Med.* 11:429–533.

Seeger, K. (1973) Die Laparoskopie, eine Technik zur Routineuntersuchung des Genitaltrakts beim Schaf. *Tieraerztl. Prax.* 1:295–299.

Seeger, K. (1977) Laparoscopic investigation of the bovine ovary. *Vet. Med. Small Anim. Clin.* 72: 1037–1044.

Semm, K. (1969) Gynaecological pelviscopy and its instrumentarium. *Acta Eur. Fertil.* 1:81–97.

Semm, K. (1970) Das Instrumentarium der Gynakolgischen Pelviskopie. *Endoscopy* 2:36–42.

Siegler, A. M., and Garret, M. (1970) Ancillary techniques with laparoscopy. *Fertil. Steril.* 21:763–773.

Silander, T. (1963) Hysteroscopy through a transparent rubber balloon in patients with carcinoma of the uterine endometrium. *Acta Obstet. Gynecol.* 42:284–299.

Smith, B. D., and Dillon, T. F. (1970) Laparoscopy. *Fertil. Steril.* 21:193–200.

Synder, D. A., and Dukelow, W. R. (1974) Laparoscopic studies of ovulation, pregnancy diagnosis, and follicle aspiration in sheep. *Theriogenology* 2: 143–148.

Steiner, O. P. (1924) Abdominoscopy. *Surg. Gynecol. Obstet.* 38:266–269.

Steptoe, P. C. (1967) *Laparoscopy in Gynecology.* Livingstone, London.

Steptoe, P. C. (1979) Extra corporeal conception in human. Special lecture. American Fertility Society, 35th Annual Meeting, San Francisco.

Steptoe, P. C., and Edwards, R. G. (1970) Laparoscopic recovery of preovulatory human oocytes after priming of ovaries with gonadotropins. *Lancet* 4: 683–689.

Stolkind, E. J. (1919) The value of pleuroscopy (thoracoscopy) in the diagnosis of pulmonary diseases, and laparoscopy in the diagnosis of abdominal diseases. *Med. Press* 107:46–48.

Stone, W. E. (1924) Intra-abdominal examination by aid of the peritoneoscope. *J. Kans. Med. Soc.* 24:63–66.

Tedesko, F. (1912) Ueber Endoskopie des Abdomens und des Thorax. *Mitt. Ges. inn. Med. Kinderheilk.* 12:323–327.

Thimonier, J., and Mauleon, P. (1969) Variations saisonnieres du comportement d'oestrus et des activities ovarienne et hypophysaire chez les ovins. *Ann. Biol. Anim. Biochim. Biophys.* 9:233–250.

van Zwaluwenburg, G. J., and Peterson, R. (1921) Pneumoperitoneum of the pelvis, gynecological studies. A preliminary report. *A.J. R.* 8:12–19.

von Ott, D. (1901) Illumination of the abdomen (ventroscopia). *J. Akush. i Zhensk. Boliez.* 15:1045–1049.

Wheeless, C. R., Jr., and Thompson, B. H. (1973) Laparoscopic sterilization—review of 3600 cases. *Obstet. Gynecol.* 42:751–758.

White, R. J., Blaine, C. R., and Blakley, G. A. (1973) Detecting ovulation in *Macaca nemestrina* by correlation of vaginal cytology, body temperature, and perineal tumescence with laparoscopy. *Am. J. Phys. Anthropol.* 38:189–194.

Wildt, D. E., Bush, M., Whitlock, B. S., and Seager, S. W. J. (1978) Laparoscopy: a method for direct examination of internal organs in zoo veterinary medicine and research. *Int. Zoo Yearb.* 18:194–197.

Wildt, D. E., Doyle, L. L., Stone, S. C., and Harrison, R. M. (1977a) Correlation of perineal swelling with serum ovarian hormone levels, vaginal cytology, and ovarian follicular development during the baboon reproductive cycle. *Primates* 18:261–270.

Wildt, D. E., Fujimoto, S., Spencer, J. L., and Dukelow, W. R. (1973) Direct ovarian observation in the pig by means of laparoscopy. *J. Reprod. Fertil.* 35:541–543.

Wildt, D. E., Kinney, G. M., and Seager, S. W. J. (1977b) Laparoscopy for the direct observation of internal organs of the domestic cat and dog. *Am. J. Vet. Res.* 38:1429–1432.

Wildt, D. E. Levinson, C. J., and Seager, S. W. J. (1977c) Laparoscopic exposure and sequential observation of the ovary of the cycling bitch. *Anat. Rec.* 189:443–450.

Wildt, D. E., Morcom, C. B., and Dukelow, W. R. (1975) Laparoscopic pregnancy diagnosis and uterine fluid recovery in swine. *J. Reprod. Fertil.* 44: 301–304.

Wishart, D. F. (1972) Observations on the estrous cycle of the Friesian heifer. *Vet. Rec.* 90:595–597.

Wishart, D. F., and Snowball, J. B. (1973) Endoscopy in cattle: observation of the ovary *in situ*. *Vet. Rec.* 92:139–143.

Witherspoon, D. M., and Talbot, R. B. (1970a) Ovulation site in the mare. *J. Am. Vet. Med. Assoc.* 157: 1452–1459.

Witherspoon, D. M., and Talbot, R. B. (1970b) Nocturnal ovulation in the equine animal. *Vet. Rec.* 87: 302–304.

Zollikofer, R. (1924) Ueber Laparoskopie. *Schweiz. Med. Wochenschr.* 104:264–265.

# CHAPTER 2

# Optical Principles of Laparoscopy

## Rochelle Prescott, B.S. Ch.

---

### INTRODUCTION

A laparoscope is almost invariably a rigid endoscope. It is introduced into the peritoneal cavity through a cannula which has been passed through the abdominal wall using a sharpened trocar to fill the cannula and pierce the abdominal wall. The purpose of the instrument is to allow visualization of the viscera for the purpose of diagnosis, biopsy, or certain surgical procedures. Laparoscopy can generally be carried out as a simple procedure under light anesthesia with a minimum of morbidity. Laparoscopy, like laparotomy, is an art which is learned through practice. Visualization of the internal anatomy from within gives an entirely different perspective and one's visual capabilities must be educated by practice to precisely diagnose, biopsy, and operate under endoscopic visualization. Endoscopes are produced in a wide range of sizes and a variety of styles. Each practitioner must decide, on the basis of personal needs and preferences, which endoscope to use. The laparoscopist is primarily interested in those characteristics which directly affect instrument effectiveness: size of telescope, visual field, and photographic capabilities. The operator should also have some understanding of the basic principles involved with optical systems. This chapter discusses the physical aspects associated with laparoscopic optics, illumination, and photography.

### Types of Laparoscopic Optical Systems

There are three basic rigid optical systems used in laparoscopy today: the thin lens system; the rod lens system of Hopkins; and the graded index (GRIN) system (Fig. 2.1). All of the systems follow the same basic optical laws insofar as their external characteristics are concerned and are simply different technological approaches to the same problem. It should be noted that flexible endoscopes, used in some fields of biomedical research and medicine, are based on entirely different optical principles which will not be presented in the present discussion.

### THIN LENS SYSTEM

This system consists of an objective, a series of relay lenses to bring the image through the channel of the instrument, and an eyepiece to provide an enlarged image for viewing. New developments in optical glass types, low-reflection coatings, and

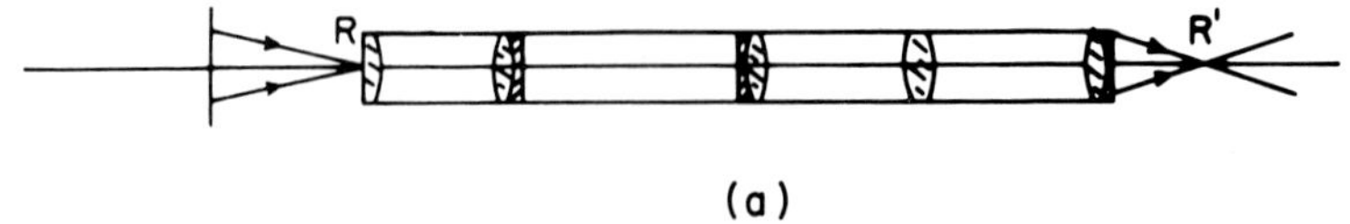

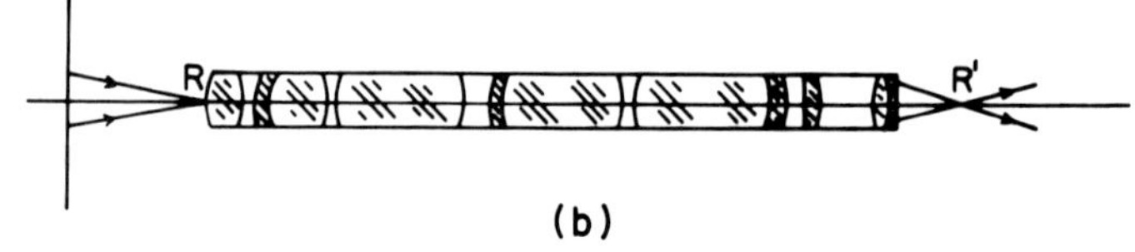

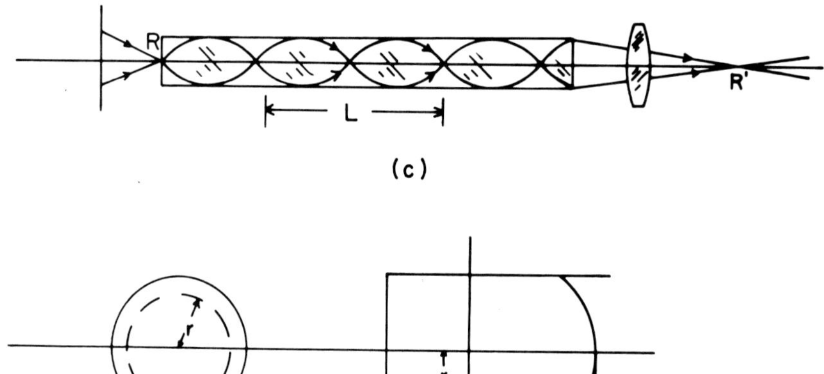

**Figure 2.1**   These are three types of optical systems used in modern endoscopes. In **(a)** is shown a schema of a classical lens system in which an eye placed at R′ views the plane on the left from the perspective of R. This type of system was used exclusively until the invention of the rod lens system **(b)** by Hopkins in the 1950s. In late 1960 the development of a new type of optical element, graded index (GRIN) lenses, made possible the development of an endoscope in which a single component, a solid rod of glass, performed the functions of the usually numerous components in the slender penetrating portion of the endoscope **(c)**. In these elements the index of refraction decreases from the axis to the periphery according to a specific mathematical formula **(d)**. The rays from any point in object space form helioid paths and relay the image along the GRIN rod. (Reproduced with permission from *Journal of Medical Primatology* 5:133–147, 1976.)

optical design have all provided continued improvement in the imaging quality of this type of endoscope.

## ROD LENS SYSTEM

Compared to the above, lenses in this system are extremely thick and the air spaces between lenses are thin. This system has certain optical and mechanical advantages over the thin lens systems and the advantages are more pronounced as the diameter of the instrument is reduced. It provides less stray light, a wider angle of view, and greater brightness and resolution.

## GRIN SYSTEM

The advantages of this system are most pronounced when the diameter is quite small; these optics are normally 1 mm in diameter but are available in a 0.7 mm diameter. This system consists of a single glass component of two glass rods fused end to end in which changes in refractory index convey the image instead of a series of lenses. A relatively long ocular is usually employed to enlarge the image for ease in viewing.

### Types of Basic Laparoscopes

A laparoscope is simply a long slender tube with an eyepiece at one end through which one can view objects as though the eye were placed at the opposite end of the tube. Most modern laparoscopes also contain, in addition to the viewing optics, a fiber optic light guide for illuminating the area viewed. Certain operating laparoscopes have an offset eyepiece and a channel through which operating instruments can be inserted directly into the area visualized.

Laparoscopes are usually characterized according to the diameter of the telescope and the direction of view through the instrument (i.e., 5 mm, 180°). When considering purchase of a laparoscope one should remember that the diameter of the cannula, through which the laparoscope will be inserted, is slightly greater than the diameter of the laparoscope itself. Thus, the opening in the tissue for the insertion of the instruments will be proportional to the diameter of the cannula and not the laparoscope. A 5 mm in diameter laparoscope requires a 6 mm in diameter cannula which has a cross-sectional area of 28.3 mm$^2$; a 10 mm in diameter laparoscope with an 11 mm in diameter cannula has a cross-sectional area 3.36 times greater, 95.0 mm$^2$. These facts should be considered when operative procedures are to be performed. A two puncture procedure using a 5 mm laparoscope with a 6 mm cannula and a 6 mm accessory cannula will have 60% of the cross-sectional area of a 10 mm laparoscope using an 11 mm cannula.

The direction of view and other parameters will be described in the following section. These parameters are of importance from an optical standpoint and procedures for their evaluation and comparison will be given. The reader will find it easier to understand these evaluation procedures if a laparoscope is available.

## OPTICAL PARAMETERS

### Terminology

Certain terms not normally familiar to the researcher or veterinary clinician must be understood to properly evaluate and compare various laparoscopes and instruments of different manufacturers. This section will familiarize the reader with these terms and describe methods of measurement.

## DIRECTION OF VIEW

The direction of view is measured by the angle between the axis of the laparoscope and a line connecting the tip of the endoscope with the center of the field of view (Fig. 2.2), or by the supplement of that angle. Depending on the manufacturer, a 0° laparoscope and a 180° laparoscope may have the same direction of view (i.e., the field of view is centered on the line made by the axis of the laparoscope). The area that can be visualized by rotating the laparoscope around its axis will be unchanged with the 180° instrument and will be significantly changed when rotating the 130° laparoscope (Fig. 2.2). The most common laparoscopes have either a 180°, 160°, or 130° direction of view. Operating laparoscopes usually produce a 170° direction of view. Instruments are available with right angle or even acute angle direction of view. Descriptive literature usually provides this information or it can be measured as described later. The following terms are based on measurements made using a 180° laparoscope (straightforward view).

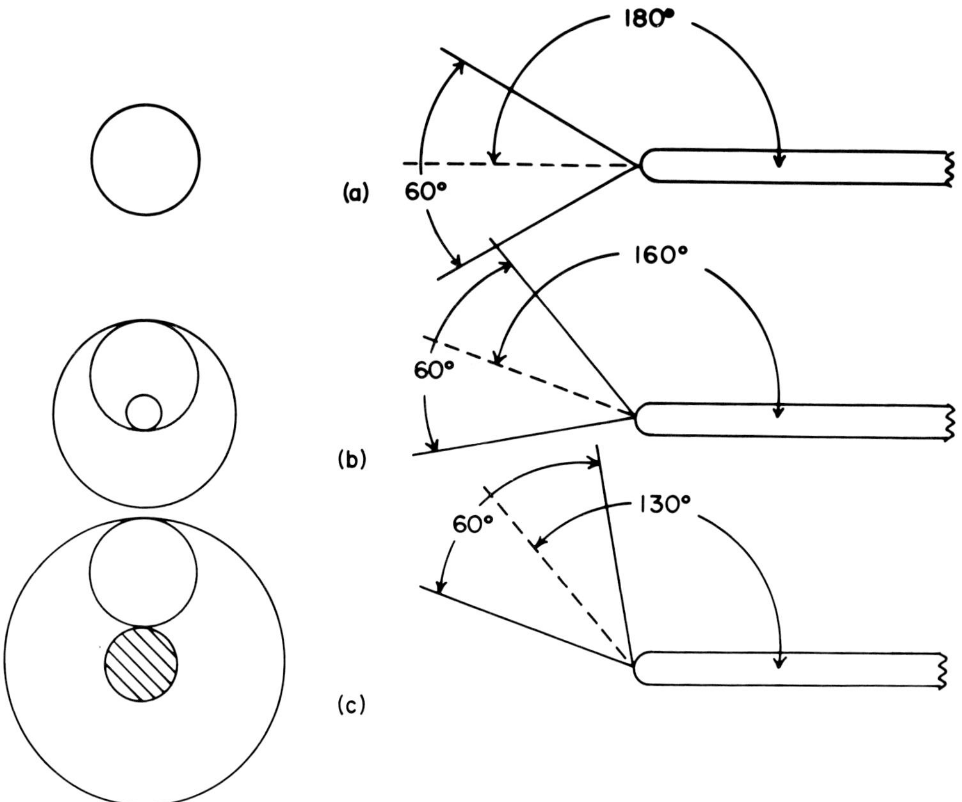


**Figure 2.2**   A comparison of the fields of view and the area viewed when the endoscope is rotated on its own axis to scan. Note that each laparoscope has a 60° angle of field of view. In **(a)** the field of view does not change due to rotation of a straight view endoscope. In **(b)** rotation of the forward-oblique endoscope scans a large field of view, as indicated by the large circle, while keeping in view a small area directly in line with the endoscope, as denoted by the small circle. In **(c)** the oblique view endoscope scans an area about seven times the instantaneous field of view but never sees the area directly ahead of it. During scanning the image does not rotate. (Reproduced with permission from *Journal of Medical Primatology* 5:133–147, 1976.)

## ANGLE OF APPARENT FIELD OF VIEW

The angle of the apparent field of view is the angle in degrees included between the two lines drawn from the eye to points at the opposite extremes of a diameter of the apparent field of view. This is the angle A subtended by dashed line A′ in Figure 2.3a. Point O′ is the center of the apparent field of view.

## ANGLE OF FIELD OF VIEW

The angle in degrees included between the lines drawn from the tip of the laparoscope to two points at the extremes of a diameter of the field of view is the angle of the field of view. The angle of field of view in Figure 2.3a is the angle B subtended by the solid line B′ with the point O in the center of the field. The relationship between field of view and magnification is indirectly proportional. A wider field of view reduces the relative scale of the viewed image.

## EXIT PUPIL

All light leaving the eyepiece of a laparoscope will pass through a circle in space behind the eyepiece. This circle is termed the exit pupil; it is also known as the eyepoint,

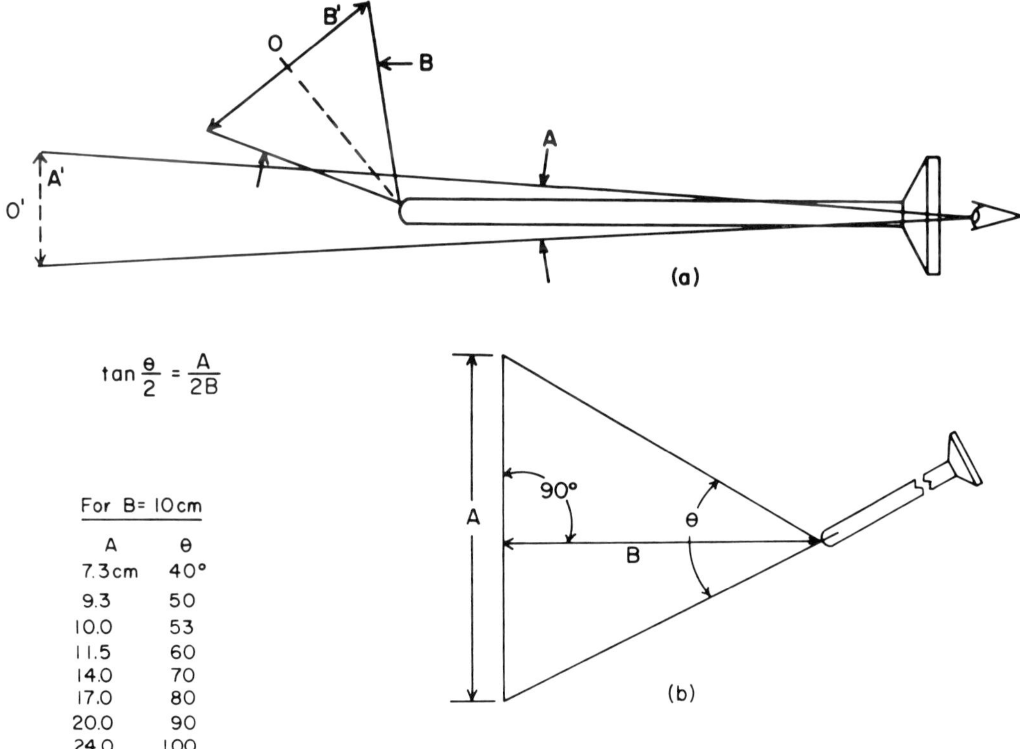


| A | θ |
|---|---|
| 7.3 cm | 40° |
| 9.3 | 50 |
| 10.0 | 53 |
| 11.5 | 60 |
| 14.0 | 70 |
| 17.0 | 80 |
| 20.0 | 90 |
| 24.0 | 100 |

**Figure 2.3** In **(a)** the diagram shows how a wide field of view as seen from the tip of the endoscope is viewed as a relatively narrow virtual image at an appreciable distance from the eye. The resulting perspective distortion requires the endoscopist to educate his visual senses for good visualization of anatomy. In **(b)** the diagram shows how an estimate of the field of view can be made by placing the tip of the endoscope at a known distance from a scale or lined paper and measuring the width of the area viewed. (Reproduced with permission from *Journal of Medical Primatology* 5:133–147.)

or Ramsden disk. The distance from the eyepiece to the exit pupil is termed the "eye relief" (Fig. 2.4). The exit pupil is an image of the entrance pupil of the instrument and all of the image forming light passes through it with the light from each point in the field of view uniformly distributed over it. The significance of the exit pupil and eye relief will be discussed later.

## ENTRANCE PUPIL

The entrance pupil is a small circle at the distal end of the laparoscope through which the light that forms the image must pass. Light entering the instrument outside the

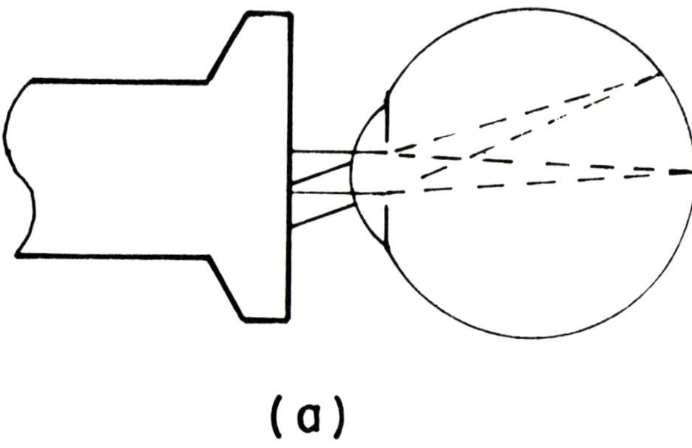


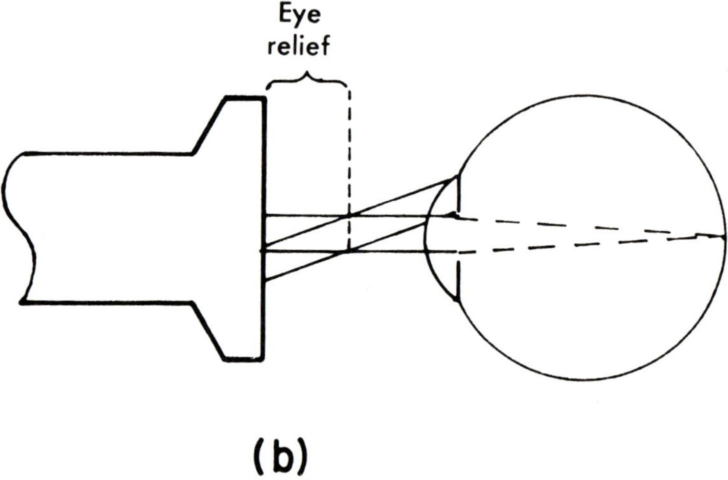


**Figure 2.4** **(a)** A schema of the eye at eyepoint of the endoscope. Light from all parts of the field passes through the iris to form an image at the back of the eye. In **(b)** the diagram shows what happens when the eye is not brought close enough to eyepoint. Only light from the central portion of the field passes through the iris. The periphery of the field is occluded, and the eye must be moved laterally to scan the entire field (i.e., "knotholed"). (Reproduced with permission from *Symposium on Arthroscopy and Arthrography of the Knee*, C. V. Mosby Co., St. Louis, 1978.)

entrance pupil is stopped by mechanical stops in the instrument. If not stopped, this nonimaging light may be reflected and "wash out" the image.

Other terms deal more with the optical parameters of the image visualized. Some of these terms have different meanings to the nonengineer. The reader should keep the following definitions in mind when reading later sections in this chapter.

## STIGMATISM OF THE IMAGE

This term is used to refer to whether all the light from a single point in the field is focused as a single point. The failure of a point in the field to be focused as an image point usually indicates faults in design or workmanship.

## DISTORTION

Distortion is an optical term meaning that a straight line in the object is not seen as a straight line in the image. Distortion is termed "pincushion" or "barrel" when the sides of a square, symmetrically situated in the field of view, are curved inwardly or outwardly, respectively. The common endoscope is afflicted with some barrel distortion.

## CURVATURE OF THE FIELD

This is usually associated with distortion, and causes the image of a plane to appear to be on a spherical surface; it is usually convex toward the viewer.

## CHROMATIC CORRECTION

An endoscope may be chromatically deficient in either or both of two respects. The images may be displaced axially as a function of color, or the images may be of different sizes for each color. Chromatic aberration is due to different colors being refracted at different angles. Correction is made by the use of specific lenses in series or by chemical formulas in the GRIN system. The chromatic correction of an instrument is much more critical for photography than for normal visual use.

## VIGNETTING

A defect due to the mechanical stops or misalignment caused by bending or displacement of the optical elements may cause vignetting. It results in a loss in brightness of the peripheral image area due to blockage of light by mounts, stops, or element cells. The field of view may appear oval instead of round.

## TRANSMISSION

An optical system never transmits all of the light that impinges on the objective surface. Each surface reflects some fraction of the light falling upon it and each element has some absorption. When it is considered that there are some 10 to 20 or more elements in an endoscopic system, even when low absorption glasses are used and antireflection coatings are placed on all glass-air surfaces, an effective transmission of only about 90% will be obtained.

## VEILING GLARE

Some image forming light is reflected by surfaces within the optical system and a part of this is in turn reflected back by preceding surfaces. Some of this light, together with scatter light due to imperfections in polish and dirt on the surfaces, falls in the image and reduces contrast. This makes it difficult or impossible for the endoscopist to resolve fine detail. The effect of antireflection coatings is probably more important in reducing the veiling glare than in increasing the transmission of light through an endoscope.

With the above definitions in mind, one can proceed with a critical evaluation of a laparoscope.

## Evaluation of the Optical Parameters

The following are procedures to qualitatively evaluate optical parameters of a single endoscope or compare two or more endoscopes. Having an endoscope in hand while reading this section will allow these procedures to be more easily understood.

### DIRECTION OF VIEW

The endoscope is held in a horizontal position, pointed toward a bright object, and looked through at the eyepiece. If the target object appears to be in the center of the field of view, then the direction of view is 180° (or zero depending on the nomenclature system). If the object appears to one side of the field of view the distal end of the endoscope should be swung until the object appears in the center of the field of view. The direction of view is the supplement of the swing angle, or the angle itself, depending on the nomenclature system.

### ANGLE OF FIELD OF VIEW

To determine the angle of the field of view requires the measurement of (1) the diameter of the field of view on a plane surface that is perpendicular to the direction of the field of view; and (2) the distance from the tip of the endoscope to the plane (Fig. 2.3b). The angle of the field of view is then twice the angle whose tangent is equal to the radius of the field of view divided by the distance. The angle of view in most laparoscopes is 60 to 70° but may range from 40 to 100°.

### ANGLE OF APPARENT FIELD OF VIEW

The angle of the apparent field of view is often confused with but is independent of the angle of the field of view. It is the angle covered by the image of the endoscope as seen by the eye. A large apparent field of view is desirable, but physical limitations in endoscope design limit the size attainable. A large apparent field of view is only obtained at a considerable cost in image brightness.

### EXIT PUPIL AND EYE RELIEF

The exit pupil, or Ramsden disk, can be seen by looking at the eyepiece (not through the eyepiece) with the endoscope held so it is pointed directly at a bright field, such as a well-lighted white sheet of paper. The diameter of the exit pupil is of great importance in determining the brightness of the image. This is of particular interest to endoscopists who are interested in photography, since the image brightness varies as the square of the exit pupil diameter. Another test can be performed to determine exit pupil position (i.e., distance from the eyepiece). This distance, known as the eye relief (Fig. 2.4), should be at least 8 mm for non-eyeglass wearers and about 20 mm for eyeglass wearers. Eye relief may be determined by looking at a bright field through the endoscope and moving one's eye to and away from the eyepiece. At the exit pupil the sharp outlines of the edge of the image field will coincide with the edges of the eyepiece opening. When the eye is not at the exit pupil the observer must "knothole" to visualize the entire field of view. The optimum amount of eye relief should be such that when the endoscope is used in the usual manner the eye is behind the optically ideal point. In this manner the endoscopist will reflexively react to keep the eye pupil centered but not so far back that the entire field of view cannot be observed at one time.

The diameter of the exit pupil is the single most important factor in determining the brightness of the image in an endoscope. All of the light transmitted through the eyepiece passes through the exit pupil and its diameter is determined by the aperture of the lenses and stops within the endoscope. Exit pupil diameters usually range from about 2 mm down to approximately 0.5 mm. Maximal theoretical resolution of the eye is achieved at the upper limit and resolution is definitely reduced at the lower value. Interestingly, reduction of the exit pupil size does not reduce the apparent brightness until the diameter is reduced below 1.5 mm. However, if the diameter is reduced to 0.5 mm, the field will appear quite dark.

## ENTRANCE PUPIL

The size of the entrance pupil is quite small, approximately 0.1 mm. It can be observed by pointing the eyepiece toward a bright light and looking at the distal lens. A small point of light will be noted; this is the entrance pupil and should be located at or near the center of the lens.

## STIGMATISM AND CHROMATIC ABERRATIONS

Stigmatism of the image is easily determined by placing a bare bulb flashlight 30 to 100 cm away and carefully maneuvering the endoscope so as to move the image from the center to the periphery of the field at 90° intervals. An endoscope giving perfect stigmatic imagery simply shows a point of white light in all parts of the field. In a well-constructed system any aberrations will be symmetric about the center of the field. Longitudinal chromatic aberration will show as a red or blue ring or halo surrounding the central point image which should be white. A radial spectral dispersion indicates lateral chromatic aberration and would occur near the edge of the field. As described earlier, chromatic aberration is due to different wavelengths (colors) being refracted at different angles. A well-corrected system will display a symmetrical white image with one or two faint rings around it. If the rings are not faint or are surrounded by a halo, spherical aberration is indicated. Images in the field may be of various shapes and indicate astigmatism. Even the best systems will display noticeable aberrations very near the edge of the field, particularly if the field of view is very large.

## DISTORTION

Distortion is a very innocuous aberration in endoscopic systems. It is readily observed by bringing an object with straight lines over toward one side of the field of view and noting the curvature of the image. The usual distortion is of the "barrel" type (i.e., outward curving).

## CURVATURE OF THE FIELD

This condition is detected by observing a field where the image at the edge of the field appears farther away than the image at the center. This condition is not usually considered serious unless it is so severe that the outer portions of the field are out of focus.

## VIGNETTING

This condition is usually due to general defects. A laparoscope should not be purchased when this condition exists. The loss of peripheral brightness can be detected by simply viewing through the instrument at an illuminated object.

## TRANSMISSION AND VEILING GLARE

These two factors are best evaluated by simply using the instrument in a routine examination. If sufficient light is transmitted so that fine detail and contrast of the area viewed are evident, there is no need to be further concerned with these factors.

### Magnification of Image

The distance of unity magnification is closely associated with the above quantities. It is usually of the order of the few centimeters and one can sometimes (again with a 180° endoscope) superimpose the image as seen with the other eye with that observed through the endoscope. The distance from the tip of the endoscope to the target is approximately the distance of unity magnification. At other distances the magnification is approximately the reciprocal ratio of that distance to the distance of unity magnification (i.e., if the distance of unity magnification is 25 mm then the magnification at 10 mm is $^{25}/_{10}$ or 2½ times; at a distance of 50 mm it is ½).

One of the most striking characteristics of the endoscopic optical system is its remarkable depth of field, or the range of distances over which the viewed objects are in acceptably sharp focus. This is true because the entrance pupil of an endoscope is extremely small, the usual diameter being of the order of 0.1 to 0.2 mm. Looking through an endoscope one is aware that objects at a great distance from the observer are greatly reduced in size, usually by a factor of approximately 10. This minification has the effect of increasing the accommodation of the eye in focusing by a factor of roughly 100 times. Thus, for example, an eye which could focus down to 25 cm can now focus down to approximately 0.25 cm. As a result, moving close to the object viewed can produce an effective magnification of 10 or more times.

### General Considerations

The choice of an endoscope is based on many factors, only a few of which come within the scope of this chapter. In general, the larger endoscopes (8 or 10 mm in diameter) are of the classical thin lens type of Figure 2.1a; the rod lens design of Figure 2.1b is generally used in medium sized endoscopes of 3 to 5 mm in diameter; and the GRIN lens is used in the smallest endoscopes down to 1.7 mm in diameter. Taylor (1975) has carried out an extensive evaluation of the 5 mm in diameter endoscope in laparoscopy. This medium-sized laparoscope requires less surgical intervention than the larger diameter instruments but produces a smaller field of view, a smaller apparent field of view, reduced image brightness, and less illumination. Furthermore, photography with the smaller endoscope requires more skill. Conversely, visualization through the smaller endoscope is remarkably good and, with arc type light sources, video, movies, and still photography (slides or prints) are possible. The small puncture wounds associated with the smaller diameter laparoscope produce less morbidity and complications and, if the view is adequate for the requirements of the procedure, medical results are not compromised.

Comfortable viewing for the operator requires that the image observed in the endoscope be in focus. The wearing of bifocals during laparoscopy may cause considerable discomfort and neck strain so it is recommended that single vision spectacles be used during such procedures.

The direction of the field of view has little effect on image brightness but one should ensure that the visualized area is adequately and uniformly illuminated. More practice is required to develop an adequate orientation for visualization and operations using endoscopes with oblique directional views. Many individuals will find the 180°, straightforward, instrument initially easier to use and will consider it their first choice. Experienced laparoscopists may find that the 130° instrument allows for a greater field of vision.

An endoscope is a delicate optical instrument. It will not withstand rough handling and its optical components are easily damaged by contact with other surgical instruments. Many endoscopes are damaged during cleaning and sterilization procedures. Consequently, these tasks should be entrusted only to carefully trained and highly responsible personnel. Details for instrument sterilization and care are provided in the following chapters.

## THE ILLUMINATION OF ENDOSCOPES

Illumination is very important in endoscopy. The small entrance pupils of laparoscopes, which are usually less than 0.2 mm in diameter, allow very little entry of light. For adequate visualization the light levels in the field of view must be in the hundreds of footcandles, several times the illumination level required for comfortable normal vision with the naked eye. For photography, with fractional second exposures, the illumination must be in the thousands of footcandles, levels comparable to noon sunlight.

Over the years a number of methods for endoscope illumination have been used but the invention of the fiber optic light guides made all previous methods obsolete. (The fibers within the flexible light cable that transmit light from the projector to the laparoscope and those within the laparoscope itself are collectively termed the light guides.) A glass fiber has a core of approximately 25 to 50 micrometers diameter and a cladding of 2 to 3 micrometers thickness. Light falling on the end of the core within a certain angle of the fiber axis is reflected internally and travels through the fiber to its terminus, leaving the fiber at approximately the same angle to the fiber axis as it entered. This phenomenon occurs in spite of any bending or twisting of the fiber. To make a light guide, bundles of these fibers are assembled and the ends brought through a stainless steel tube where the fibers are set in epoxy cement, ground flat, and polished. Similar fibers are also packed in the annular space around the optical viewing system of the endoscope with one end of the fibers at the distal end of the endoscope and the other end of the fibers brought out to a sidearm. The latter is connected to the flexible light cable from the light source placed at a convenient distance from the endoscope.

The separation of the light source from the endoscope itself is very important. Early model endoscopes have consisted of a lens system with an incandescent light bulb incorporated at the terminus of the laparoscope. Energy applied to this incandescent bulb is converted to light and heat. The amount of energy converted to light is the luminous efficiency of the bulb. The luminous efficiency of an incandescent light source can never exceed about 14% and for sources in the range of temperatures feasible for tungsten light sources the efficiency ranges from about 0.1% to a maximum of perhaps 5%. It is practically impossible to direct more than about 10% of the light produced to the area to be illuminated. Thus, this earlier type light source dissipates as heat or wasted illumination from 200 to 10,000 times the amount of energy given off as useful illumination. Almost all of this wasted energy ends up as heat at the point of light production. With fiber optics most of the nonuseful energy can be kept out of the body and nearly all of the energy brought into the body can be concentrated as light on the desired area.

Fiber optics are also extremely functional in construction, as the fibers may be made to efficiently occupy narrow annular spaces in the penetrating portion of the endoscope and are one of its most trouble free components. They are nonconductive and hence do not contribute a hazardous electrical connection between the endoscope and ancillary electrical instruments used, nor will they furnish an electrical circuit to ground which may also constitute a hazard to the endoscopist and to the patient.

Figure 1.8 illustrates how a tungsten lamp in a reflector is used to illuminate the end of the light guide which is composed of thousands of fibers. In the arrangement shown, a joint usually exists where the light cable attaches to the endoscope so that a damaged light cable can be replaced without replacing the expensive endosope. It is important that the diameter of the flexible light cable be greater than the diameter of the endoscope light guide to ensure illumination of all of the fibers of the latter when the two are joined. Usually the maximum number of light guide fibers possible are placed into the penetrating section of the endoscope to produce the maximum illumination available.

One can quantitatively characterize the illuminating tip of an endoscope by its candlepower and its numerical aperture. It is desirable that the angle of light projected be equal to the angle of the field of view so that the area viewed is fully illuminated. Candlepower is determined by the area of the cross section of the light guide bundle.

In general, brightness (candlepower per unit area) is equal to the brightness of the original source multiplied by the product of the reflectance of the mirror and the transmittance of each of the components in the train. Light is lost at each end of the light fibers, reducing transmittance to about 65 to 70%. Additional loss in transmission is approximately 5% per foot. The losses of light from the ends of the fibers are due to reflection at the surface and also to the area of the light conducting cores being less than the total area (due to space between fibers). As a result of these losses the brightness at the distal end of the endoscope is usually less than 40% of the brightness with which the proximal tip of the light cable, adjacent to the light source, is illuminated. The primary light source, being in a separate cabinet, can be as large as desired and may be operated at the highest possible brightness. (Tungsten-halogen lamps usually operate at temperatures up to 3450° Kelvin.) For even greater illumination, mercury or xenon arc lamps may be used. Due to greater intrinsic brightness, these sources increase the illumination by three or more times and are especially valuable for photography or video recording.

The spatial characteristics of the illumination are a function of the light source design, the light cable numerical aperture, and the characteristics of the light guide within the endoscope itself. In general it is desirable to place as many optical fibers as possible into the space around the viewing optics; this is usually the limiting factor in the illumination provided. Straight view endoscopes can usually be packed more efficiently with optical fibers so the illumination is generally greater in these instruments than in oblique angle endoscopes.

Magnified examination of the distal end of several endoscopes with the sidearm connector of the light guide pointed at a fluorescent ceiling light is very informative. If the area of the light guide is to be measured, it can best be done at the sidearm with the tip pointed at the light. In some endoscopes the fibers are tapered so one can only compare overall illumination as described below. The flexible light cable should also be well packed and have very few broken fibers. This can be determined by a similar examination. In any case the flexible light cable should be somewhat larger than the integral light guide of the endoscope so that the latter is fully illuminated.

The overall illumination provided by a fiber optic system can only be accurately measured by careful photometric measurements at the distal end of the endoscope for the entire system. Side by side comparison of various endoscopic fiber optic systems reveals some significant differences. It is most important that the illumination fill the entire visual field because, in laparoscopy, very little light is reflected from one part of the field to another. Additional light may be provided by the specialized equipment discussed in the following section.

## PHOTOGRAPHY THROUGH THE ENDOSCOPE

The eye has the ability to focus on one area in a field, to move so as to see the entire field, to accommodate over six magnitudes of brightness, and to detect color differences. A camera cannot select the field of view and even the fastest color film requires more light than the eye for an acceptable image. Photography with the laparoscope becomes an art requiring much careful preparation and usually much practice.

Cameras used for laparoscopic photography are of the single lens reflex (SLR) type for reasons that will be obvious in this discussion. The adapter attaching a laparoscope to the camera should be designed so as to put the exit pupil of the laparoscope at the entrance pupil of the camera. If one looks into the front of a camera lens when the lens is "stopped down" the image of diaphragm that is seen is the entrance pupil of the camera. Most, if not all, SLRs have an automatic diaphragm, which means that the diaphragm remains wide open except during the exposure.

## Adapters to Mate Camera and Endoscope

One problem common to most laparoscopic photography is that the entrance pupil of the camera is usually about 2 cm behind the first lens surface, and the exit pupil of the endoscope is 1 cm or less behind the eyepiece (Fig. 2.5). Two solutions to this optical problem exist. One is to couple the camera as close as possible to the endoscope and open the camera lens to its maximum aperture so that the exit pupil of the endoscope becomes the entrance pupil of the camera lens. If the camera lens is stopped down (higher f-numbers) it may cause vignetting of the image. The second, and more practical, solution is to utilize a camera adapter that securely holds the camera to the endoscope in such a position that the exit pupil of the endoscope is in the designed position of the camera entrance pupil. All laparoscope manufacturers make such adapters.

## Focal Length and Focusing

The f-number of the photographic system is determined by the diameter of the exit pupil of the endoscope and focal length of the lens. The selection of the focal length of the lens is important because it, together with the angle of the apparent field of view, determines the size of the image and the effective exposure. In this regard, an image diameter of approximately 8 mm has been more or less accepted as standard. For apparent fields of view of 6 and 10° this image diameter would require focal lengths of 76 and 46 mm, respectively. Naturally, if the image in the endoscope is not at infinity but at a relatively short distance, then, due to the extension of the camera lens in focusing, the photographic image will be enlarged by about 10%. The camera should be focused prior to the laparoscopic procedure using a suitable target and never during the procedure.

When highly specialized electronic flash units are used for photographic exposure with large diameter endoscopes (having large exit pupils of 2 mm in diameter) and large fiber optic light cables (of 6 mm in diameter), it is possible to adequately expose, with lenses of more than 100 mm focal length, most, if not all, of a 24 × 36 mm film format. It should be remembered, however, that the total light falling on the film is the same and thus doubling the diameter of the image will require a fourfold increase in exposure which is not feasible in many instances.

## Focusing Screens

An additional problem in the adaptation of a camera to endoscopic photography is the internal focusing screen of SLRs. The ground glass of the ordinary focusing screen scatters light and makes the image appear a great deal darker than when viewed directly through the endoscope eyepiece. This may be avoided by replacing the ground glass focusing screen with a clear glass screen which may or may not have a reticle (a line or lines which give a reference plane for the eye to focus on). To assure that these desired changes in the lens and the focusing screen can be made, the potential laparoscopic

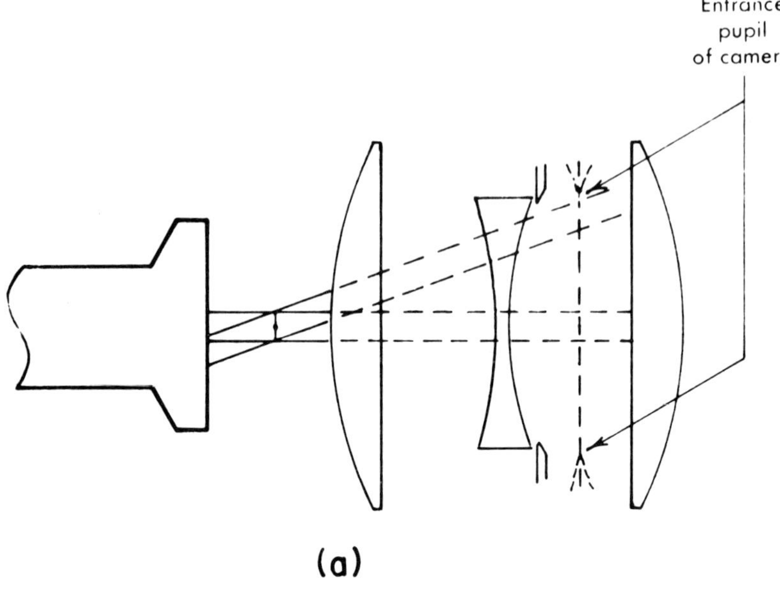


**(a)**

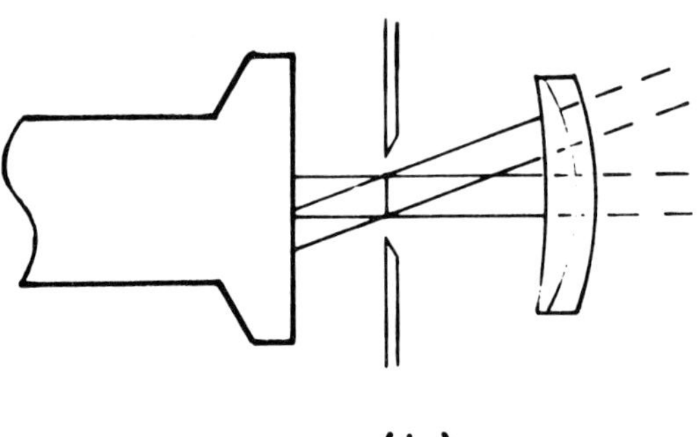

**(b)**

**Figure 2.5**   **(a)** The entrance pupil of an ordinary camera lens is well inside the front of the lens and hence cannot be brought up to the eyepoint of an endoscope. Unless it is very large it will vignette the image. **(b)** A camera lens design with an entrance pupil in front of the lens can be brought up to the eyepoint of the endoscope. In both cases the exit pupil of the endoscope becomes the entrance pupil of the camera lens. (Reproduced with permission from *Symposium on Arthroscopy and Arthrography of the Knee*, C. V. Mosby Co., St. Louis, 1978.)

photographer should carefully check that the camera being considered allows for such modifications.

### Supplemental Light for Photography

Due to the importance of photography in clinical documentation and in scientific publication, a number of specialized aids have been developed to assist the laparoscopic photographer.

The arc type light source, either of enriched mercury or xenon, has a much higher intrinsic brightness than the tungsten-halogen lamps. Their use provides an increase in illumination at least three times that of the latter lamps and are useful for slides, movies, or videorecording. The light approximates "daylight" quality and a daylight balanced color film should be used. These arc type light sources frequently have a tungsten-halogen lamp in the same cabinet which may be used for simple diagnostic observation and not photography. The tungsten-halogen lamp also serves as a convenient reserve lamp in case of lamp failure.

Xenon electronic flash systems are generally of two types. In the first, the xenon flash tube is in the projector cabinet and its light transverses the same light guides as the viewing light. This is made possible by optical or mechanical arrangements in the light projector. In the second type, the xenon flash tube is in a small housing which attaches directly to the light guide on the endoscope. In this case, a flexible light cable is attached to the housing from a tungsten-halogen source in the cabinet which also houses the electrical power supply for the flash tube. This second unit is supposedly more efficient as the light from the flash does not transverse the long flexible light cable nor the connection of the light guide at the endoscope. Both types give extremely good results with no worries about movement, as the exposures are only of a few milliseconds duration. These flash systems are undoubtedly superior for slides but are not suitable for movies or videorecording.

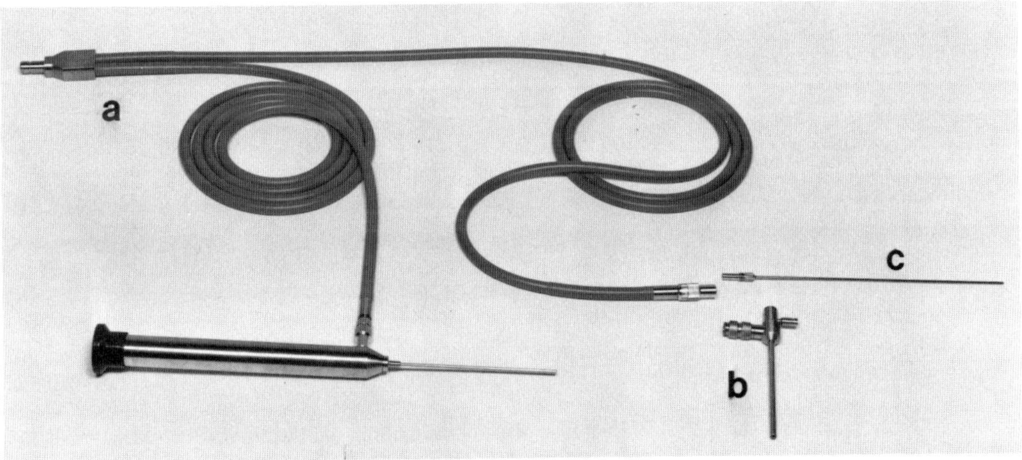

**Figure 2.6**  A bifurcated light cable **(a)** can be used to replace the usual light cable and allows the use of auxillary illuminators such as the halo light **(b)** or a light wand **(c)** which is introduced through a separate cannula.

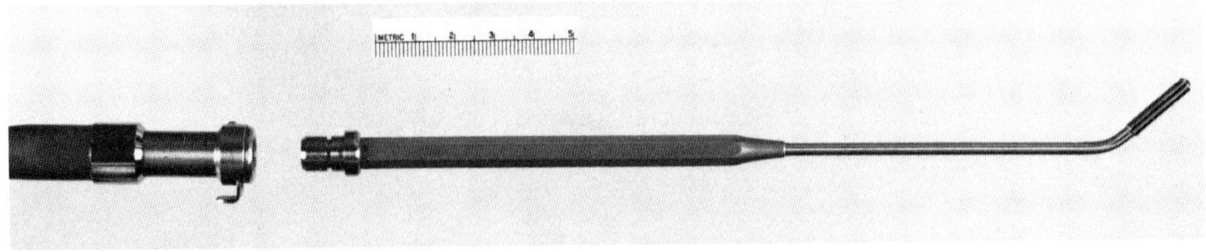

**Figure 2.7**  Light wand designed to attach to light cable. Can be inserted through a separate puncture site to provide supplement lighting. (Reproduced with permission of D. J. Dierschke.)

Other methods of augmenting the illumination for all types of photography are the use of a "light wand," a separate light guide introduced through a second puncture wound, or a "halo light," which is a light guide built into the laparoscope (Figs. 2.6 and 2.7). As a result of the added light guides the cannula will have a somewhat thicker wall and hence a larger diameter than the usual cannula. With the smaller endoscopes, either of these systems will usually provide approximately an order of magnitude more light than the light guide attached to the endoscope itself. The increase will be less dramatic when large diameter endoscopes are used. These units can, by means of a special bifurcated light guide, be supplied from the same light source as the endoscope with no significant loss in brightness. The light wand has the advantages of providing "modeling" or side light for improving the depiction of anatomic morphology or transilluminating internal structures.

## CONCLUSIONS

Successful endoscopy in animals requires patience and an understanding of the principles involved. It is the author's hope that this chapter has aided in providing the latter requirement.

**References**

Prescott, R. (1976) Optical principles of endoscopy. *J. Med. Primatol.* 5:133–147.

Taylor, H. W. (1975) A comparative evaluation of the 5 mm laparoscope in gynecological laparoscopy. *J. Reprod. Med.* 15:65–68.

# CHAPTER 3

# Laparoscopy in the Dog and Cat*

## David E. Wildt, Ph.D.

### INTRODUCTION

The dog and cat play an integral role in veterinary medical science and serve as valuable animal models in biomedical research. In these professions, direct examination and/or alteration of the contents of the abdominal and pelvic cavities have generally required major invasive surgical intervention. Until most recently, there has been little consideration of an alternative, endoscopy, for use in canine and feline veterinary medicine and research. Lettow (1972) reported the first clinical findings on laparoscopy for evaluation of hepatic disease in the dog, but discussed no procedural details on technique. In 1975, our laboratory initiated a canine and feline reproductive research program primarily using laparoscopy as a tool for monitoring ovarian function. These investigations gave rise to related experimental and case studies designed to determine the efficacy of laparoscopy as a diagnostic procedure in clinical veterinary medicine. In 1977, the technical details and applicability of this technique in the male and female dog and cat were first published (Wildt et al., 1977a). This report demonstrated that laparoscopy was a simple, accurate, and practical technique for observation of internal organ anatomy and function. Preliminary results indicated that endoscopy provided considerable clinical potential with respect to health care of these two species. In support of this supposition, Johnson and Twedt (1977) demonstrated the effectiveness of laparoscopy in veterinary oncology for the detection and management of certain intraabdominal neoplasms.

Laparoscopy in canine and feline veterinary medicine and biomedical research remains in infancy. One primary reason has been that laparoscopy techniques and instrumentation have been oriented and promoted only to the human medical profession. This practice shows indications of changing; recently various manufacturers of endoscopy equipment have become aware of the vast veterinary market and have realized the need to develop fiber optic instruments designed specifically for clinical or research animal use. Another reason for the delayed practice of veterinary laparoscopy

* The author acknowledges Paul Guthrie for his expertise in photographing the details of laparoscopic techniques and Richard S. Hall for drawing the medical illustrations.

Thanks are also due to Dr. S. W. J. Seager for advice and critical evaluation of the manuscript, and G. M. Kinney, S. Charman Guthrie, and P. Schmidt for their very capable technical assistance and support.

This work was supported in part by research grants provided by the Ralston Purina Company, Checkerboard Square, St. Louis, Missouri.

has been the lack of a comprehensive description of various techniques and previous experiences by practitioners of the art. This chapter seeks to provide such an inclusive review for the dog and cat.

### General Impressions and Comments on Laparoscopy

Fiber optic technology has advanced considerably in recent years to the extent that most laparoscopes provide optically superior visual fields. For this reason the novice is generally surprised in his first endoscopic viewing experience. Present lens systems provide a variety of panoramic views which encompass large areas of the abdominal cavity without the need to excessively maneuver the laparoscope. Such systems produce varying degrees of magnification which, in many instances, actually allows clearer and more accurate visualization than can be achieved at surgical laparotomy. Unlike the latter procedure, laparoscopy is rarely accompanied by tissue hemorrhage capable of obscuring the visual field. Compared to laparotomy the optical and magnification capabilities of the laparoscope provide a far improved method of documenting certain physiologic events. For example, in research and clinical studies, laparoscopy has allowed the diagnosis and photographic documentation of both subtle and dramatic alterations in ovarian morphology. Many of these investigations have involved the cat in which the vesicular ovarian follicle and mature corpus luteum average only 2.5 and 4.0 mm in diameter, respectively. When one considers that laparoscopy allows accurate distinction of ovarian structures 1 mm or less in diameter, it is difficult to imagine similar success using laparotomy and normal unassisted vision.

The endoscopic examination will never completely replace the need for major abdominal surgery. The technique as developed for human clinical medicine was never intended to eliminate the surgeon or the surgical suite. However, the concept of laparoscopy was initiated to aid and provide a suitable alternative to (or prior to) laparotomy when the clinical or research circumstances accorded such a minor invasive procedure.

### Uses of Laparoscopy

The uses of laparoscopy as performed in our laboratory in the dog and cat can be classified into two major categories: (1) Diagnosis of internal events (Table 3.1); (2) Intraabdominal surgery and manipulation or treatment of disease or injury (Table 3.2). It should be emphasized that the most advantageous characteristic of laparoscopy is that it allows direct examination of the abdominal cavity with only superficial surgical intervention. Of equal importance, laparoscopy, unlike laparotomy, can be performed repeatedly and at frequent intervals within the same animal. The various endoscopic and ancillary procedures included in the tables will be discussed in detail later in the chapter. These lists are not inclusive. Many diagnostic and surgical procedures have

**Table 3.1**
**Laparoscopy for Diagnosis of Internal Events**

1. Direct examination of the abdominal cavity with minor surgical intervention (singular or repeated examinations)

2. Diagnosis of
   a. internal organ hemorrhage or rupture
   b. neoplastic tumors or pathological lesions
   c. adhesions or hernia
   d. reproductive tract disease or infection
   e. early pregnancy or ectopic pregnancy
   f. number of embryos *in utero*
   g. ovarian events and assessment of hormonal therapy

**Table 3.2**
**Laparoscopy for Intraabdominal Surgery, Manipulation, or Treatment of Disease or Injury**

1. Tissue biopsy (liver, kidney, spleen, ovary, adrenal, lesions, tumor).
2. Surgical breakdown of adhesion formation or damage following surgery or pharmacologic treatment.
3. Surgical alteration of the ovarian bursa for ovarian exposure.
4. Aspiration of ovarian or parovarian cysts.
5. Aspiration of follicular oocytes for subsequent *in vitro* culture.
6. Collection of reproductive tract fluids and secretions.
7. Insemination directly into the uterus, uterine horn, or oviduct.
8. Direct intraperitoneal administration of medicinal agents.
9. Uterine horn/oviductal ligation or occlusion, and ovarian coagulation in the female.
10. Vas deferens occlusion in the male.

not, to the author's knowledge, been attempted. As an illustration, there would appear to be a substantial need to determine the efficacy of laparoscopy in the dog and cat for the study, diagnosis, and treatment of gastrointestinal dysfunction, including gallbladder and pancreatic disorders. Both of the latter organs can be viewed easily through an endoscope. As another example, preliminary investigations have been completed in which both dogs and cats have been sterilized laparoscopically. However, considerable contributions remain to be made by the further development of surgical laparoscopy techniques for reproductive control in pets.

In addition to these clinical and research uses, laparoscopy affords a powerful and unique educational device. Recent advances in still photographic capabilities and videotape cassette recording, in combination with laparoscopic instrumentation, provide the student interested in physiology and veterinary science with a new and more detailed perspective of internal organ anatomy and function. At present, several academic institutions have initiated lectures, including laparoscopic photographs and/or videotape recordings of gross organ morphology, pathology, or dynamic internal events such as the structural processes associated with follicular rupture and ovulation. The potential of laparoscopy as an adjunct teaching device deserves further investigation.

### Background

The following information is based on studies conducted over a 3½ year interval using primarily colonized research dogs and cats. A number of the laparoscopic examinations have been performed on privately owned animals and data from these animals have been included in the overall results. A total of 112 dogs and 103 cats have been subjected to one or more laparoscopic examinations. The age and size of the animals have varied widely. Random source cats of mixed breed have been utilized and include kittens weighing 0.2 kg at 18 days of age to adults weighing 4.5 kg at 1 to 9 years of age. In canine studies, dogs weighing 0.5 to 32 kg and 10 days to 9 years of age have been used. Although the dogs vary widely in breed, the majority of animals examined have been purebred beagle, Labrador retriever or mixed breed. Basic laparoscopic technique has not varied among breeds. As will be discussed, size of the animal to be examined does dictate the type of laparoscope and insufflation volume used.

## ANIMAL PREPARATION AND EQUIPMENT

### Animals, Anesthesia, and Restraint

Food is withheld from dogs for 24 hours before laparoscopy. In clinical circumstances, cats should also not be fed; however, in our research situation, fasting has been found unnecessary. On the day of the examination, water is withheld from both species. Routinely, the bladder is not catheterized. Rarely does an enlarged bladder inhibit normal laparoscopic observation or ancillary manipulation. In the event that urinary volume is sufficient to cause inconvenience, a superpubic puncture procedure is performed. This involves the insertion of a 20 gauge, 1.5 inch sterile needle through the abdominal wall and then, with direct laparoscopic observation, into the bladder lumen. A syringe is attached to the needle externally and used to aspirate the urinary fluid.

Laparoscopy in the dog and cat is performed with the animal in a surgical plane of anesthesia. Examinations have been reportedly performed under local anesthesia, but in conjunction with tranquilizers or narcotic analgesics (Johnson and Twedt, 1977). The drug induction regimen to be used depends on the purpose of the laparoscopy and the experience of the laparoscopist. Because many of our studies are concerned with reproductive function and since barbiturates have been implicated to impair ovulation in certain species, such drugs have been avoided for producing anesthesia.

The drug combination of choice for the dog has been ketamine hydrochloride (Ketaset, Bristol Laboratories, 11.0 mg/kg) and xylazine (Rompun, Haver-Lockhart Laboratories, 2.2 mg/kg) given intramuscularly. Induction is rapid (5 minutes or less) and the surgical plane of anesthesia lasts approximately 30 minutes, which is generally sufficient for the experienced laparoscopist. The ketamine-hydrochloride-xylazine mixture has induced a short period of tetany (usually less than 1 minute in duration) in approximately 20% of the dogs weighing less than 11.5 kg body weight. This occurrence, which has not been observed in larger dogs, has not produced any other adverse behavioral or physiologic effects. Dogs appear fully recovered 1½ to two hours after drug administration. The combination of ketamine hydrochloride (20.0 mg/kg) and acepromazine (Ayerst Laboratories, 0.18 mg/kg), injected intramuscularly has been used in cats. Induction time averages 10 to 12 minutes and the surgical plane of anesthesia lasts approximately 30 to 45 minutes. Cats appear fully recovered five to seven hours after administration.

Neither of the above anesthetic regimens has produced drug tolerance, even after frequent administration during studies requiring serial laparoscopy. These particular drug combinations have been administered, for the most part, to clinically healthy animals. It should be emphasized that these drugs may not be the most appropriate for use in animals in a diseased state, particularly those with hepatic or renal dysfunction. In addition, although producing excellent results in our laboratory, neither drug combination would be ideal for situations in which a prolonged laparoscopy examination is required. This would be particularly true for the novice laparoscopist who requires additional anesthesia time for anatomical orientation and the development of various ancillary skills. In this situation, it is more expedient to insert an endotracheal tube and administer inhalation anesthesia (halothane, Fluothane, Ayerst Laboratories).

After anesthesia induction, it is vitally important to correctly position and restrain the animal properly for the forthcoming examination. A standard surgical table with variable tilt is ideal for most average to large sized dogs and cats. Our laboratory generally utilizes a portable, adjustable restraint board (20 × 100 cm, Fig. 3.1) placed on a surgical table for cat and small dog (less than 4.5 kg body weight) laparoscopy. This convenient device allows easier restraint of average sized cats, small kittens and puppies and, when performing a large number of laparoscopies one after the other, eliminates the need to repeatedly adjust the surgical table.

For insertion of the laparoscopic instruments, the surgical table or restraint board should be adjusted so that the animal lies in a supine, head-down position at an angle of approximately 30° (Trendelenburg position). Positioning the animal in this manner allows the abdominal organs to voluntarily shift cranially, closer to the diaphragm. Two advantages are provided by such a maneuver. First, there is a lessening of the danger of traumatizing an organ with a sharp trocar point when inserting the laparoscopic trocar-

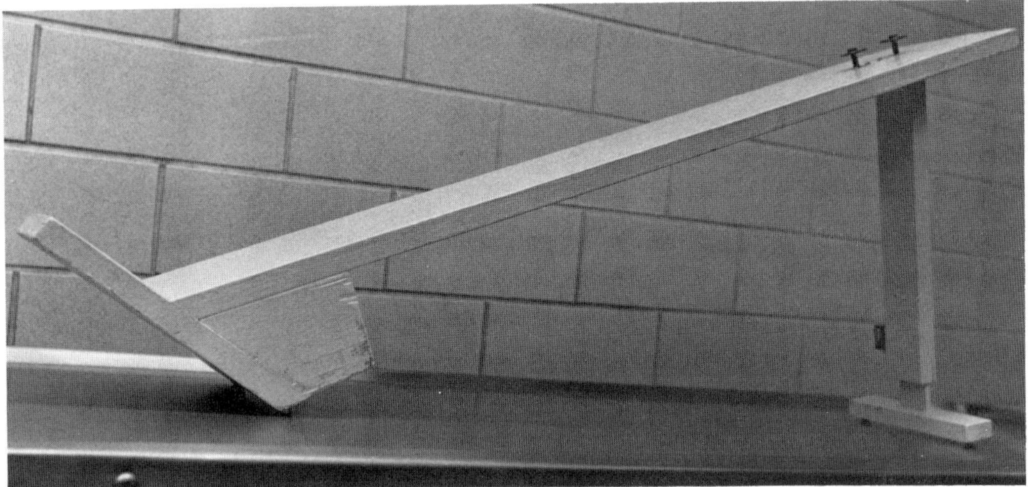

**Figure 3.1** Portable restraint board for examination of cats and small dogs.

cannula unit. Second, the repositioning of the abdominal cavity organs cranially improves the visualization of the pelvic cavity contents, particularly the reproductive organs, colon, and bladder. For viewing the abdominal organs (liver, gallbladder, stomach, spleen) the restraint table is readjusted to a flat 180° plane or 20° with the head elevated.

## Equipment

### LAPAROSCOPES

All of the companies described in Chapter 12 produce instrumentation suitable for canine and feline laparoscopy. The beginner can easily become confused over the variety of sizes and angles of vision provided by various laparoscopic telescopes. After experience with a number of telescopes, the author recommends using a laparoscope providing either a 170° or 180° direction of view. Our laboratory has had particular success with the latter instrument which provides a wide directional view directly from the end of the telescope. This particular type of laparoscope allows rapid visual orientation within the abdominal cavity. Unlike other telescopes which provide an oblique angle of vision which can be initially confusing, the 180° laparoscope provides the "expected normal" field of view. However, before purchase, one should experiment with various instrument types. Oblique angle telescopes are preferred by certain investigators who have criticized the 180° instrument for allowing the terminal viewing lens to become easily contaminated with blood or tissue, thus hindering observation. We have not encountered such a problem.

The range and size of laparoscopes used in the dog and cat vary from 2.7 to 10 mm in diameter. Figure 3.2 illustrates the three laparoscopes (Richard Wolf Medical Instruments Corp.) available in our laboratory. Figure 3.2a is a 10 mm in diameter, 180° laparoscope which provides a superior field of vision. However, because this instrument requires insertion through at least a 2 cm incision site, its use is restricted to dogs weighing more than 10 kg. This size instrument is not recommended for cats. Figure 3.2b shows the 5 mm in diameter, 180° telescope which requires a 1 cm incision site and provides an excellent visual field. The 5 mm in diameter laparoscope is the most versatile, being suitable for cats and dogs regardless of body size. Since the average

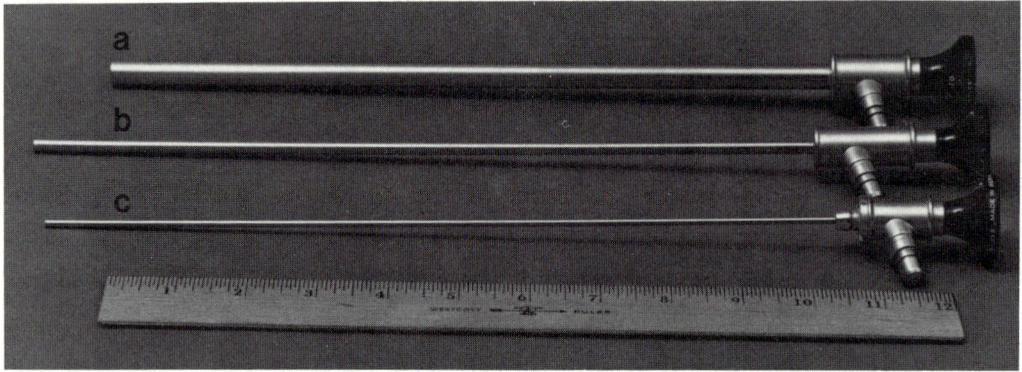

**Figure 3.2**   Three 180° laparoscopes used in the dog and cat: **(a)** 10 mm in diameter; **(b)** 5 mm in diameter; **(c)** 2.7 mm in diameter.

clinic or laboratory will purchase a single telescope, those interested in dog and cat laparoscopy should strongly consider a similar size instrument. Laparoscopes of comparable size, which have been found equally suitable for the dog and cat, include the 4 mm in diameter laparoscope (Dyonics, Inc.), 5 mm in diameter laparoscope (Eder Instrument Co., Inc.), and 4 or 7 mm in diameter laparoscope (Karl Storz Endoscopy-America, Inc.). If a single laparoscopic telescope is to be purchased, it should vary from 4 to 7 mm in diameter.

Our laboratory also has available an endoscope 2.7 mm in diameter (Fig. 3.2c). This instrument is a modified arthroscope and has been found useful only in examination of very small kittens or puppies. The incision length for insertion is small (0.5 cm); however, the field of vision is limited, making the use of this particular endoscope for routine canine or feline examination rather complicated and time consuming.

Reference should also be made to the operating laparoscope (Fig. 3.3). The eyepiece of this instrument is offset to the body of the telescope barrel, the latter containing a channel for the insertion of accessory instruments. The operating laparoscope is designed to allow internal organ biopsy or surgical manipulation without the insertion of a secondary accessory cannula. Although effective for obtaining tissue samples in large sized dogs, the diameter of this instrument excludes routine diagnostic use in small dogs and cats. The insertion cannula is large in diameter (11 to 12 mm) due to the additional space required for the operating channel. Most laparoscopists generally consider that the two puncture accessory cannula technique provides versatility not capable of being achieved with a single puncture operating laparoscope.

## LAPAROSCOPIC TROCAR-CANNULA ASSEMBLY

Trocar-cannula units must correspond in size to the type of laparoscope used. Most assemblies resemble that shown in Figure 3.4. Trocar tips are conical or pyramidal (Fig. 3.4) in shape. The latter is generally preferred in dogs and cats since the cutting edge allows easy perforation through the muscle and peritoneal wall. Although the conical tip trocar requires more force for insertion, there is less danger of injuring internal organs than when using the pyramidal type. However, both trocar designs are satisfactory and safe when used correctly. The cannula generally consists of a channel with a trumpet (Fig. 3.4a) or clip valve to prevent insufflation loss when the laparoscopic trocar is withdrawn. Most cannulae contain an insufflating sleeve and valve situated perpendicular to the channel (Fig. 3.4b). The insufflating hose is attached to the sleeve and gas is passed through the channel to maintain a pneumoperitoneum. The cannula with insufflation sleeve is very useful when performing dog and cat laparoscopy.

## ILLUMINATION SOURCE AND LIGHT CABLE

The total expense of the laparoscopy unit depends considerably on the type of light source purchased. A variety of such devices exists capable of providing illumination suitable for diagnostic procedures alone or combined diagnostic and photographic use (see Chapter 12). Relatively inexpensive units are available which are compact in size and usually contain a single 150 watt lamp. These units are suitable for diagnostic examination but are inadequate for providing sufficient illumination for laparoscopic photography. The latter can be achieved using a light source similar to that illustrated in Figure 3.5 which consists of a heavy duty light projector with an alternating light source (150 watts for diagnosis and 1000 watts for photography). A variety of other such units exists which contain sophisticated lamp or synchronous electronic flash systems capable of allowing laparoscopic photography.

The decision on the type of illumination source to purchase should be examined carefully. In research, it is obviously important to document observation; consequently, investigators should consider the purchase of a light unit with photographic capability. Veterinary clinicians may have well-founded reservations concerning the added expense of a photographic illumination source. Discussions with clinicians who have purchased these units have been favorable. Veterinarians have cited numerous advantages of laparoscopic photography, including documentation of interesting clinical case observations for later consultation with colleagues or clients or for illustration at scientific meetings.

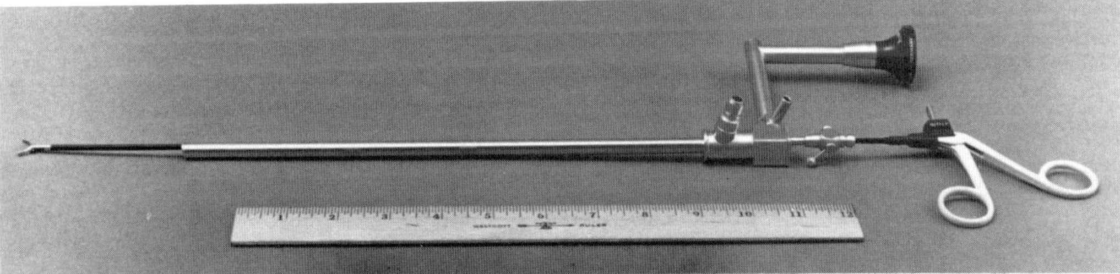

**Figure 3.3** Operating laparoscope for single puncture technique. This instrument contains a channel for insertion of an ancillary device. A manipulatory forceps is inserted as an example.

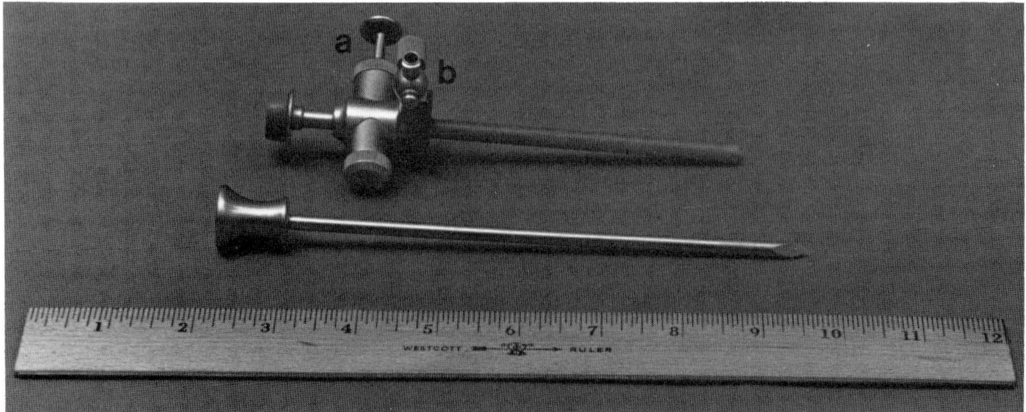


**Figure 3.4** Trocar with pyramidal tip and cannula with trumpet valve **(a)** and insufflating sleeve **(b)**.

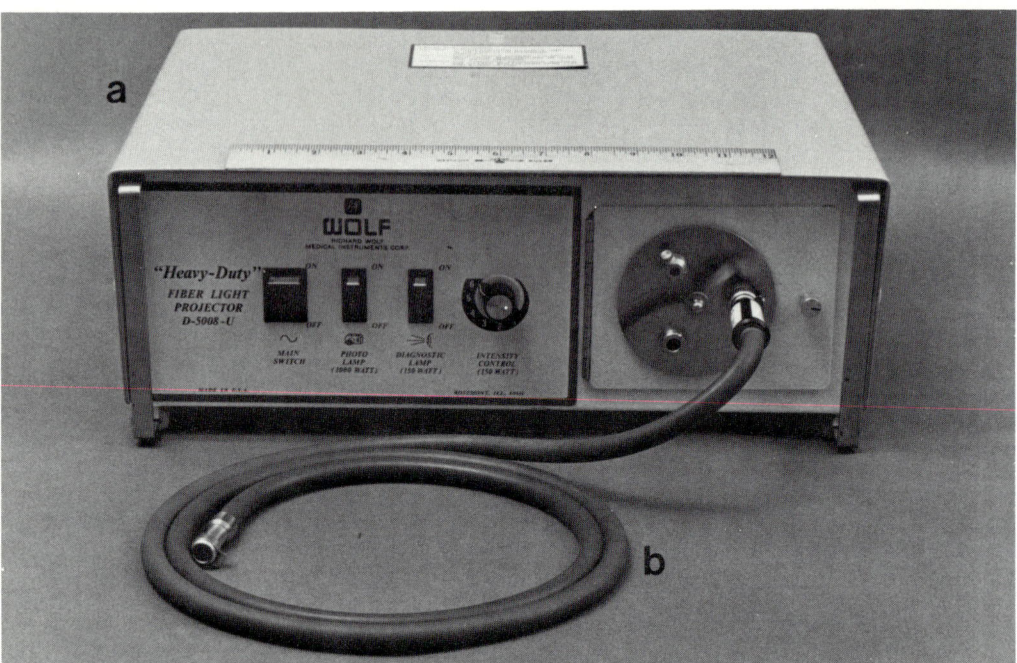

**Figure 3.5**  Heavy duty light source **(a)** with diagnostic and photographic capability and 6 mm in diameter fiber optic cable **(b)**.

A fiber optic cable is required to transmit the light from the illumination source to the laparoscopic telescope. Cables can be purchased in a variety of diameters. For dog and cat laparoscopy, a large diameter cable (6 mm) is preferred (Fig. 3.5). Although more bulky, the greater sized cable provides more light transmission and, hence, better internal illumination.

## PNEUMOPERITONEUM INSTRUMENTATION

For routine laparoscopy, the abdominal cavity must be insufflated to create an intraabdominal air space. The pneumoperitoneum is produced before insertion of the trocar-cannula assembly, since the added internal air space lessens the possibility of puncturing organs with the trocar tip. A hollow Verres needle with a spring loaded, blunt tip that protrudes beyond the needle bevel when the abdominal cavity space is entered is used for producing the initial pneumoperitoneum (Fig. 3.6). In the dog and cat, a Verres needle approximately 120 mm in length and equipped with an on-off valve should be used. Four different types of equipment may be utilized for supplying gas to the Verres needle.

**1. Automatic Insufflators.** Most manufacturers of fiber optic systems produce these devices (Fig. 3.7). Generally, the insufflator is attached to a commercial tank of gas by means of a yoke and cable apparatus. The device contains an internal chamber, which is filled with gas from the external tank, and a sleeve with hose attachment which transfers the gas to the Verres needle. Gauges and flowmeters on the insufflator record external tank pressure, internal tank volume, intraabdominal pressure, and gas flow rates into the animal. From this information, one can accurately determine the degree of pneumoperitoneum, thus avoiding the problems of excessive insufflation. In short, although adding expense, automatic insufflators provide convenience and safety. In the

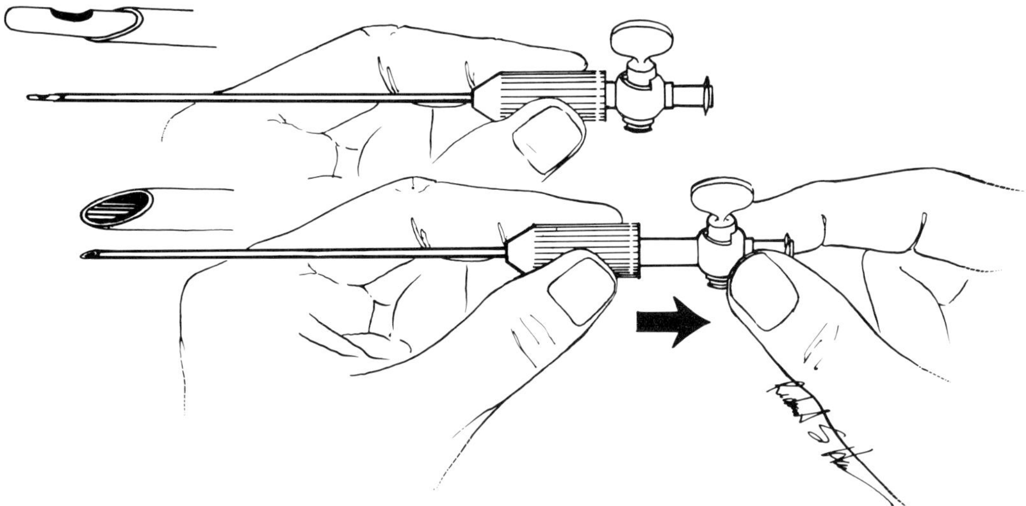

**Figure 3.6** Verres needle for insufflation and manipulation. The blunt tip of the needle can be retracted, producing a sharp outer tip which facilitates insertion through the abdominal wall.

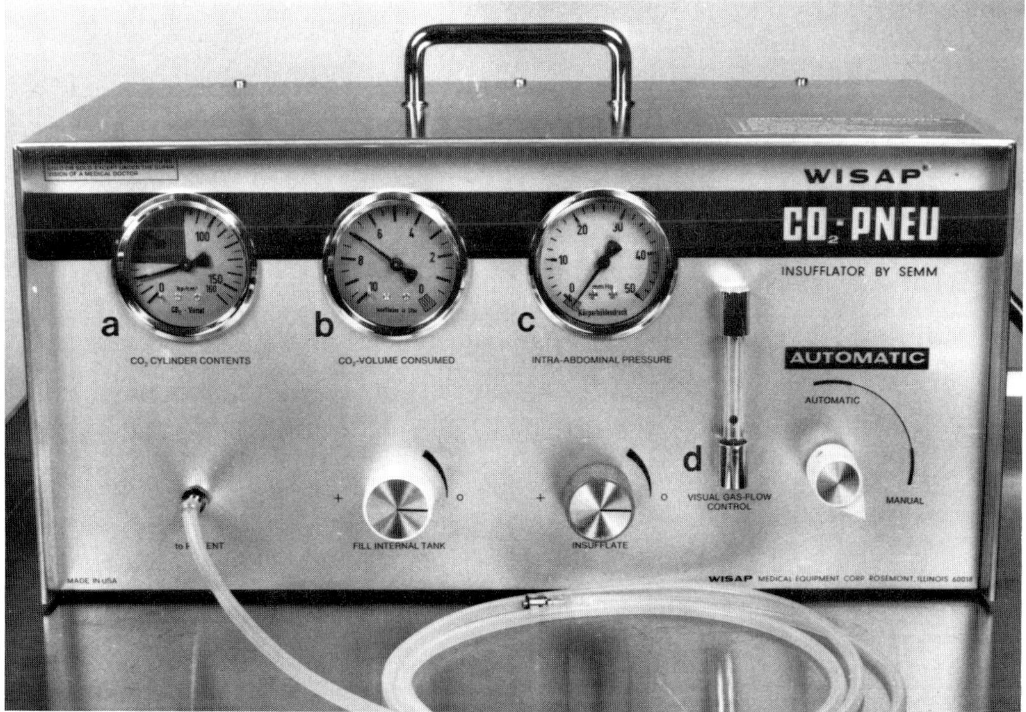


**Figure 3.7** Commercial insufflator with gauges to indicate $CO_2$ cylinder contents **(a)**; $CO_2$ volume consumed **(b)**; intraabdominal pressure **(c)**; visual meter to indicate gas flow **(d)**; and attached insufflatory hose.

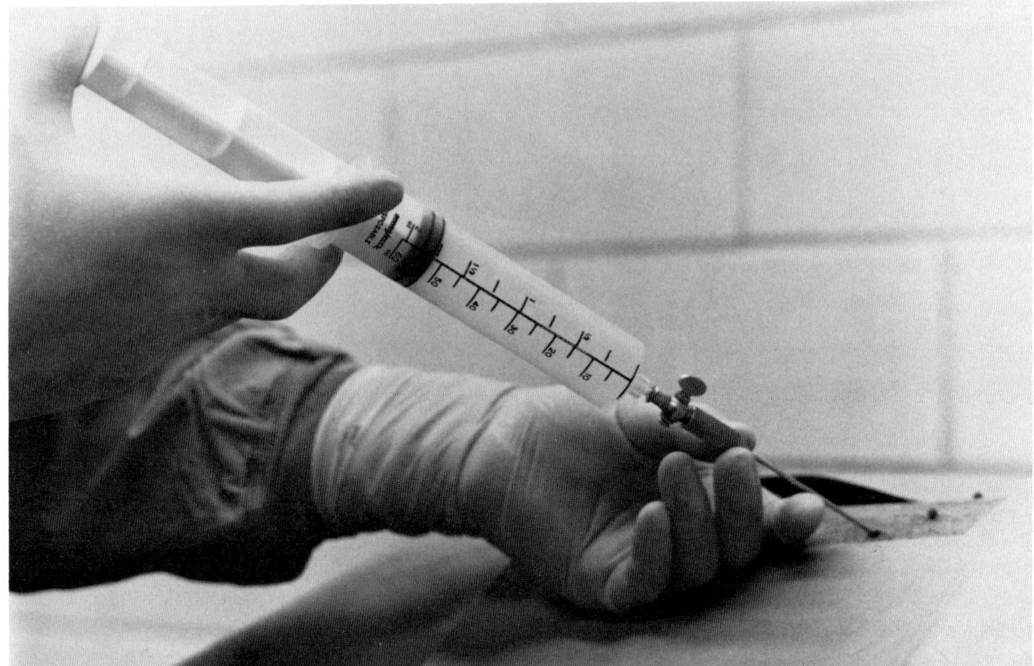

**Figure 3.8**   Insufflation using the hand syringe technique. Syringe (60 ml) is attached to the Verres needle inserted through the abdominal wall.

author's opinion, the automatic insufflator is an important addition to the laparoscopy instrumentarium.

**2. External Gas Tanks.** Commercial tanks of various sizes have been equipped with regulatory valves, a gas hose attached and the animal insufflated with gas directly from the tank. This technique has been used effectively, but requires regulator valves which allow *slow* gas release at *reduced* pressure. Caution is required to avoid overinsufflation of the animal when using this system.

**3. Hand Syringe or Bulb Pump.** A sterile syringe (20 to 60 ml volume) can be directly attached to the Verres needle and used to introduce room air into the abdominal cavity (Fig. 3.8). This technique is not efficient, since to produce an adequate pneumoperitoneum the syringe must be removed from the needle, refilled with room air and the procedure repeated a number of times. During some laparoscopy examinations, gas will escape from the abdominal cavity, necessitating further insufflation. The hand syringe technique is inconvenient since the examination must be momentarily stopped to allow reattachment of the syringe and further transfer of gas via the Verres needle.

An alternative hand method involves using a hand bulb pump similar to those used to inflate a blood pressure cuff. Such a device can also be attached to the Verres needle, is inexpensive, and also portable.

**4. Carbon Dioxide Dispenser.** Several investigators have reported the successful use of a hand carbon dioxide ($CO_2$) dispenser (Corkmaster-Leland Industries, Inc., or The British Oxygen Co. Ltd.). This unit contains a small $CO_2$ pressurized cartridge and can be directly attached to the Verres needle by means of a short length (2 to 5 cm) of flexible hose. This device is convenient and effective for use in the dog and cat. However, caution should be exercised in cats and small dogs since gas can be easily released too rapidly from the cartridge, producing excessive pneumoperitoneum.

Air, carbon dioxide (Wildt *et al.*, 1977a), or nitrous oxide (Johnson and Twedt, 1977) have been successfully and safely used for insufflation of the dog and cat. Currently, our laboratory prefers a mixture of 5% $CO_2$ in air or 100% $CO_2$. Since $CO_2$ is a product of natural biological metabolism it is, therefore, open to the lowest possible rate of complications. Following the examination, this gas is readily absorbed by the tissue of the abdominal cavity. This lessens postoperative discomfort reportedly experienced by women subjected to insufflation (Loffer *et al.*, 1978). Neither nitrogen, due to its insolubility, nor oxygen, due to its combustibility, is an acceptable gas for creating the pneumoperitoneum.

## SURGICAL INSTRUMENTS

Standard surgical instruments required include scalpel, scalpel blade (no. 10), thumb forceps, needle holder, and suture material. Our laboratory utilizes 3-0 Dexon absorbable suture (American Cyanamid Co.) for repairing the peritoneum and skin incision sites.

## ACCESSORY LAPAROSCOPIC INSTRUMENTS

A variety of ancillary instruments exists to perform various internal manipulations under direct laparoscopic observation. Only three general type instruments are required for most clinical or research procedures in the dog and cat. These include a manipulatory forceps, biopsy forceps, and scissors device (Fig. 3.9). Most of these devices are insulated and equipped for use in conjunction with electrocoagulation units, thus allowing dual function. Further details on preferred instrument types will be discussed later in the chapter.

Insertion of these devices into the abdominal cavity is preceded by the insertion of an accessory trocar-cannula unit 3 or 6 mm in diameter (depending on the size of the corresponding forceps). Accessory cannulae are generally not equipped with trumpet valves, although some contain internal clip valves to prevent loss of gas.

## PHOTOGRAPHY INSTRUMENTATION

For still photography an SLR camera with standard 50 or 100 mm lens or specialized laparoscopic lens system is generally used. The design of a laparoscope adapter by one manufacturer (Richard Wolf Medical Instruments Corp.) allows use of most standard

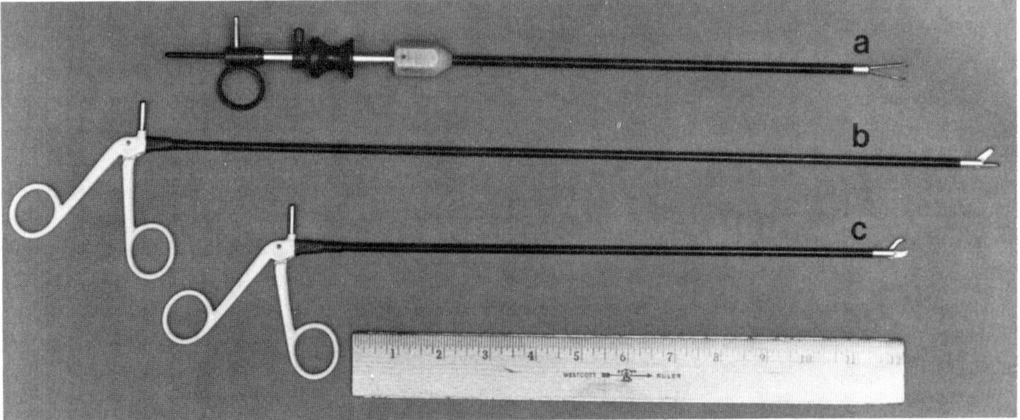

**Figure 3.9**  Three accessory instruments: **(a)** Palmer forceps for manipulation, electrocoagulation, or biopsy; **(b)** grasping biopsy forceps; **(c)** hook scissors.

SLR cameras routinely used in the research laboratory or clinical practice. These cameras can be readily adapted for endoscopic photography by using a special laparoscopic ring adapter which screws into the lens and allows the camera to be easily attached and removed from the eyepiece of the laparoscope.

In the event that a camera body and lens must be purchased, one should carefully consider size and weight. Some cameras are bulky and require both hands to steady the unit while photographing. Our laboratory prefers use of a small lightweight camera such as the Olympus OM-1 (Olympus Corp. of America). This particular unit provides improved picture quality since the laparoscopist can easily operate the camera with one hand while holding the laparoscope with the other hand. Film for still photography should be of the high speed type. In our studies, excellent results have been obtained with Kodak Ektachrome color film (daylight, ASA 200 or 400). Movie and videotape systems, to the author's knowledge, have not yet been utilized in dog and cat laparoscopy programs. Since these devices have been successful in laparoscopically documenting internal events in zoo mammals (see Chapter 10) and in birds and reptiles (see Chapter 11), it is logical that such systems would be equally effectual in domesticated mammals.

## MOBILE UTILITY CART

In our laboratory facility, laparoscopic examinations are performed in various surgical suites. It has been convenient to maintain the light source, automatic insufflator, and accessories (photographic equipment, surgical gloves, syringes, etc.) on a mobile utility cart (Fig. 3.10). This allows equipment to be easily transferred from room to room and closely situated to the surgical table. Specialized laparoscopy carts with space for insufflating tanks are available or standard laboratory carts may be modified accordingly.

### Equipment and Surgical Preparation

The laparoscope and accessory instruments require sterilization or chemical cleansing prior to use. Autoclavable laparoscopes are available but are not recommended. Previous investigators have had the unfortunate experience of determining that some telescopes fail to withstand repeated steam autoclavings. Lens seals within the endoscope have deteriorated, allowing internal moisture formation and necessitating costly repairs and delay. In addition, often several animals are scheduled to undergo laparoscopy at approximately the same time. This is particularly true in a laboratory situation in which two to five animals are subjected to laparoscopy one after the other. It would be impractical to autoclave the laparoscope between examinations. Gas autoclaving can also be performed but is not feasible for this same reason.

Cold or "wet" sterilization of instruments is the method of choice. A germicidal solution, Nolvasan-S (chlorhexidine, Fort Dodge Laboratories, Inc.) is mixed in a deep plastic or metal pan of sufficient length to allow total immersion of the laparoscope and accessory instruments. If desired, one may also sterilize the gas hose and fiber optic cable in this manner. Equipment is kept in this solution for 20 minutes prior to use. With the exception of the eyepiece of the telescope, it is not necessary to rinse or dry the instruments before performing the examination.

Controversy has existed over the degree of sterility which must be maintained in performing a rather minor surgical procedure such as laparoscopy. Infection is really related to the degree of peritoneal contamination which is minimal at laparoscopy. Large areas of open tissue and large amounts of necrotic tissue predispose to infection problems. These conditions are not found at laparoscopy. There is no question that the veterinarian should exercise the same precautions to achieve sterile conditions for laparoscopy that would be used for routine laparotomy. This would include utilization of sterile drapes and surgical clothing. Due to financial limitations and the large number of animals requiring examination in our laboratory studies, the majority of laparoscopic

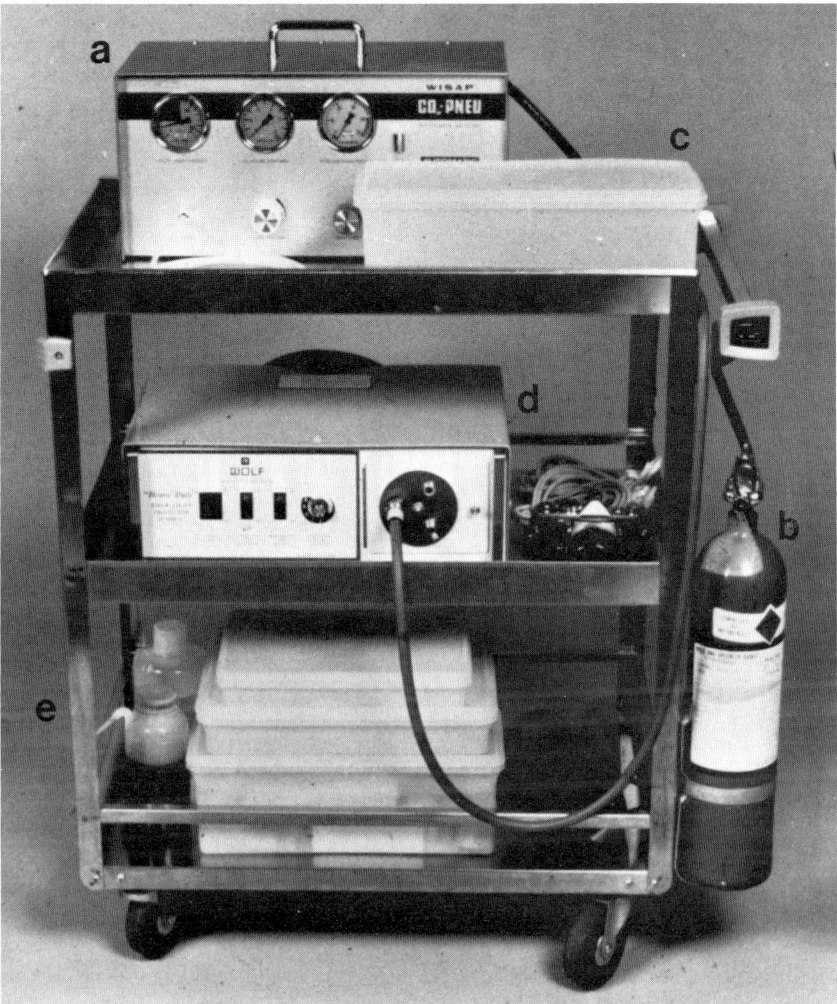

**Figure 3.10** Standard laboratory cart modified for transfer of laparoscopy equipment: **(a)** insufflator; **(b)** CO$_2$ tank; **(c)** plastic pan for immersion of instruments; **(d)** light source and fiber optic cable; **(e)** miscellaneous, including drugs, surgical preparation solutions, surgical gloves.

examinations have involved only "wet" sterilization of instruments and surgical preparation of the animal. Sterile surgical drapes and clothing have not been routinely used.

Following restraint of the animal in a supine position, the abdominal region from the pubis to the point of the xiphoid process is clipped. This area is scrubbed and disinfected with a povidone-iodine (Betadine, Purdue Frederick Co.) solution. At this time, if sterile surgery is required, the animal should be draped.

## LAPAROSCOPIC TECHNIQUES AND ANCILLARY PROCEDURES

### Insufflation and Laparoscope Insertion

The surgical table or restraint board is tilted to the previously described angle (Fig. 3.11). In the dog and cat a pneumoperitoneum should be established *before* insertion of the laparoscopic instruments. This is accomplished by retracting the internal blunt tip of the Verres needle, thus producing a sharp point to allow easy instrument insertion. This maneuver can be performed with one hand, simultaneously inserting the needle through the abdominal wall while using the other hand to grasp the skin and steady the animal (Fig. 3.12). Generally, the Verres needle is inserted in the lower right abdominal quadrant, 4 to 8 cm lateral to the midline. The laparoscopist can reasonably detect when the Verres needle has perforated the internal peritoneal wall. The spring of the needle is released, adjusting the Verres needle back to a blunt instrument. It is essential that the insufflator needle penetrate all layers of the abdominal wall to avoid false placement into the skin, fat, muscle, fascia, or peritoneum.

The gas hose from the automatic insufflator or commercial tank is fixed to the Verres needle, the valve on the latter opened and the gas transferred into the abdominal cavity (Fig. 3.13). Insufflation volume varies with body size. Table 3.3 illustrates gas volumes commonly used for various sized dogs and cats. Unless an automatic insufflator is available, the laparoscopist will be unaware of the exact volume used. One can subjectively judge that a sufficient volume of gas has been incorporated when the ventral abdominal wall becomes slightly distended and turgid to touch (Fig. 3.14). If the animal appears quite "ballooned," too much insufflation has been used and normal respiration could be adversely affected. The gas hose from the Verres needle should be immediately removed, leaving the valve open to allow escape of excessive abdominal gas. This can be facilitated by pressing the abdominal wall.

After obtaining a proper pneumoperitoneum, a 1 to 2 cm (depending on trocar-cannula size) midline incision is made in the skin 2 to 4 cm cranial to the umbilicus (Fig. 3.15). Incision or blunt dissection of the muscle layer is unnecessary. The trocar and cannula are removed from the sterilization pan and assembled. The trocar-cannula unit is held so that the base of the trocar abuts against the heel of the hand with the fingers grasping the cannula unit (Fig. 3.16). The trocar-cannula is held at 30° to the longitudinal plane of the animal. The animal is supported by the laparoscopist's free hand which is used to grasp the ventral abdominal wall adjacent to the insertion site (Fig. 3.17). The trocar-cannula unit is inserted with a steady twisting motion of the hand and wrist (Fig. 3.17). Due to the cutting edge of the pyramidal trocar tip, the latter maneuver lessens resistance and thus permits easier insertion. Ramming or repeated short stabbing motions with the trocar-cannula assembly should be avoided.

Upon piercing the peritoneal wall, the laparoscopist will detect an audible "pop" and should immediately stop further insertion until the trocar tip is withdrawn inside the cannula. Once assured the cannula is within the abdominal cavity, the trumpet valve is depressed, the trocar removed (Fig. 3.18) and the valve immediately released and allowed to shut to avoid insufflatory loss (Fig. 3.19). The gas hose is removed from the Verres needle and attached to the insufflatory sleeve of the cannula (Fig. 3.20). The laparoscope is removed from the sterile solution and the eyepiece lens dried with sterile gauze. The laparoscope is inserted into the anterior end of the cannula and the trumpet valve depressed, thus allowing insertion into the peritoneal cavity (Fig. 3.21). The flexible light cable is then attached to the sleeve of the laparoscopic eyepiece. The lamp

**Table 3.3**
**Insufflation Volumes Used for Laparoscopy of the Cat and Dog***

| Animal body weight (kg) | Volume of gas (L) |
|:---:|:---:|
| <2.5 | <0.5 |
| 2.5–4.5 | 0.5 |
| 4.6–14 | 1 |
| >14 | 1–2 |

* Reproduced with permission from the *Am. J. Vet. Res.* 38(9):1429–1432, 1977.

within the illumination source is switched on, thus transferring light to the cable and laparoscope. If the animal is properly positioned, and an adequate pneumoperitoneum has been established, the laparoscopist should be able to immediately identify internal organs.

## Technique Problems Encountered During Laparoscopy

The inexperienced operator should be aware of several techniques to allow rapid anatomical orientation and skill development. Correct positioning and support of the laparoscope while inserted into the abdominal cavity is one critical factor. Due to the patient's size, it is necessary in human endoscopy for the laparoscopist to take a standing position to the side of the surgical table. However, during laparoscopic examinations of most dogs and cats, size of the animals allows them to be positioned on the surgical table so that the laparoscopist can sit on a laboratory stool at the end of the table. This permits the endoscopist to rest the elbows on the table as shown in Figure 3.22, providing additional instrument support. Most beginning laparoscopists tend to hold the laparoscope near the eyepiece (Fig. 3.23), a mistake which allows the telescope to descend dorsally into the abdominal tissue, thus prohibiting visualization. To alleviate this problem, the laparoscope should be supported by the cannula, which is grasped and elevated slightly ventrally (Fig. 3.24). In effect, this maneuver both prohibits tissue from obstructing the viewing field and assists in maintaining the intraabdominal space.

A related problem is sometimes encountered during the early stages of the laparoscopic examination and is due to omentum hindering visualization. This occurs when the Verres needle initially becomes inserted under the omental fold and insufflation elevates the omentum vertically to the ventral abdominal wall. Since at this time the omentum is supported only by air, it is rarely pierced by the trocar-cannula. When the laparoscope is inserted, one discovers the inflated omental fold lying against the end lens of the endoscope (Fig. 3.25). This can be corrected by utilization of the Verres needle as a manipulatory probe. Maneuvering the probe onto the omentum and applying slight pressure will deflate this tissue, allowing clear visualization.

A laparoscopist will sometimes discover that the end lens of a telescope becomes contaminated with fat or body fluids, or the view appears hindered by fog. Although sometimes required, it is not always necessary to remove the laparoscope from the cavity and clean the lens with sterile gauze. Often, the lens can be cleared simply by touching the end of the telescope against internal tissue (Fig. 3.26). Fogging may result due to temperature differences from inserting a laparoscope sterilized in cold solution into the warm abdominal cavity. This problem is usually alleviated by using a warm germicidal soaking solution or by allowing the laparoscope a short equilibration time to achieve the same temperature as the peritoneal cavity.

It is rare that one can perform a diagnostic laparoscopy without manipulation of some internal organ or tissue. For example, in the cat it is generally necessary to use an accessory probe to view the ovaries. Each ovary is located slightly dorsally, usually under a portion of the small intestine and generally covered by the fimbria. Depending on the exact situation, ovarian exposure may require only slight to rather extensive manipulation. The laparoscopist should not be overly concerned with traumatizing the internal organs of the dog and cat with the accessory probe or forceps. The beginning laparoscopist tends to fear such an occurrence, thus avoiding the proper utilization of accessory instruments designed to facilitate the examination.

## Diagnostic Capabilities of Laparoscopy

The laparoscope provides a panoramic view of the abdominal cavity contents. Specific procedures required for observing various organs will be described later. The

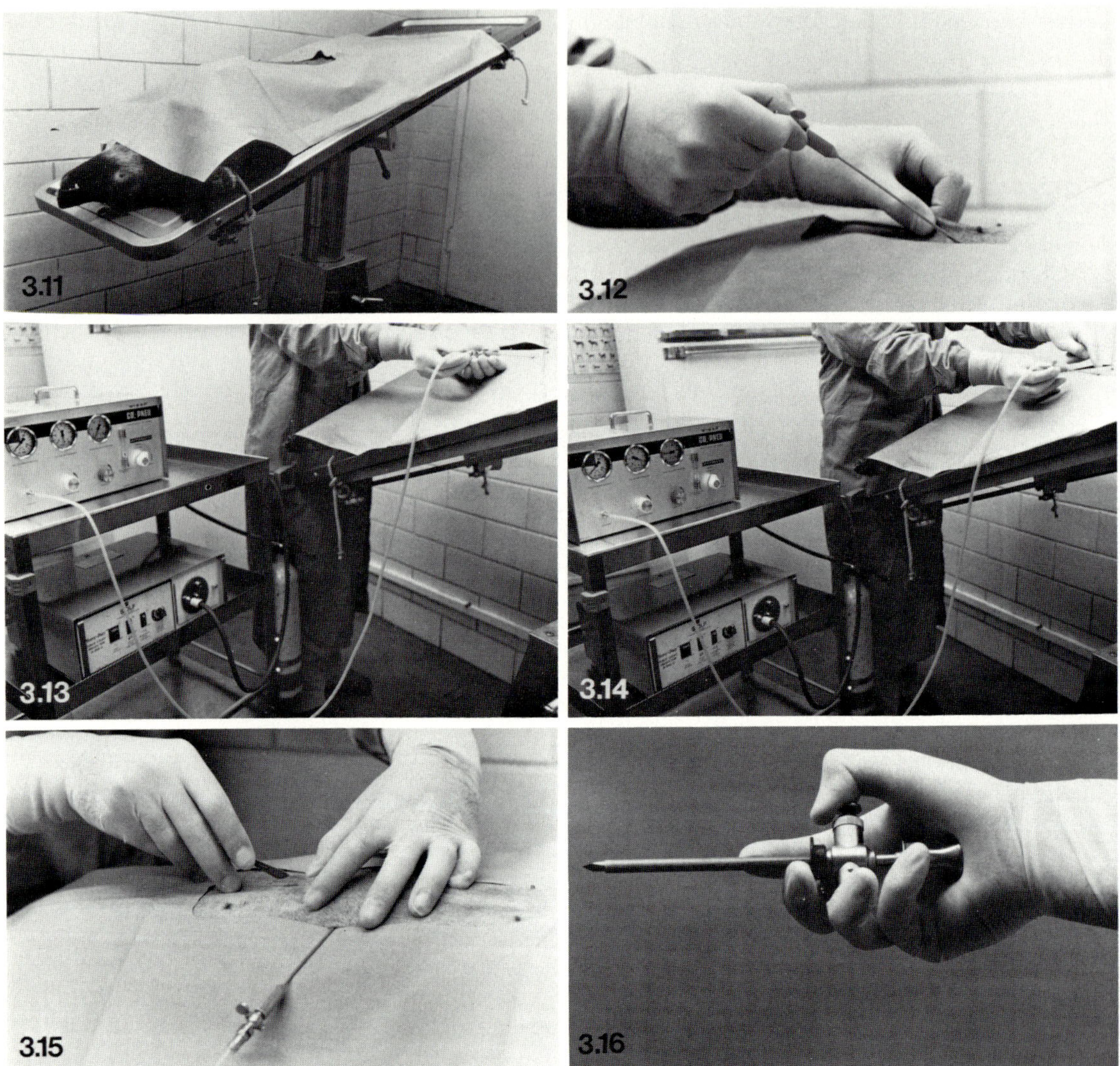

**Figure 3.11**   Animal surgically prepared in a Trendelenburg position.
**Figure 3.12**   Inserting the Verres needle through the abdominal wall. The left hand is used to grasp the skin and support the abdominal wall. The right hand is used to retract the blunt tip of the needle, simultaneously inserting the device.
**Figure 3.13**   Attaching the gas hose from the insufflator to the inserted Verres needle.
**Figure 3.14**   Determining the distension of the abdominal wall during insufflation. The intraabdominal pressure gauge and the visual flowmeter of the insufflator indicate that gas is being passed into the peritoneal cavity.
**Figure 3.15**   Site and length of midline skin incision.
**Figure 3.16**   Method for holding the assembled trocar-cannula during insertion. The base of the trocar abuts the heel of the hand.

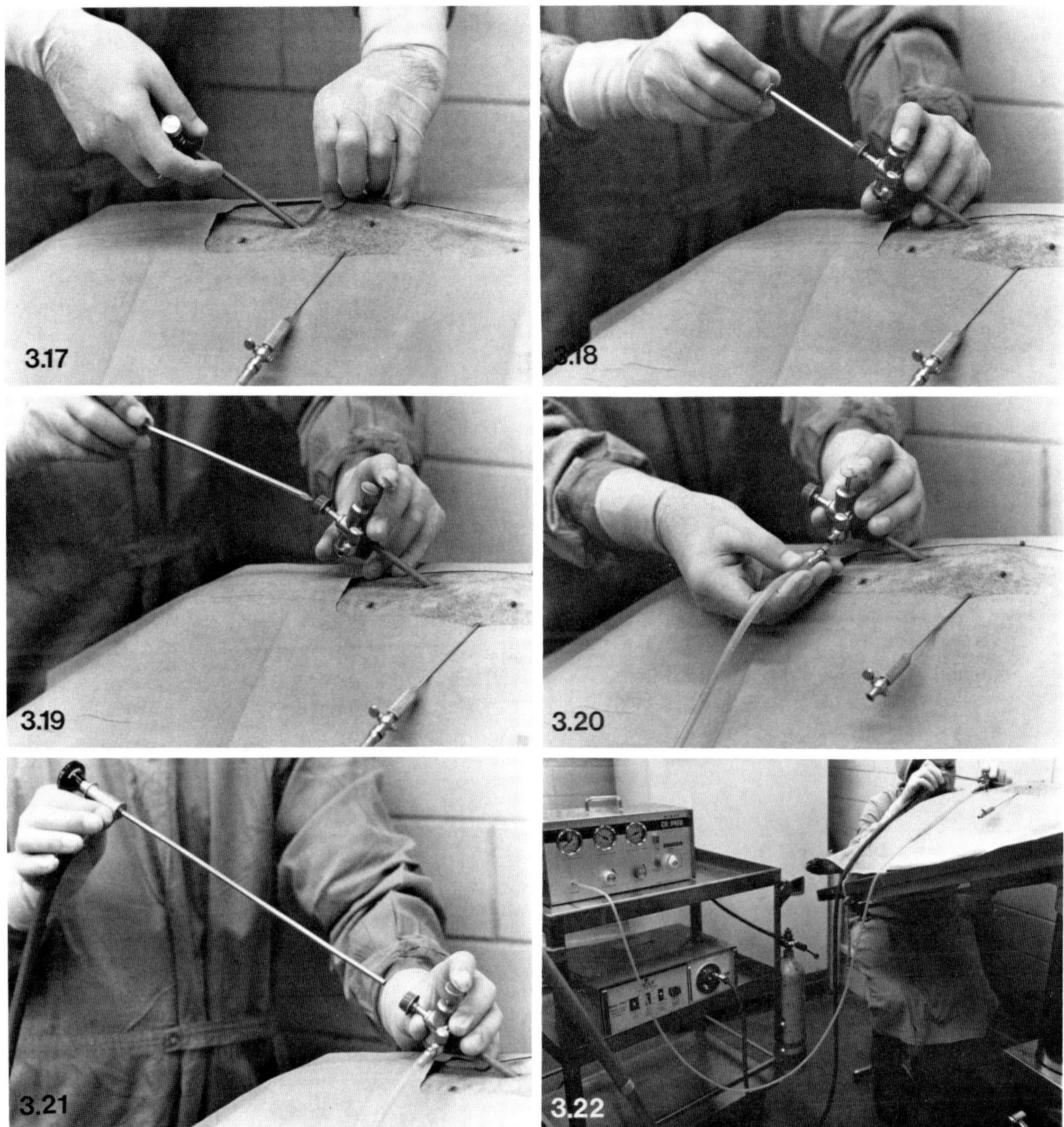

**Figure 3.17**  Insertion of the midline trocar-cannula. The left hand is used to support the abdominal wall; the right hand is used to twist the trocar-cannula for easy insertion.
**Figure 3.18**  Trumpet valve of the cannula is depressed, allowing removal of the trocar.
**Figure 3.19**  Trumpet valve of the cannula is immediately released after trocar removal, prohibiting insufflatory loss.
**Figure 3.20**  Attachment of the gas hose to the insufflatory sleeve of the cannula.
**Figure 3.21**  Insertion of the laparoscope (with cable attached) through the midline cannula.
**Figure 3.22**  Examination with the operator in a sitting position.

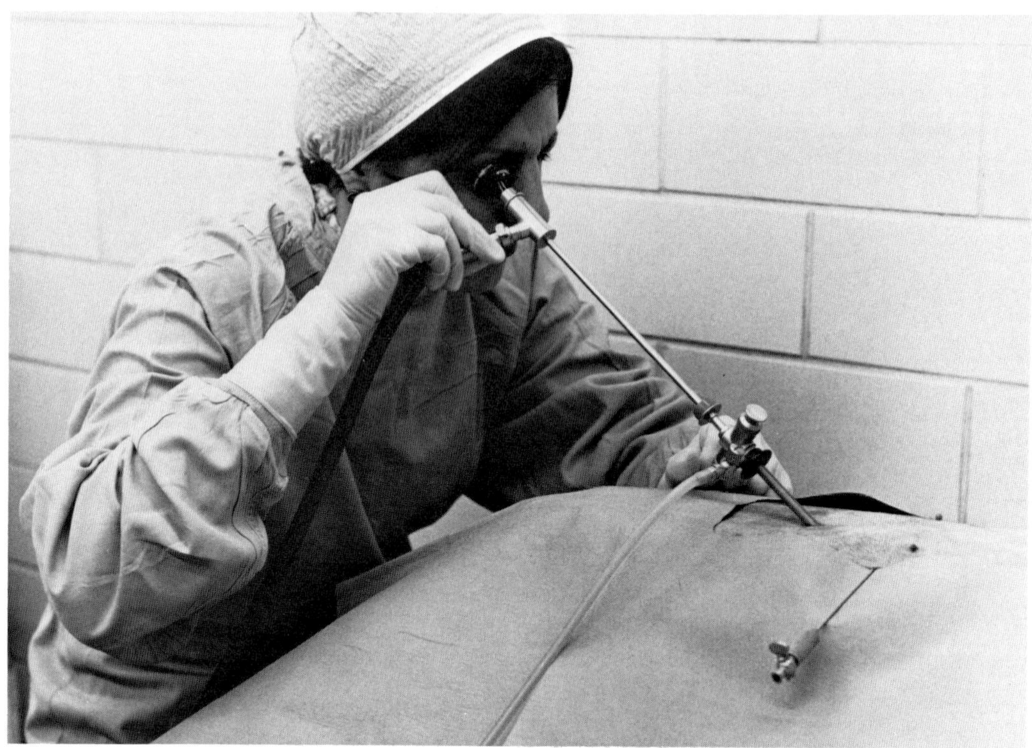

**Figure 3.23** Incorrect support of the laparoscope-cannula assembly. Holding the instrument near the eyepiece allows the terminus of the endoscope to descend dorsally into the abdominal tissue.

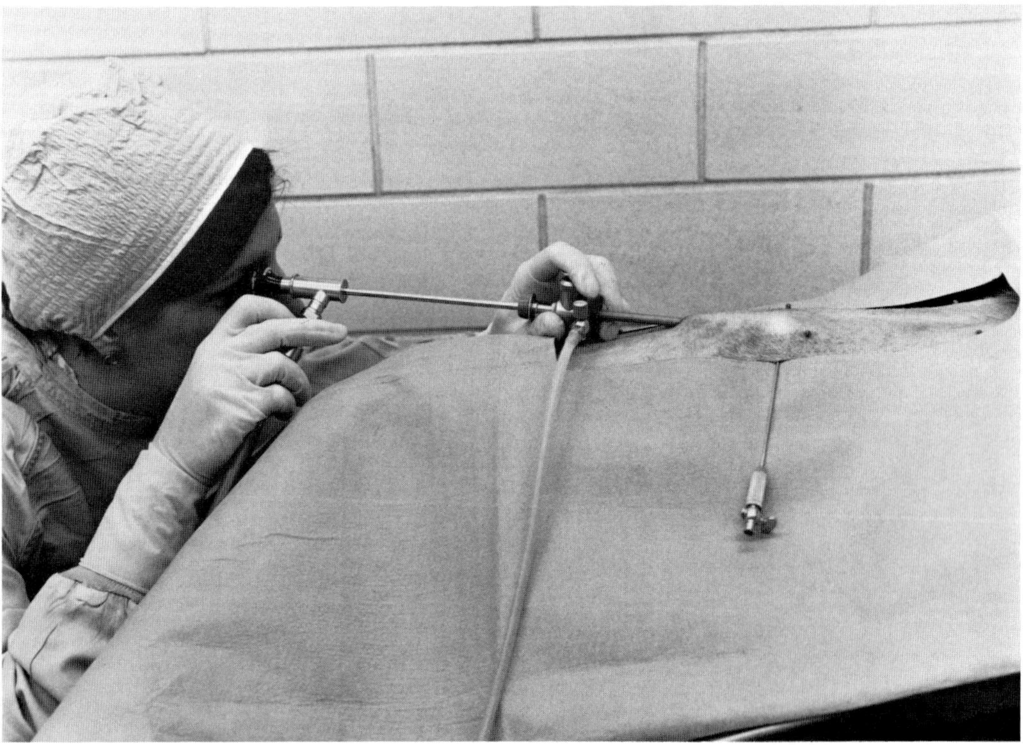

**Figure 3.24** Correct support of the laparoscope-cannula assembly. Most of the weight of the instrument is supported by the left hand holding the cannula. The entire assembly is elevated ventrally to allow visualization.

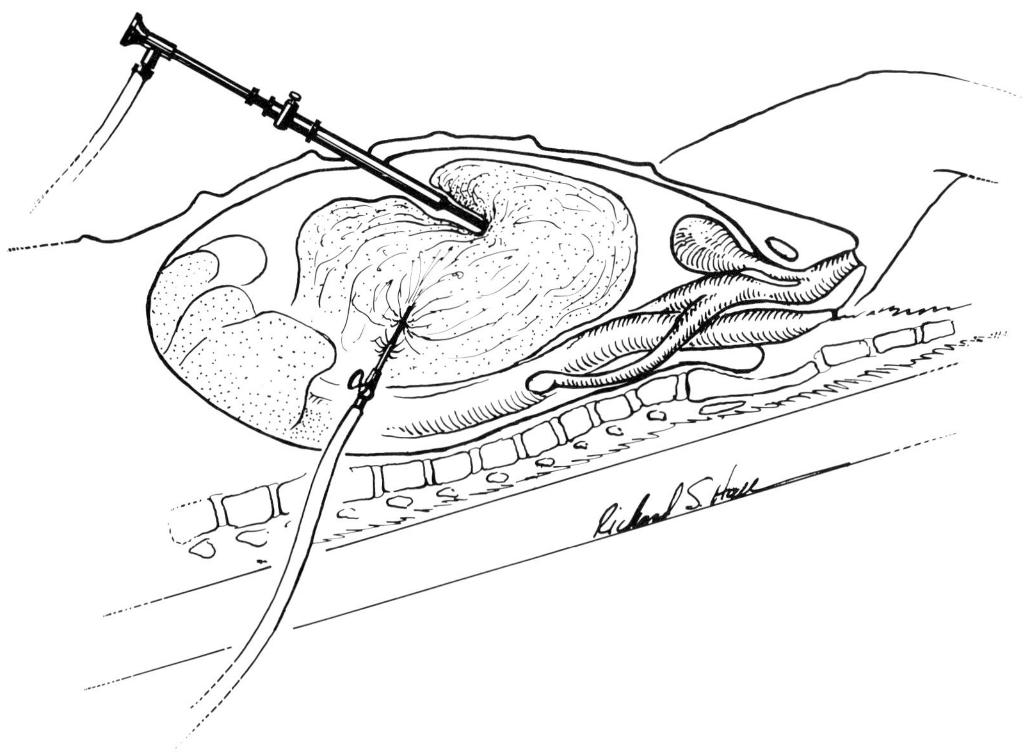

**Figure 3.25** When the Verres needle is initially inserted under the omental fold, the omentum can be elevated by insufflation, thus inhibiting visualization through the laparoscope.

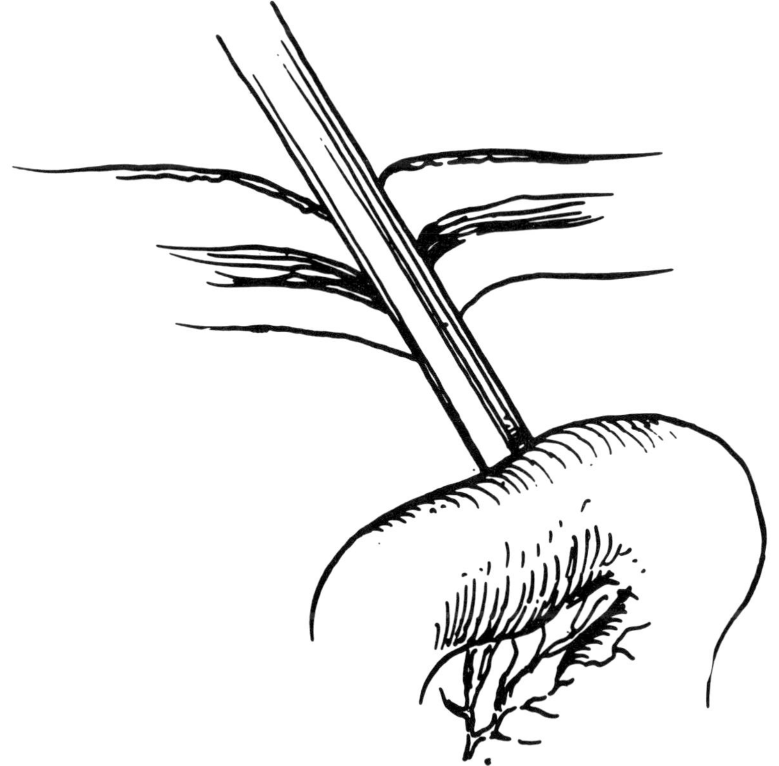

**Figure 3.26** A contaminated or foggy lens can often be cleared by simply touching the end of the telescope against internal tissue.

technique provides a powerful diagnostic tool for simply determining if major internal organs appear morphologically healthy or abnormal.

In the dog and cat, most aspects of the urinary bladder, spleen (*Color Atlas*, Pl. 1, Fig. 1), liver (Pl. 1, Fig. 2), gallbladder (Pl. 1, Fig. 2), and pancreas are readily observed. Much of the jejunum, lower colon (Pl. 1, Fig. 3), and ventral surface of the stomach (Pl. 1, Fig. 4) are visible when accessory probe manipulation is used. The duodenum is not easily visible because observation requires accessory probe displacement of the jejunum and colon. The diaphragm can be partially visualized by probe manipulation of the liver to one side. Observation of the kidney is possible in both species but necessitates slight repositioning of the animal. The kidneys of the cat are located retroperitoneally and, consequently, cannot be observed directly. However, the ventral contour of the feline kidney can be visualized which is sufficient to allow accurate biopsy.

Details concerning specific reproductive organ function and events visible by laparoscopy will be discussed later. In the male dog and cat, each vas deferens is easily located and fully observed from its origin at the ejaculatory orifice of the urethra to its descent through the abdominal inguinal ring (Pl. 1, Fig. 5). The spermatic artery-vein plexus as located along the dorsal lateral abdominal wall is also clearly visible (Pl. 3, Fig. 1). The prostate is difficult to distinguish due to its anatomical location which varies with the position and volume of the bladder.

In the bitch and queen, the genital system is readily visible, including the uterine body and horn (Pl. 1, Fig. 3, 6), oviduct and ovarian bursa (Pl. 1, Fig. 7, 8). The laparoscopist with probe manipulation can also easily discern the feline ovary (Pl. 2, Fig. 1, 2) and adjacent ovarian vasculature.

Neoplastic tumors, gross pathological lesions or obvious structural deformities are perceptible. Laparoscopy has recently been implemented for diagnostic use in canine and feline oncology (Johnson and Twedt, 1977). In many types of cancer, laparotomy is of little benefit and may be detrimental to compromised animals. These forms of cancer include metastatic liver disease, lymphoma, mast cell tumor, and myeloproliferative diseases. Laparoscopy in these clinical cases appears to be less stressful on the patient and still offers documentation and monitoring of the disease necessary for further management.

## Insertion and Use of Accessory Instruments

As indicated previously, a variety of techniques have been utilized in the dog and cat for intraabdominal surgery, organ manipulation, and treatment of disease or injury. Such procedures require the utilization of accessory instruments.

### SIMPLE MANIPULATION

The most useful tool for assisting diagnosis and performing simple manipulation in the dog and cat is the Verres needle. Although originally developed only for establishing the pneumoperitoneum, the Verres needle is of sufficient size to perform most reasonable manipulation, even in larger dogs. In some instances, two such instruments inserted at slightly different locations can be used together to assist in performing an internal maneuver. This is generally facilitated by the presence of a laparoscopic assistant who may be required to provide support of one or more instruments during the examination.

The Verres needle can be easily modified to allow measurement of internal tissue or organs. We have mechanically etched distinct marks (at 2 mm intervals) on the lower one-quarter of the needle barrel (Fig. 3.27). During the examination, the Verres needle can be inserted into the cavity at the position which allows the target site to be most accurately measured. This device has been particularly useful in reproductive studies for observing changes in size of the uterine horns and ovarian structures, including

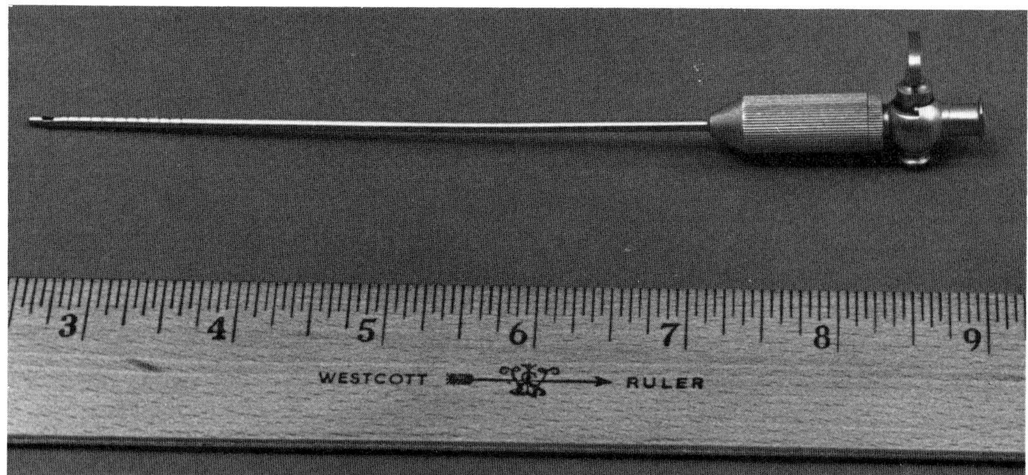

**Figure 3.27**   Verres needle cannula with mechanically etched marks (at 2 mm intervals) for internal measuring.

follicle and corpus luteum diameter (Pl. 2, Fig. 2). It has been found equally useful for determining the dimensions of internal lesions and monitoring alterations in size of tumor growths.

Several manufacturers of laparoscopic instruments produce an elongated metal probe which contains measurement indicators. This instrument was developed for humans, requires insertion through an accessory cannula, and because of its size is not recommended for use in the dog and cat.

## EXTENSIVE MANIPULATION

In some instances, it may be necessary to extensively maneuver or support heavy organs. Such action will necessitate the insertion of an accessory trocar-cannula, the 6 mm in diameter cannula being preferred in the dog and cat.

The accessory-trocar cannula unit is inserted through a skin incision made 6 to 8 cm lateral to the midline site. Complications in connection with the second puncture are generally confined to possible perforation of one of the abdominal wall blood vessels. This can be avoided by transillumination of the abdominal wall from within, using the already in place laparoscope (Semm, 1977). By this means, the vascular patterns in the layers of the abdominal wall can be clearly visualized. The insertion technique used is the same as previously described for the laparoscopic trocar-cannula assembly. As intromission is initiated the trocar-cannula unit is held at a 30° angle to the plane of the body with the tip of the trocar pointed at a 45° angle to the animal's ventral midline (Fig. 3.28). If the laparoscopist is right handed, it is preferable to insert the accessory cannula to the right of the midline (the laparoscope pointed in a caudal direction). The left handed endoscopist may be more comfortable with the accessory cannula on the left side; however, caution must be exercised since the insertion site of the trocar approximates the internal locale of the spleen.

Following removal of the trocar from the accessory cannula, the second instrument is introduced (Fig. 3.29). The beginning operator occasionally has difficulty locating it within the cavity. To facilitate location, Rioux (1978) has described the "chopstick method," which consists of crossing the telescope with the newly inserted instrument and then sliding them against one another until the latter suddenly appears in front of the telescope (Fig. 3.30).

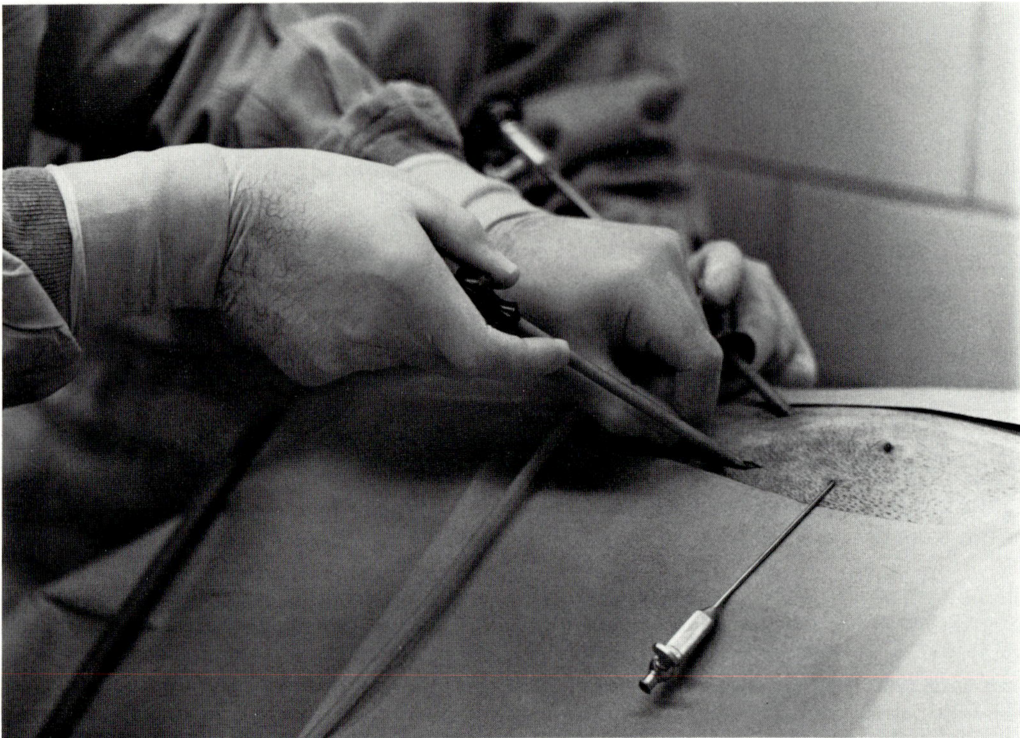

**Figure 3.28**   Insertion of the accessory trocar-cannula through the lateral skin incision.

The grasping forceps are useful for extensive manipulation. A variety of suitable devices exists for the dog and cat. Instruments in which the jaws of the forceps can be broadly expanded allow the laparoscopist to grasp and support sizable organs. One should also consider overall length of the forceps. Excessively long forceps are manufactured which are impractical for use in small dogs and cats.

## BIOPSY

Biopsy specimens of internal organs can be readily obtained by laparoscopy. Two techniques have been generally used for obtaining tissue samples. The first involves use of a biopsy needle apparatus, several of which are commercially available from laparoscopic equipment manufacturers. Some controversy has developed concerning the usefulness of these particular devices in laboratory species. Our laboratory has had limited success in utilizing such biopsy needles and prefers the use of the needle instrument and technique developed by Bush *et al.* (1978, see Chapter 10). The latter device consists of a 13 gauge, 8 cm spinal trocar-cannula needle (special needle, Becton, Dickinson and Co.), particularly beneficial for kidney biopsy purposes.

Kidney biopsies may be obtained in the dog and cat relatively easily using laparoscopy. Due to the dorsal location of the kidney in these two species, collecting a tissue specimen requires a slight alteration in animal position. Observation of the kidney is facilitated by the animal remaining in a head-down supine position but with the body rotated slightly laterally to elevate the desired kidney (Fig. 3.31). Laparoscopic location of this organ generally requires some manipulation of the small intestine and/or colon toward the midline away from the kidney site. In the dog, the kidney can be completely visualized. The skin above the kidney location site is surgically prepared and the needle

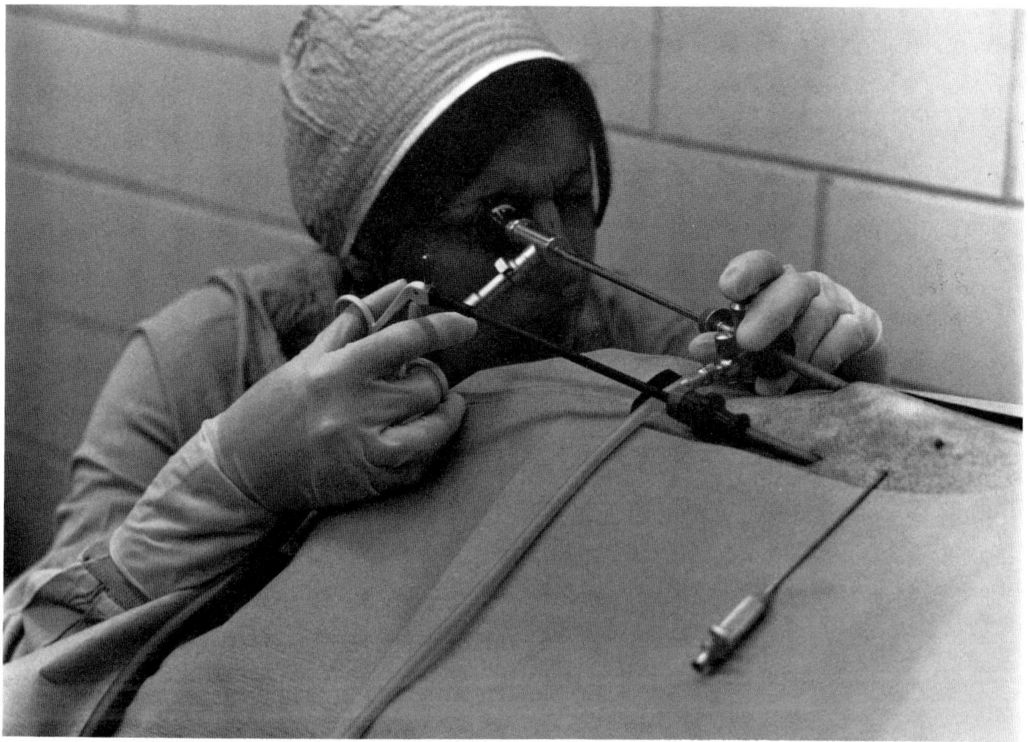

**Figure 3.29** Following removal of the trocar, the accessory instrument is directed through the cannula.

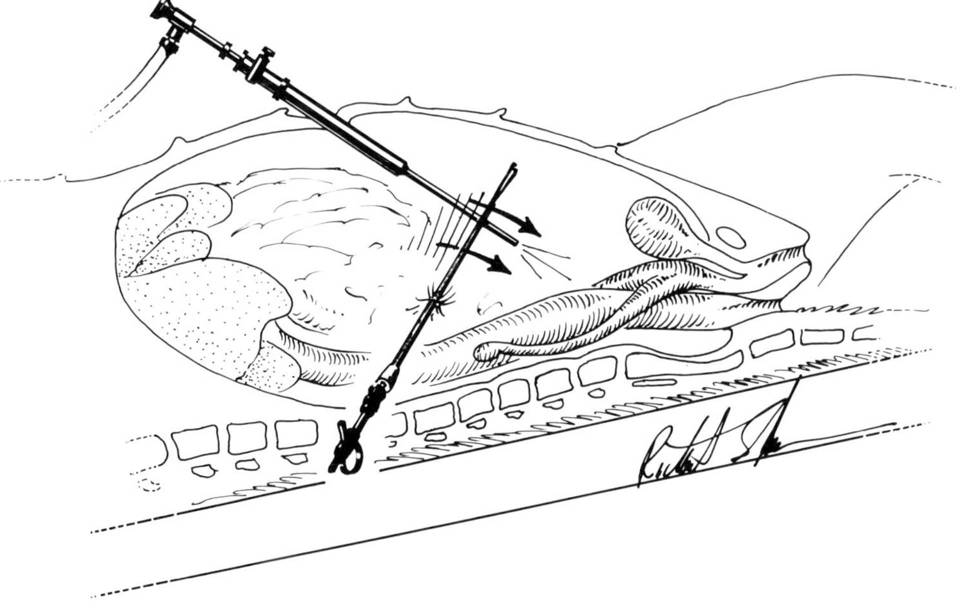

**Figure 3.30** The "chopstick method" is used to help locate and visualize the accessory instrument. The latter is crossed with the telescope and both are slid against each other until the accessory instrument appears in view.

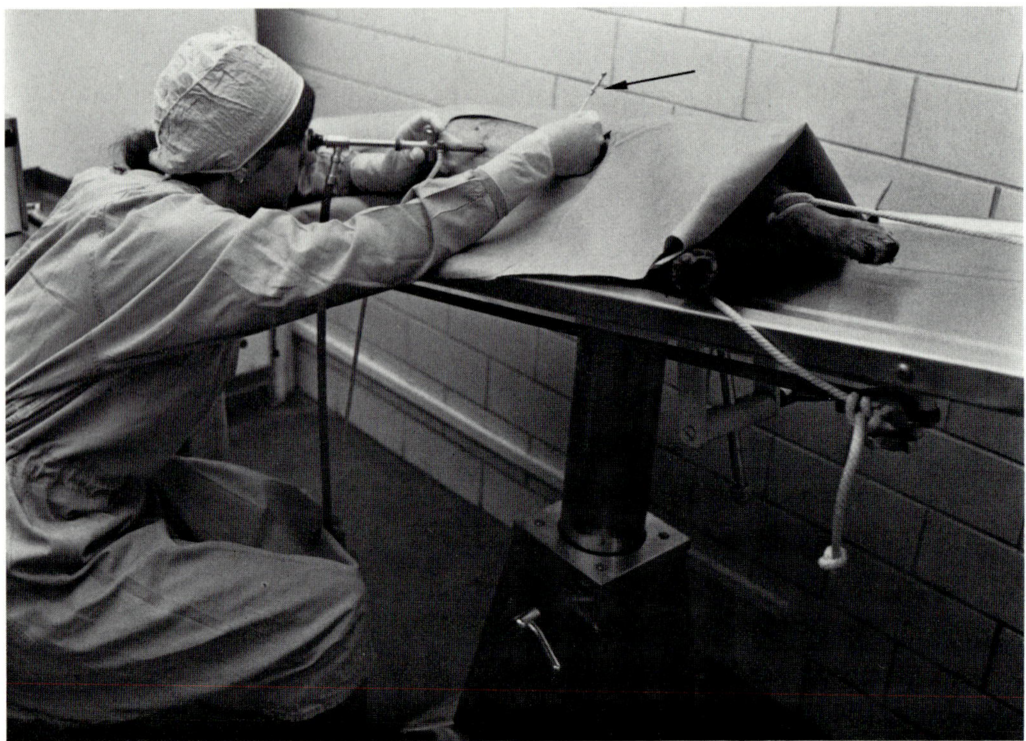

**Figure 3.31**   For kidney biopsy, the animal is restrained with the body slightly rotated. This position allows visual access to the kidney and permits the biopsy needle (arrow) to be directed to the organ.

with trocar inserted percutaneously. Under direct laparoscopic visualization, the needle assembly is directed into the kidney capsule. After perforation of the cortex, the trocar is removed and the cannula inserted slightly further. A 10 ml syringe containing 4 to 6 ml of physiological saline is attached to the cannula hub. Moderate suction will generally produce a renal tissue specimen adequate for pathological/histological evaluation. Slight to moderate hemorrhage usually results after withdrawal of the cannula from the kidney. Blood loss has not appeared excessive and no subsequent adverse effects have resulted from using such methods, even in circumstances necessitating multiple biopsy from the same organ. The anatomical location of this organ in the cat is retroperitoneal. Nevertheless, the contour and underlying tissue of the kidney can be completely visualized, allowing accurate biopsy using the above procedure.

Similar needle techniques have been reported in clinical evaluations of the gallbladder (Johnson and Twedt, 1977). These investigators determined that laparoscopy in conjunction with small gauge needle puncture enabled the clinicopathological analysis of bile which permitted cholecystocholangiography for evaluation of gallbladder and bile duct status.

The second technique for collecting tissue specimens involves use of a grasping biopsy forceps. Like the grasping manipulatory forceps, the biopsy forceps must be inserted through an accessory cannula, the insertion site for the latter varying depending on the organ to be sampled. The grasping forceps appear to be more effective and to provide a larger specimen sample than the commercial needle biopsy device. They are particularly useful for rapid hepatic or splenic biopsy procedures. For example, in the dog, required time for combined laparoscopic diagnosis and hepatic biopsy (excluding induction of anesthesia) usually varies from five to ten minutes.

For splenic biopsy, insertion of the laparoscope and accessory cannula unit is performed according to the techniques previously described (i.e., laparoscope directed caudally, accessory cannula inserted laterally to the right of midline). To avoid organ damage, the trocar-cannula assemblies are never initially inserted in a cranial direction. To adequately view the splenic surface the surgical table is returned to a flat 180° plane. The laparoscope is rotated counterclockwise until the spleen is visible (Pl. 1, Fig. 1). The biopsy forceps are then directed to the splenic surface and the tissue sample obtained from the desired site. Following collection, moderate hemorrhage is inevitable, but generally negligible. Excessive bleeding can be remedied by external abdominal compression, tamponade with a blunt probe, or electrocautery. As previously indicated, most ancillary forceps are equipped for fixation to a suitable electrosurgical unit. If necessary the biopsy site can be coagulated using the biopsy forceps attached to the cautery system.

For observation and sampling of hepatic tissue, routine positioning of the animal and instrument insertion techniques should be performed as previously described. Following laparoscope-midline cannula intromission, the animal should be repositioned in a flat 180° plane (Fig. 3.32). The laparoscope-cannula unit should then be slowly rotated counterclockwise (Fig. 3.32) until the laparoscope is directed cranially and the liver is visible (Pl. 1, Fig. 2). Biopsy of this organ is facilitated by introduction of the accessory trocar-cannula on the animal's left side (operator's right when facing *cranially*) (Fig. 3.33). The operator should recall that since the spleen is located approximate to this site, the accessory trocar-cannula unit should be directed caudally for insertion and then redirected and rotated cranially before receiving the biopsy forceps. The latter

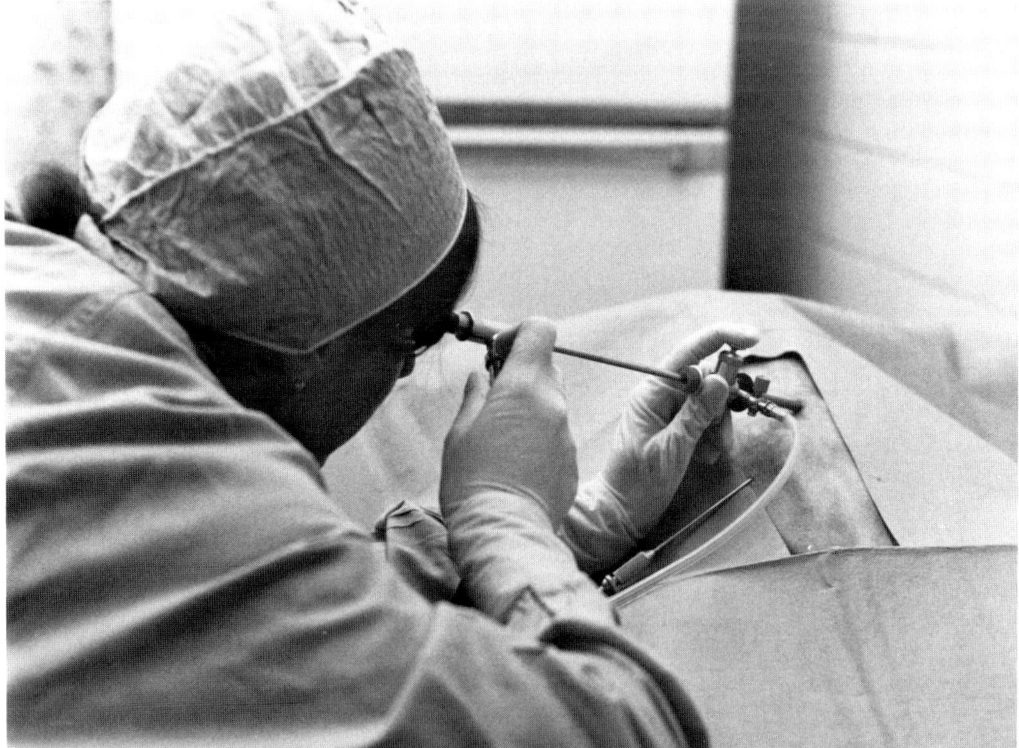

**Figure 3.32** For examination of the cranial abdominal contents the surgical table is returned to a 180° plane and the laparoscope-cannula assembly rotated counterclockwise.

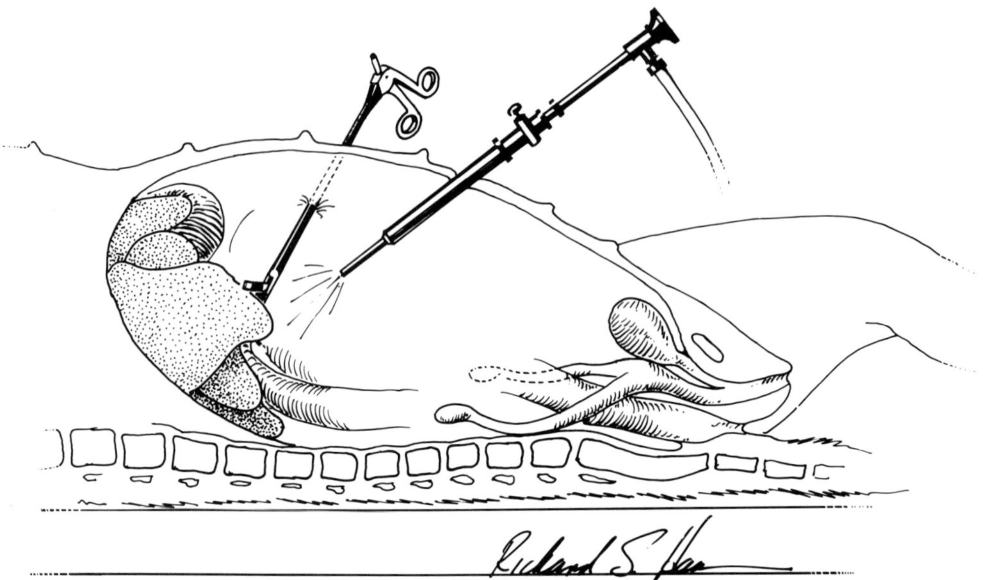

**Figure 3.33** For liver biopsy the animal is placed in a flat supine position, the laparoscope rotated and pointed cranially and the accessory cannula and biopsy forceps inserted on the animal's left side.

instrument can be guided to the organ and the specimen obtained (Fig. 3.33). A Verres needle may be useful as a manipulatory probe to displace the various hepatic lobes if multiple samples are desired. The degree of hemorrhage following biopsy of the liver ranges from nonexistent (Pl. 2, Fig. 3) to modest. Electrocoagulation of the biopsied hepatic site has rarely been required.

Information on biopsy techniques of other major abdominal organs is limited and requires further investigation. Our preliminary attempts at prostatic biopsy in male dogs have been unsuccessful. Further study is necessary in the dog and cat to establish the feasibility of using endoscopic procedures for acquiring tissue samples from the gastrointestinal and reproductive tracts.

## INTERNAL SURGERY

Certain internal surgical alterations can be performed using an ancillary scissors device. We have used this instrument to alter the reproductive tract for ovarian exposure, produce sterilization (see **Laparoscopy for Reproductive Study** section), or surgically break down adhesion formation. The latter operation has been particularly useful in animals developing adhesions following laparotomy which are used in subsequent studies requiring visualization of abdominal cavity contents by laparoscopy. The accessory trocar-cannula is inserted into the peritoneal cavity, at a site dependent on the location and type of structural adhesion, and the adhesion simultaneously cauterized and severed with the scissors.

### Termination of the Examination and Postoperative Care

Following laparoscopic examination, the laparoscope and accessory unit (if used) are removed, rinsed in tap water and returned to the germicidal soaking solution. To obviate the possibility of creating internal postoperative pain, it is important to evacuate the pneumoperitoneum. This can be accomplished by depressing the trumpet valve and allowing the $CO_2$ to escape via the cannula. Deflation can be facilitated by gentle massage of the ventral abdominal surface.

The cannula is removed, rinsed of body fluids, and returned to the sterilizing solution. Generally, in both the dog and cat, a single suture is placed in the peritoneal layer and two to four sutures in the skin. The absorbable suture has provided excellent tissue repair results in both species. In the cat, it is particularly important to accurately suture the peritoneum. In several cases from our colony, failure to properly repair this tissue layer has allowed the formation of a small diameter (2 to 4 cm) omental hernia. Although not a grave health risk, such an occurrence is esthetically unappealing, which emphasizes the importance of proper suturing procedures to the clinical veterinarian practicing feline laparoscopy.

The need to apply topical ointment or spray to the puncture sites or to administer prophylactic antibiotic is questionable. Such actions depend on the measure of sterility maintained during the endoscopic examination. The author is familiar with laboratories which use neither and report no postoperative complications. Our laboratory employs a preventative approach; following suturing, the incision sites are treated with a topical antibacterial dressing or spray and penicillin (150,000 to 600,000 units) is injected intramuscularly.

Further postoperative attention is minimal. During the anesthesia recovery interval, the animal is positioned on a heating pad or towel with heat furnished via a heat lamp. Using the anesthetic regimens previously described, the recuperative phase in both species has been relatively smooth and uneventful.

Following laparoscopy, equipment is removed from the soaking solution, rinsed with tap or distilled water and dried with clean gauze sponges. Instrumentation is best protected by storing in a padded case (Fig. 3.34).

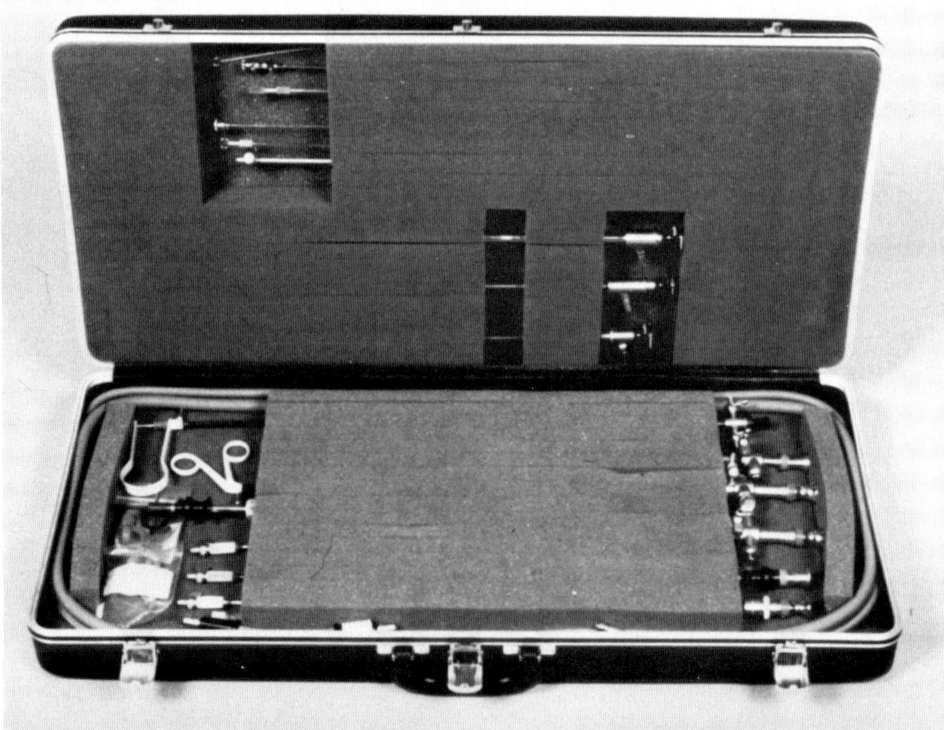

**Figure 3.34**   Storage/carrying case for laparoscopy instruments.

## GENERAL CONSIDERATIONS

### General Results, Complications, and Contraindications

Many of our colonized animals have been subjected to laparoscopy repeatedly. During a 40 month period, a total of 800 and 1400 laparoscopic examinations have been performed on 112 dogs and 103 cats, respectively. Seven dogs have been examined 30 or more times and six cats have been examined 50 or more times. With respect to the maximum number of laparoscopies performed in an individual of each species, one bitch and each of two queens have undergone 38 and 62 examinations, respectively. This information may not be of relevance to the veterinary clinician who would rarely perform laparoscopy more than once or twice in an individual dog or cat; however, the data do illustrate the general innocuous effect of this minor surgical technique. Furthermore, the results demonstrate the value of laparoscopic methods to certain research investigators who in the past have had to utilize laparotomy in dogs and cats for obtaining experimental results. Certainly, in situations of this nature, endoscopy permits more efficient and protracted research use of valuable experimental animals.

Certain research or clinical studies have necessitated conducting laparoscopy at frequent intervals. A healthy dog or cat can generally tolerate the described anesthetic and diagnostic examination well when performed at 48 hour intervals for 7 to 12 days. Daily laparoscopy has also been performed in most species for 3 to 5 day intervals without creating a health risk. More frequent endoscopic schedules have been employed but not tested thoroughly. For example, one 9 year old beagle bitch has been examined laparoscopically 16 times over a 16 day interval with no apparent adverse physical effects. Obviously, in veterinary medicine, the overall clinical condition of the animal will dictate the number of laparoscopic examinations feasible.

When laparoscopy is conducted at 48 to 96 hour intervals, different midline incision sites for trocar-cannula insertions should be used. The same midline site can be employed when the endoscopic examinations are made at more frequent intervals (24 hours or less). In the latter case, sutures are removed and the trocar-cannula inserted through the previous perforation.

In our laboratory, no deaths have resulted in dogs from the anesthesia or laparoscopic technique used. Two deaths have occurred in cats, one attributed to an anaphylactic response to prophylactic penicillin, the other due to an anesthetic accident. Interstitial herniation at the midline insertion site has not occurred in the dog. As discussed previously, it occurred in six feline cases when suture was improperly inserted in the peritoneal layer following examination. Infections or other adverse physical effects have not been observed in any animal subjected to laparoscopy, using sterile or nonsterile techniques. No internal adhesion development attributable to laparoscopy has resulted, even in animals subjected to 20 or more examinations.

Certain contraindications are associated with laparoscopy. The procedure should not be performed in animals with coagulopathies or peritonitis (Johnson and Twedt, 1977). As discussed earlier, laparoscopy may be used to break down abdominal adhesions. However, whenever such formations develop extensively between the bowel and the ventral abdominal wall, there is an increased hazard of visceral perforation during introduction of the trocar-cannula. Complications may also be associated with the insufflatory procedure in animals prone to respiratory or cardiovascular distress. In such cases, even an average pneumoperitoneum, when combined with the attendant Trendelenburg position, may result in excessive pressure on the diaphragm and respiratory or cardiovascular arrest. Johnson and Twedt (1977) reported that gas embolism or subcutaneous emphysema during induction of pneumoperitoneum is a potential complication. In addition, a preperitoneal emphysema is possible which may result in the separation of the peritoneum from its adjacent tissues and cause it to bulge into the abdominal cavity, making visualization of the abdominal cavity impossible. These occurrences are certainly conceivable, but are extremely rare with proper utilization of the Verres needle technique. The size of the dog and cat does not appear to limit the capabilities of laparoscopy in these two species. However, obese animals are more difficult to evaluate due to excessive intraabdominal fat. Diagnostic examination of this animal type by the inexperienced laparoscopist is often frustrating. Most skilled endoscopists can compensate for obesity by repositioning of the restrained animal and the use of accessory instrumentation.

## Laparoscopy for Reproductive Study

Laparoscopy has been used most extensively in animal species for reproductive studies. Until recently, little specific data existed in the dog and cat on basic reproductive parameters already established for years in other common domestic animals. Realization of this deficiency was the impetus for the initiation of laparoscopy into our laboratory's ongoing research program. This technique has been used primarily to assist in determining correlations between normal parameters of the reproductive cycle of the bitch and queen. Laparoscopy has also been utilized experimentally in these species to develop the following eight ancillary methods for further reproductive research and clinical evaluation.

### DOCUMENTATION OF OVARIAN ACTIVITY

These studies have been concerned with the relationship of ovarian morphology to other reproductive factors which can be measured during various stages of the reproductive cycle. Of particular interest has been determining the onset of ovulation with respect to pituitary release of luteinizing hormone (LH), ovarian secreted steroids, and day of sexual receptivity (estrus).

Laparoscopy has provided a simple but effective means of studying such relationships in the female cat, an induced ovulator. In the queen, the ovaries can be located by first distinguishing the uterus and then observing each uterine horn (Pl. 1, Fig. 3) cranially and laterally to the horn terminus. The ovary of the cat is located in a pocket of peritoneum, the ovarian fimbria (Pl. 1, Fig. 8). This tissue is attached laterally to the dorsal suspensory ligament of the ovary. The translucent fimbria is highly vascular and normally completely encompasses the ovary. Since the fimbria is not attached to the medial portion of the suspensory ligament, it can be easily removed using the Verres needle probe to expose the ovarian surface (Pl. 2, Fig. 1). The ovary can then be completely viewed to determine onset of follicle development and ovulation (Pl. 2, Fig. 2). The latter phenomenon can be detected simply by observing sequential changes in vascular patterns around and on the ovarian follicle, changes in the shape of the follicular dome, and alterations in both coloration and translucency of the follicle. Details of ovarian morphology in the cat, as documented by laparoscopy have recently been published (Wildt and Seager, 1979). The availability of this method for accurate monitoring of feline ovarian activity has allowed other investigations, including development of exogenous gonadotropin regimens for inducing sexual receptivity (Wildt *et al.*, 1978c) and ovulation (Wildt and Seager, 1978); determining the LH response following mating (Wildt *et al.*, 1979c) or gonadotropin-releasing hormone (GnRH) administration (Chakraborty *et al.*, 1979); and establishing the relationship of ovarian activity to sexual behavior (Wildt *et al.*, 1978b; Wildt *et al.*, 1979b). Frequent laparoscopy appears to have no adverse effect on the ability of the adult queen to cycle normally or exhibit normal ovarian function. At present, data on the results of recurrent laparoscopy on serum hormone titers in the cat are incomplete.

Laparoscopic reproductive investigations have been conducted in the domestic bitch.

The reproductive anatomy of this species precludes easy visualization of the ovary. Unlike most other species, the ovary of the bitch is completely encapsulated and concealed in a bursa ovarii. Fat and smooth muscle forms the layers of this pouch which continue to the cornua of the uterus constituting the ovarian ligament and mesosalpinx. In most cases, the bursa, which has a slit-like ventral opening (1 to 2 cm in length), effectively inhibits direct examination of the ovary. It should be noted that, in the author's experience, one or both bursa slits are inexplicably elongated in approximately 20% of the dogs examined. In these animals accessory instruments can be utilized to manipulate a portion or the entire ovary into view.

In our studies designed to document ovarian morphology in the bitch, it was necessary to develop a technique for exposing the ovary by laparoscopy. These procedures have been published in detail elsewhere (Wildt *et al.*, 1977b). In brief, this technique involves insertion of a cautery scissors instrument through the accessory cannula during routine laparoscopic examination. By observation through the laparoscope, the jaws of the scissors can be inserted into the posterior edge of the bursa slit nearest the anterior terminus of the uterine horn (Pl. 1, Fig. 7). The jaws of the scissors are closed on the bursa tissue and after a period of electrocautery discharge ranging from 3 to 30 seconds, the tissue is cut. This technique effectively lengthens the bursa slit 1.0 to 1.5 cm and allows immediate and chronic exposure of the ovary (Pl. 2, Fig. 4). This procedure performed in a group of multiparous bitches allowed frequent laparoscopic ovarian observation during proestrus and estrus. Cutting the bursa at the described site had no apparent effect on ovarian blood supply since ovarian cyclicity including follicle development, ovulation, and corpora lutea formation occurred (Pl. 2, Fig. 5).

Bitches with laparoscopically exposed ovaries have been used in more detailed studies dealing with the anatomical events associated with ovulation (Wildt *et al.*, 1977b), the relationship of ovarian activity to reproductive behavior, serum hormone concentrations (Wildt *et al.*, 1978a; Wildt *et al.*, 1979a), and vaginal cytology (Kinney *et al.*, 1979, unpublished results).

These investigations have been designed to determine if frequent laparoscopy adversely affects reproductive function. Reproductive parameters have been measured in bitches subjected to laparoscopy at 48 hour intervals during the proestrous and estrous intervals and compared to values obtained in control animals undergoing no laparoscopy. Frequent induction of anesthesia followed by endoscopic examination failed to affect the onset of sexual receptivity or inhibit ovarian activity. In a collaborative study with Drs. Chakraborty, Panko, and Seager of our laboratory, blood samples were obtained twice daily from proestrous-estrous bitches and the serum analyzed for hormone concentrations by radioimmunoassay. Figure 3.35 illustrates the mean hormone profiles of serum LH, estradiol-17$\beta$ and progesterone in these animals. Frequent laparoscopy had no discernible effect on the concentrations of these critical hormones in the peripheral circulation. It can be concluded that, to date, laparoscopy has had an innocuous influence on ovarian and reproductive-endocrine functions in the bitch.

Some question exists on the possible use of the laparoscopic ovarian exposure techniques to aid in clinically diagnosing ovarian disorders in the bitch (i.e., infantile ovaries, cystic follicles, Pl. 2, Fig. 6) without adversely affecting reproductive potential. Surgical alteration of the ovarian bursa could produce two undesirable results: (1) loss of ovulated ova into the peritoneal cavity (the probable evolutionary intent of an encompassing type ovarian bursa in the bitch is to assure ova passage into the oviduct); (2) damage or severance of the oviduct. The oviduct in the domestic bitch courses through the bursa tissue, usually from the lateral to medial ovarian pole. Because the bursa tissue is rather thick, it is difficult to distinguish the oviduct proper, thus increasing the potential of laparoscopic injury. Neither of these hypotheses has been extensively tested. In our laboratory, we have attempted to produce pregnancy in only three bitches with bilaterally exposed ovaries. These animals were artificially insemi-

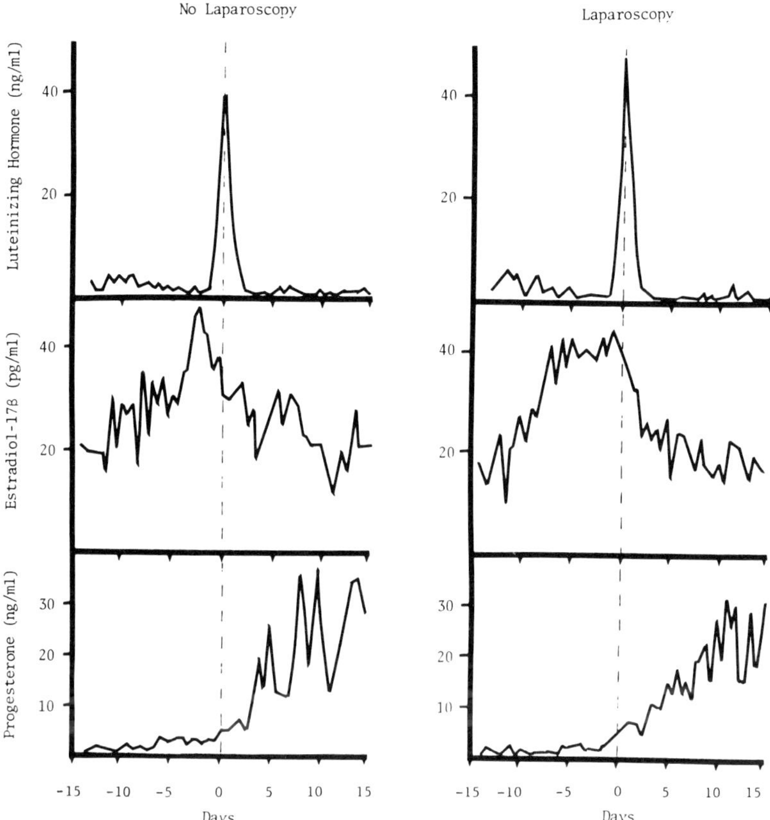


**Figure 3.35** Serum hormonal profiles in bitches undergoing laparoscopy (n = 15) or no laparoscopy (n = 10) during the proestrous-estrous interval. Hormones (luteinizing hormone, estradiol-17β, and progesterone) were normalized to day 0 (day of the LH peak).

nated with previously frozen spermatozoa on the first, third, and fifth days of estrus. One of three bitches conceived and delivered a single live born puppy following a gestation of normal duration.

The possibility of lowering fertility by laparoscopic ovarian exposure should exclude current use of laparoscopy in most clinical cases of suspected canine ovarian dysfunction until further studies are conducted. In critical cases, a frustrated owner/breeder may insist that there is "nothing to lose" from laparoscopic-surgical exposure in order to diagnose an ovarian problem. In this event, it is suggested that the laparoscopist expose and observe only a single ovary. Leaving the remaining bursa ovarii intact will still allow normal conception in the event that the reproductive disorder is ultimately diagnosed and successfully treated.

## ASPIRATION OF OVARIAN OR PAROVARIAN CYSTS

Laparoscopy can be readily used in the queen to aspirate ovarian cysts often responsible for alterations in reproductive behavior or general animal health. Ovarian cysts in the cat anatomically appear as extremely large vesicular follicles on the ovarian surface. These cysts are considered to result from gonadotropic hyperpituitarism or inadequate gonadal production of steroids to inhibit normal tonic pituitary secretion of gonadotropins. Queens experiencing this disorder demonstrate prolonged and intense periods of sexual behavior for as long as 12 months. Laparoscopy reveals the presence of surface ovarian cysts varying from 6 mm to 6 cm in diameter. Attempts to luteinize or artificially induce ovulation in large diameter follicles using gonadotropin therapy (human chorionic gonadotropin, HCG) have been unsuccessful. For an inexplicable reason, follicles of such proportion are incapable of responding to varying dosages of this drug.

Follicles can, however, be mechanically manipulated by laparoscopy. The cyst is located using routine, previously described methods. Aspiration is performed by the insertion of a sterile 20 gauge, 4 cm needle through the abdominal wall at a site contiguous with the location of the cyst (Fig. 3.36). Following intromission, the needle point is laparoscopically visualized and guided to the ovarian surface. The wall of the follicular cyst generally contains numerous small vascular patterns which should be avoided during needle penetration. The needle is inserted near the follicular dome, a syringe attached to the needle hub and the follicular fluid withdrawn until complete follicular collapse occurs. The needle may be removed from the ovary and abdominal cavity, respectively. To prevent recurrence, it may be desirable to cauterize the cyst site with an accessory forceps. Follicular aspiration (without subsequent electrocoagulation) rarely results in hemorrhage and does not interfere with subsequent reproductive cyclicity or fertility. Queens in our colony have returned to normal behavioral and reproductive patterns shortly after the aspiration procedure.

Parovarian cysts of unknown etiology exist in both the bitch and queen and can be similarly treated.

## UTERINE OBSERVATION AS AN INDICATOR OF NORMAL REPRODUCTIVE FUNCTION

The physical appearance of the uterus as viewed laparoscopically can reveal significant information on the reproductive status of the bitch and queen. Circulating reproductive hormones, which vary with the stage of the reproductive cycle, are responsible for dictating uterine appearance. For example, the uterine horns in the prepubertal or adult anestrous queen or bitch are narrow in diameter, light pink in coloration, and generally very smooth and flaccid (Pl. 1, Fig. 6). At these times, reproductive steroid hormones are at nadir concentration. In contrast, during estrus the ovaries are actively secreting profuse quantities of steroids which dramatically alter gross uterine morphology. The uterine horns, in this case, become enlarged in diameter and more avascular and grayish in coloration. In addition, the uterine horns often coil slightly, appear to contain small sequential bulges, and are turgid when manipulated with an accessory probe or forceps. These characteristics are particularly pronounced near or soon after ovulation when the ovary initiates significant progesterone secretion. These physical attributes are conspicuously absent in bitches or queens failing to ovulate during the estrous period. Therefore, one can estimate with relative accuracy whether ovulation has occurred by simply observing uterine horn appearance. This information may be of clinical relevance to the veterinary practitioner faced with a bitch which demonstrates estrous and mating behavior, but fails to conceive. Following estrus, the physical appearance of the uterus, as observed laparoscopically, would provide an estimate of whether ovulation occurred. If the uterine horns were morphologically characteristic of a normal postovulatory bitch, one might suspect that infertility is likely due to some other anatomical or endocrine anomaly.

## DIAGNOSIS OF PREGNANCY AND CONCEPTUS NUMBERS

Transformations in the gross appearance of the uterine horns allow early pregnancy diagnosis in the bitch and queen. Both female dogs and cats will experience a pseudo-

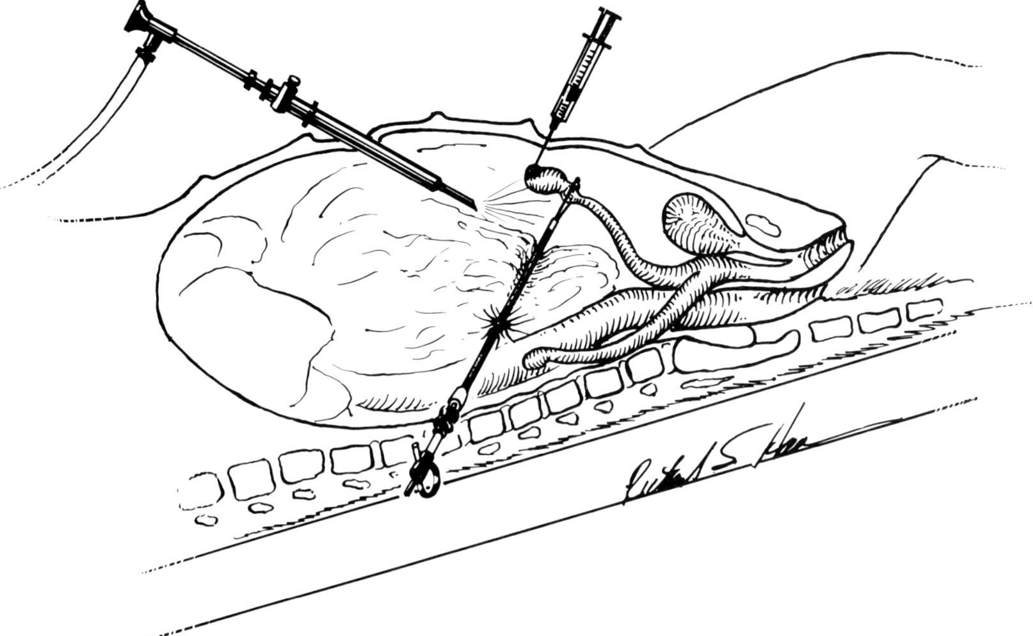

**Figure 3.36**  Ovarian follicle or cyst aspiration. The uterine horn is grasped with the accessory forceps and the aspiration needle inserted through the abdominal wall and directed to the ovary.

pregnancy condition after sterile mating. In this case, the uterus will become swollen and take on the physical characteristics of a postovulatory state as described in the previous section. However, in the gravid state, the uterine horns become comprised of segmental swellings (conceptus sites) which are initially discernible at 21 to 25 days of pregnancy. At day 28 of gestation, these individual swellings are distinct and are often characterized by large diameter vascular patterns randomly transversing the length of the segment (Pl. 2, Fig. 7).

Laparoscopic pregnancy diagnosis is performed using previously discussed techniques. The laparoscopist should obviously be extremely careful during the trocar-cannula insertion phase in a suspected pregnant animal. During later stages of pregnancy one should allow for the extra pressure of added abdominal weight against the diaphragm during restraint positioning. At this time, the surgical table should be tilted no more than 15 to 20° to avoid respiratory or cardiovascular distress.

In our laboratory studies, five bitches have been detected as pregnant by laparoscopic observation of uterine sequential swellings on days 21 to 28 of gestation. All whelped normal sized litters, including one bitch subjected to six such examinations during pregnancy. In the latter bitch, routine laparoscopic examinations were initiated approximately two weeks after conception and were conducted at five to seven day intervals through the sixth week of gestation. Similarly, laparoscopy has been used in two queens to diagnose pregnancy on the basis of uterine morphology. These animals also produced normal sized litters following average gestation periods.

Laparoscopy also affords the opportunity to determine the number of embryos *in utero* and thus potential term litter size. This is simply accomplished by performing routine laparoscopy and counting the number of sequential swellings in each uterine horn. Establishing the conceptus number using this technique is best performed before day 40 of the approximately 63 day pregnancy. After this time advanced fetal development is accompanied by significant fetal fluid volume and can result in difficulty in manipulating each horn to achieve an accurate count. In experimental studies, the gravid uterus has been manipulated extensively by laparoscopy without inducing abortion or other adverse effects. Maneuvering of the pregnant horn after day 21 should be performed using manipulatory forceps, grasping the uterine tissue between apparent conceptus site swellings.

Laparoscopic determination of embryo numbers *in utero* has provided an accurate indicator of the number of offspring to be expected. One hundred percent precision should not be anticipated, particularly in animals diagnosed during early pregnancy. One must account for the effect of *in utero* embryonic mortality, which appears to occur throughout the gestation interval in both species.

## THE STUDY OF PREGNANCY AND FETAL DEVELOPMENT (FETOSCOPY)

Little data exist in the literature concerning the events associated with normal fetal development and the incidence and causes of fetal mortality in the bitch and queen. Preliminary results would indicate that laparoscopy provides a safe procedure for serial observation of gross uterine morphology in the gravid bitch and queen. Certainly this direct access to the uterus provides the opportunity for a multitude of research and clinical investigations involving the study of pregnancy and fetal development.

Our laboratory has recently initiated preliminary trials into the use of laparoscopy and fetoscopy for direct *in utero* visualization in the bitch and queen. Fetoscopy is modified laparoscopy in which a laparoscope is inserted into the abdominal cavity and then into the gravid uterus to visualize the fetal-placental complex. As in the development of laparoscopy, fetoscopy was not utilized initially in experimental animals but was performed first in pregnant women (Valenti, 1972). To date, the majority of these human fetoscopic examinations have been experimental and designed to determine the efficacy of such a procedure for direct *in utero* diagnosis and management of genetic and acquired fetal disease.

The details of fetoscopy, as performed in our preliminary experiments, are beyond the scope of this text; however, a broad description is pertinent. In brief, pregnant bitches have undergone routine laparoscopy, and the uterus has been diagnosed gravid on the basis of distinct segmental swellings along each uterine horn. A second small trocar is inserted through the abdominal wall and then, with laparoscopic guidance, to a desired avascular location of the uterine horn (Fig. 3.37). The trocar-cannula is inserted into a segmental swelling, the trocar removed and a 2.7 mm in diameter laparoscope inserted into the uterine lumen. The canine fetus has been observed, particularly the fore and hind limbs, the tail, hindquarters, and fetal placenta. After removal of the fetoscope, uterine hemorrhage has been rare or negligible, although some amniotic fluid loss into the peritoneal cavity through the uterine puncture site has occurred. Pregnant animals subjected to fetoscopy have progressed to term pregnancy uneventfully. Puppies examined by fetoscopy near midgestation have been live born following gestations of normal duration.

Certainly the successful adaptation of fetoscopy to the bitch and queen produces broad implications on the usefulness of this procedure in genetic, reproductive, and endocrine investigations. Its success would stimulate considerable interest in the development of fetoscopic ancillary procedures (i.e., sampling fetal blood and tissue, altering intrauterine environment, providing direct fetal therapy). Fetoscopy appears to provide considerable potential for future study in both biomedical and veterinary medicine.

## DIAGNOSIS OF REPRODUCTIVE TRACT DISEASE

Laparoscopy has been found readily effective for both the detection and confirmation of pathological uterine states. Both subtle and dramatic alterations in uterine morphol-

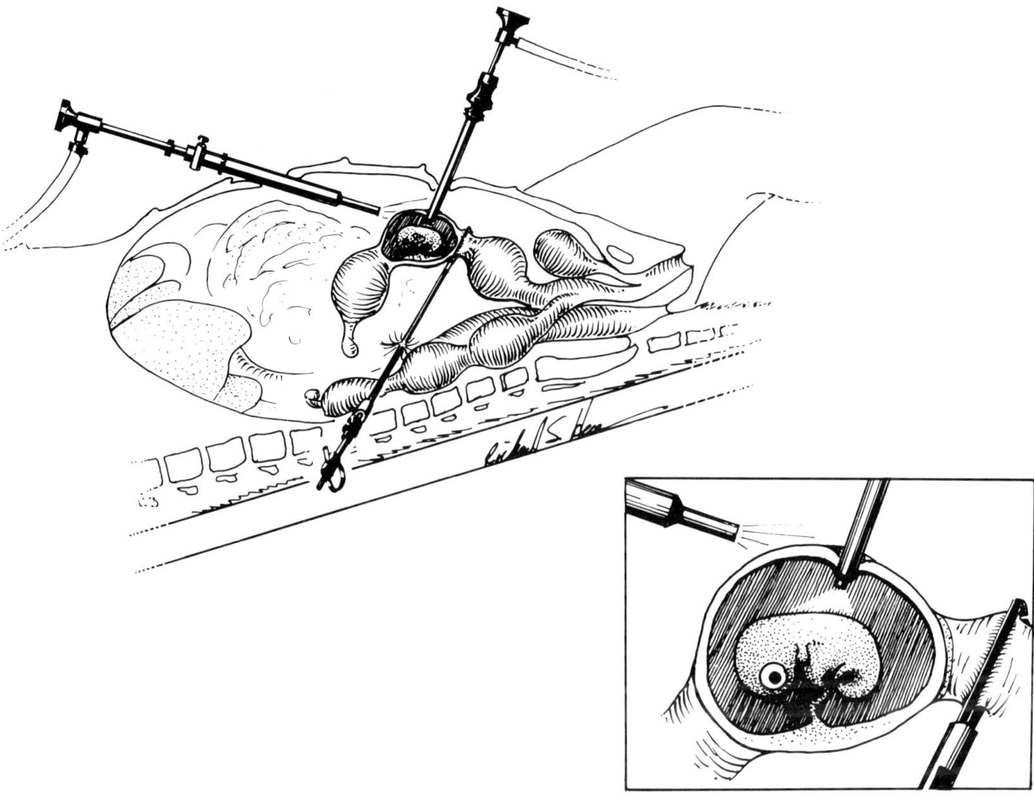

**Figure 3.37** Combined laparoscopy-fetoscopy. The uterine horn is stabilized with an accessory forceps and a small diameter laparoscope inserted into the uterine lumen to directly view the fetus.

ogy are early indicators of pyometra, metritis, or cystic glandular hyperplasia. Routine laparoscopic techniques have been used to confirm the presence of uterine pyometra (open type, cervix patent) in the queen following observation of vulvular discharge. In other cases, colony bitches or queens have displayed anorexia, depression, and elevated temperature, but have demonstrated no discharge (closed type, nonpatent cervix). In these animals if the uterine mass is palpable, laparoscopy has been useful to substantiate the diagnosis and determine the extent of uterine infiltration. In two queens laparoscopy has been used to initially detect pyometra (closed type) prior to advanced signs of typical clinical behavior and before an enlarged uterus was palpable.

## UTERINE INFUSION, INSEMINATION, AND FLUSHING

Laparoscopy can be used to administer foreign agents into the uterine lumen. This capability is more research oriented than clinically relevant, although the technique could be useful to the veterinarian for administering medicinal agents directly *in utero*. Attempts to inject into the uterine lumen using only a needle inserted through the abdominal wall are suspect. Using this technique, it is difficult to determine whether the needle tip is in the uterine stroma or in the lumen. In the bitch, a technique has been successfully adapted from endoscopic methods first described in the pig (Wildt et al., 1975). Diagrammatic illustration of this technique is provided in Chapter 7. A laparoscopic assistant is required for this procedure. The animal is subjected to routine laparoscopy and accessory forceps insertion. The latter instrument is used to grasp and stabilize a uterine horn. In the bitch, one should secure the horn by grasping near the uterine bifurcation. A sterile 16 gauge, 6 cm long needle is inserted through the abdominal wall at a site directly vertical to the desired insertion site in the uterine horn. The latter is elevated slightly with the grasping forceps. This provides stabilization and allows the needle to be inserted at a 20 to 45° angle with the plane of the horn. After sufficient needle penetration of the uterus is suspected, the assistant cannulates the uterine lumen by the insertion of a small diameter sterile tubing through the 16 gauge needle. If the tubing resists insertion, the needle is likely not in the uterine lumen and should be manipulated until a reasonable length of tubing has been inserted to suspect intraluminal placement. With the assistant stabilizing the external end of the tubing, the needle can be removed from the uterus leaving the uterine lumen cannulated. A syringe can be attached to the external end of the tubing to administer the desired drug or agent.

Although the procedural steps appear complicated, the uterine cannula technique is routine in skilled hands, requiring 5 to 15 minutes. Our laboratory has utilized this methodology for infusing drugs and *in utero* artificial insemination. Canine experimental studies have been designed to determine if sperm require vaginal exposure to achieve capacitation. Sperm have been deterred from vaginal exposure by direct deposition *in utero* using the laparoscopic uterine cannulation technique. The procedure is also used to obtain uterine flushings in the dog. Most studies of this type have been concerned with the biochemical analysis of fluid constituents secreted into the uterine lumen. Flushings can be achieved in the bitch by the injection and then the immediate aspiration of a suitable medium through the uterine cannula. Recovery of flush media in the bitch ranges from 45 to 80%.

Slight to moderate hemorrhage (estimated at 2 to 8 ml) has been observed following removal of the needle and tubing from the uterine wall. Blood loss appears to be mostly external into the peritoneal cavity since uterine flushings are uncontaminated with red cells. No problems have been encountered with the healing of uterine puncture sites, nor is any postoperative uterine disease attributable to the procedure. To date, no attempts have been made to cannulate the feline uterus. The author suspects that this technique would be equally feasible in this species although a smaller diameter needle and cannula tubing may be required.

## STERILIZATION

One of the greatest inducements for veterinary laparoscopy would be the use of this procedure for sterilization of the dog and cat. As discussed in Chapter 1, laparoscopy has been used extensively for producing infertility in women, usually by mechanical alteration of the oviduct. In women, this procedure has been shown to be simple, safe, relatively economical, and an aid to this country's current status of zero population growth. The similar use of laparoscopy to assist in alleviating the pet overpopulation problem does not permit simply adapting existing methods, used in humans, immediately to the dog and cat. Sterilization of male and female animals by laparoscopic alteration of the oviduct, uterine horn, or vas deferens will not eliminate the nuisances associated with intact gonadal systems. Specifically, the bitch and queen would still exhibit the annoyances characteristically demonstrated during periods of estrus (attraction of males, vocalization of the queen, sanguinous discharge of the bitch), and the males of each species would still tend to roam. The fact that these animals would be infertile and no longer contributing to the fecund population may offset the disadvantage of intact gonadal systems. However, most responsible owners who want no offspring from their pet also desire elimination of the problems associated with sexual receptivity. Therefore, two philosophies exist: (1) reducing the fertile population by adapting existing human laparoscopic techniques to produce infertility; (2) developing new laparoscopy procedures which will inhibit both fertility and ovarian activity, thereby effectively neutering sexual behavioral, reproductive and endocrine function.

Our laboratory has determined that a distinct need exists for each of these policies. In response, extensive experimental studies have been initiated to determine the efficacy, practicality, and safety of various laparoscopic sterilization techniques. The early studies have been concerned with simply adapting various laparoscopic ligation methods, as developed for use in humans, to dogs and cats. Studies have been designed to examine the feasibility of uterine horn or oviductal ligation in the bitch and queen and internal vas deferens occlusion in the male dog and cat. Such procedures, while permitting gonadal function, would serve as an invaluable potential means of sterilization on a massive basis, possibly through urban pet adoption agency programs. Our preliminary results would indicate several potential advantages of laparoscopic sterilization on a mass basis versus the more conventional ovariohysterectomy (spay) program. These would be associated with the short time interval required for laparoscopic sterilization; the requirement for only minor surgical intervention; ease of procedure regardless of animal age or sex; and possible reduced need for veterinary manpower through the use of highly skilled laparoscopic technicians working under veterinary supervision (Wildt and Seager, 1977). The primary advantage of such a program would be that *all* animals adopted from such programs would be infertile.

As in the extensive testing of chemical pet contraceptives, new surgical means of inducing infertility also require comprehensive experimentation. Our studies have been concerned with the chronic effects of laparoscopic sterilization on reproductive function and general animal health. Routine laparoscopy and accessory cannula procedures are performed as described previously. A variety of accessory devices are being tested. One device worthy of mention is a bipolar Kleppinger forceps (Fig. 3.38) and corresponding bipolar coagulation unit (Richard Wolf Medical Instruments Corp.). The jaws of this forceps serve as electrodes and only tissue between the forceps jaws is subjected to the electrical current (Fig. 3.38). Thus, this instrument dispels the need for a ground plate and avoids heat damage to tissues located adjacent to the cautery site.

In the male each vas deferens is easily identified (Pl. 1, Fig. 5), grasped with the forceps (Pl. 2, Fig. 8), and electrocoagulated (Pl. 3. Fig. 1). Bilateral cauterization of

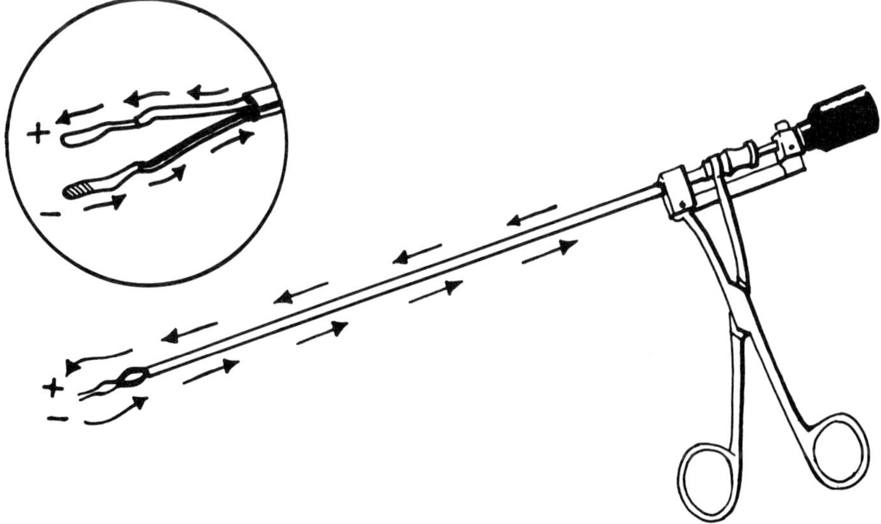

**Figure 3.38**  Bipolar forceps in which the jaws serve as electrodes.

approximately 1.5 cm of vas has resulted in permanent sterility and, to date, no adverse physical or behavioral effects. In the female, a portion of the reproductive tract, generally the uterine horn, is altered by electrocoagulation, cutting, or a combination of these procedures. Current investigations are concerned with the absolute surgical need to produce sterility (i.e., cautery versus cutting versus cautery and cutting); the preferred site to be altered (i.e., caudal horn, cranial horn, oviduct); and the long term effectiveness and safety resulting from such procedures. Both adult and prepubertal male and female dogs and cats are being utilized. Examination of preliminary data reveals that the site of laparoscopic alteration along the uterine horn dramatically affects results, particularly in female dogs. In several cases, improperly altered reproductive tissue has resulted in fluid retention within the uterine horn. *For this reason and since these studies in general are incomplete, laparoscopic sterilization cannot currently be recommended as a proven, safe method of sterilization in the dog and cat.*

These results should, however, illustrate and provide impetus for other similar investigations needed to determine the efficacy of laparoscopic sterilization. For example, several endoscopy companies manufacture sterilization devices previously proven effective in women. One, termed a lay loop applicator, allows a constricting Silastic band to be placed over a loop of oviduct, thereby occluding it. Another instrument is termed a Hulka Clip applicator, used to attach a plastic occlusive spring clip (Pl. 3, Fig. 2) to the oviductal channel. Further laparoscopic studies may be concerned with the structural modification of these devices to determine their adaptability as canine and feline fertility control methods.

Even further clinical research investigations are necessary to develop laparoscopic methods to eliminate ovarian function. Since the ovary of the queen is quite accessible, future studies of significance may involve complete ovarian cautery, intraovarian injection of sclerosing agents, or electrocoagulation of the ovarian blood supply. Recently, Semm (1978) has described a laparoscopic technique for ovariectomy in women which could have valuable application in animals. Additional ingenuity will be required to conduct similar studies in the bitch since the ovary of this species is encapsulated in an ovarian bursa. All of these possibilities illustrate the research efforts yet required to determine the all inclusive capabilities of laparoscopy in canine and feline clinical medicine.

## Laparoscopic Photography

Laparoscopic still photography is an effectual medium for documenting and illustrating internal observation. In the laboratory it serves an an invaluable aid in recording research. In the classroom, photolaparoscopy is beginning to play a useful role as an instructional tool.

Obtaining photographs does not simply entail attachment of the 35 mm camera to the laparoscope eyepiece and clicking the camera shutter. Photographic quality is directly proportional to the type of instrumentation used and the skills of the laparoscopist.

As discussed in the equipment section, to achieve quality photographic documentation in the dog and cat, the following are required: a laparoscope 5 mm or larger in diameter; an SLR camera with suitable lens adapter; a light source with high intensity illumination or electronic flash capabilities.

Adequate light is the most important factor in successful photolaparoscopy. The only light available at the desired photographic site within the abdominal cavity is the amount produced and transferred from the illumination source to the fiber optic cable and laparoscope. For this reason, the larger the cable and telescope the greater the capability of providing a brighter abdominal cavity. Although sufficient for normal visualization, most commercial diagnostic lamps (150 watts) produce inadequate incandescence for photography. The problem is compounded by the presence of numerous dark colored internal organs and tissue which tend to absorb transported light. Numerous reports in human endoscopy literature have praised illumination sources with the synchronous electronic flash systems (Kott, 1978). We have had no experience with these types of devices in the dog and cat but have achieved very satisfactory success using the heavy duty projector lamp capable of providing chronic intense photographic illumination (1000 watts).

The details for laparoscopic photography in the dog and cat are direct. Upon deciding to document an observation, the laparoscopist should evaluate the situation to determine if the target site to be photographed requires stabilization or elevation within the abdominal cavity air space. Often the normal respiratory movements of the animal produce some internal motion at the target site, resulting in a blurred photograph. Organs may be partially secured by the Verres needle probe or accessory forceps which is then held by the operator's assistant. The photographic lamp within the light source is activated and generally requires 30 to 60 seconds to achieve maximal brightness. Camera settings are examined before attaching the camera body to the laparoscope. The camera is focused at infinity and the f-stop adjusted to its most reduced numeration (for the Olympus OM-1, the preferred f-stop setting is 2.8). The shutter speed setting is a subjective judgment based on the operator's skill, size of laparoscope, target tissue coloration, and the distance between the laparoscope and the tissue being photographed. In general for the dog and cat, the exposure time for the 10 mm and 5 mm in diameter laparoscopes is initially adjusted to $^1/_{125}$th and $^1/_{60}$th of a second, respectively.

Cameras are fixed to the endoscope by a variety of adapters. The technique in our laboratory is one of the simplest, whereby a specialized ring eyepiece adapter is screwed into the 100 mm camera lens (at the site where a filter would normally fit). The ring adapter is equipped with a retractable bearing apparatus which permits the camera to be tightly mounted to the laparoscopic eyepiece.

After attaching, the target organ is located by viewing through the camera lens (Fig. 3.39). It is difficult to precisely determine how close one has positioned the end of the telescope to the desired photographic site. The author recommends that the camera-laparoscope combination be maneuvered until the target site constitutes 70 to 80% of the viewing field. Attempts at documenting panoramic views of a large portion of the abdominal cavity should be avoided. Even sophisticated illumination sources are generally incapable of providing sufficient light for this type of photography. In addition, clarity and minute detail are often lacking in resulting pictures. Immediately prior to taking the actual photograph, the laparoscopist should position himself to avoid minor movements. Optimum stabilization is achieved by using one hand to grasp the midline cannula and the other (elbow resting on the surgical table) to hold and operate the camera shutter (Fig. 3.39).

Because of light, movement, and distance variabilities, the laparoscopist should take at least three individual photographs of the target site. Exposure time varies with each picture. Using the 10 mm in diameter laparoscope, the shutter speeds are bracketed from the initial $^1/_{125}$th second speed down to $^1/_{60}$th and $^1/_{30}$th second. A similar system is used with the 5 mm in diameter instrument which is adjusted from $^1/_{60}$th to $^1/_{30}$th and $^1/_{15}$th for the remaining two photographs. After 20 to 25 hours of use, the high intensity photographic lamp of the light source will lose some intensity. The operator will then need to adjust camera shutter speed accordingly. The skilled laparoscopist can achieve quality photographs utilizing exposure times as long as $^1/_4$th to $^1/_8$th of a second.

Precise recording of photographic data is a prerequisite for avoiding confusion when processed photographs are returned to the laboratory. During each laparoscopy, one should note the film used, number of pictures taken, and the precise organ or event photographed. It is particularly advantageous to record exposure speed utilized for each individual photograph taken. Comparative analysis of this data to actual picture quality would provide an indication of the most effective shutter speed to use.

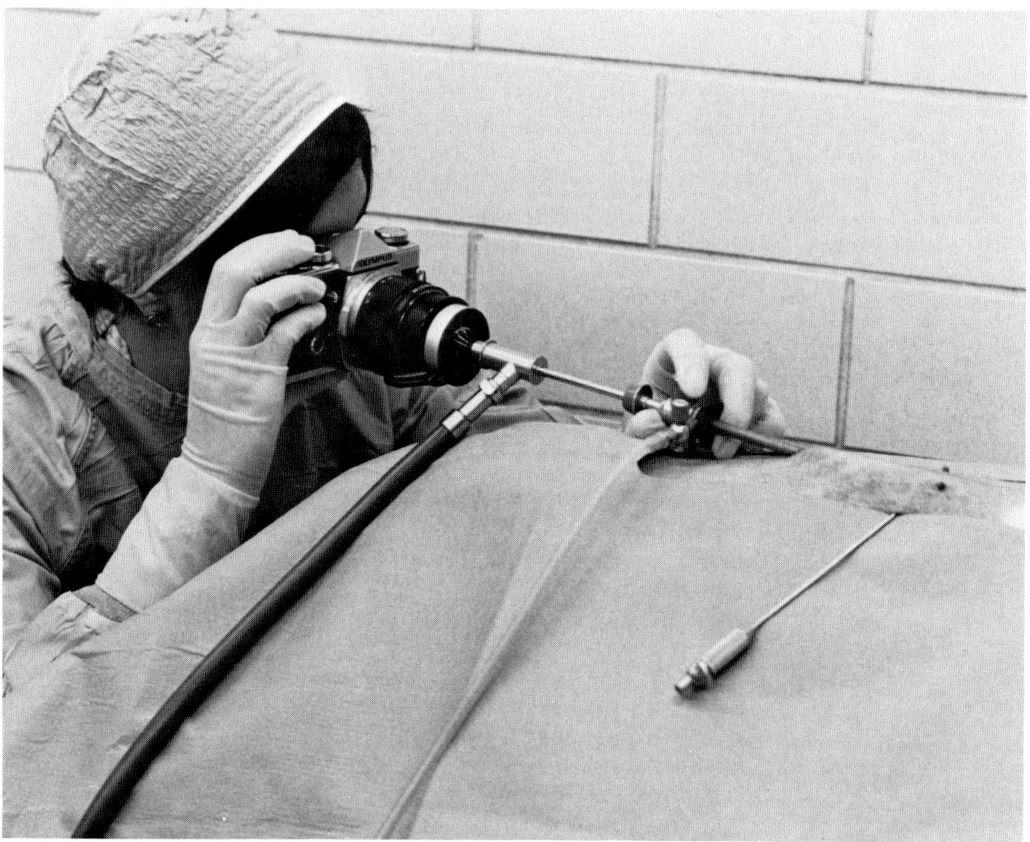

**Figure 3.39**   Camera attached to the laparoscope. Operator is correctly positioned by supporting the camera and cannula. Both elbows are on the table.

### Laparoscopic Records

It is imperative to record the information utilized and obtained during each diagnostic or surgical laparoscopy. Figure 3.40 illustrates a reporting form employed in our laboratory primarily for reproductive examinations, but with space available to note pertinent clinical diagnoses.

### Future Implications of Laparoscopy

Considerable detail has been presented in this chapter to provide the researcher and veterinary clinician with a working knowledge of canine and feline laparoscopy. In addition, an attempt has been made to emphasize or allude to specific areas where little or no potentially valuable endoscopic information for the dog and cat is available. These have included the future use of laparoscopy as a diagnostic tool in gastrointestinal dysfunction and research; as an instrument for the direct study of fetal development and the intrauterine environment; and as an alternative method for the clinical sterilization of dogs and cats.

Although these areas provide widespread potential, the present prerequisite is the education of professionals desiring to learn and develop the skills associated with canine and feline laparoscopy. It is the author's hope that this chapter has contributed to this need.

LAPAROSCOPY REPORTING FORM

Date_____________  Species___________ ID#_________
Purpose of Examination_______________________________  Laparoscopist(s)_______________

| Animal Information: | Anesthetic Information: | Laparoscopy Technique: |
|---|---|---|
| Breed ____________ /Sex ☐ F ☐ M | Premedication____________ | Laparoscope used________ |
| Weight________ ☐ kg ☐ lb | ________ ☐ IM ☐ IV or___ | Site of puncture________ |
| History and stage of cycle________ | Anesthetic________ ☐ IM ☐ IV or___ | Insufflation volume________ |
| | Concentration________ | Other: |
| | Dosage________ | Blood sample________ cc ________ hr |
| | Total mg.________ | Cervical examination________ |
| | Time of Administration________ | |
| | Onset of laparoscopy________ | |
| | End of laparoscopy________ | Antibiotic________ Dosage________ |

OBSERVATIONS:

Uterus:_______________________________________________

Left ovary:___________________________________________

Right ovary:__________________________________________

Other:________________________________________________

PHOTOGRAPHIC RECORD:
    no. speed comment          File_______________________

GENERAL COMMENTS:_____________________________________

FORM 1401L ICM/BCM

**Figure 3.40**  Reporting form useful for maintaining laparoscopy records.

## References

Bush, M., Wildt, D. E., Kennedy, S., and Seager, S. W. J. (1978) Laparoscopy in zoological medicine. *J. Am. Vet. Med. Assoc.* 173:1081–1087.

Chakraborty, P. K., Wildt, D. E., and Seager, S. W. J. (1979) Serum luteinizing hormone and ovulatory response to luteinizing hormone-releasing hormone in the estrous and anestrous domestic cat. *Lab. Anim. Sci.* 29: 338–344.

Johnson, G. F., and Twedt, D. C. (1977) Endoscopy and laparoscopy in the diagnosis and management of neoplasia in small animals. *Vet. Clin. North Am.* 7:77–92.

Kinney, G. M., Chakraborty, P. K., Seager, S. W. J., and Wildt, D. E. (1979) Relationship of vaginal cytology to ovulation and serum LH and estradiol-17$\beta$ in the bitch (unpublished data).

Kott, D. F. (1978) Photography, cinematography, and television in endoscopy. In: *Endoscopy in Gynecology.* J. M. Phillips, ed., American Association of Gynecologic Laparoscopists, Dept. of Publications, Downey, Calif., pp. 481–493.

Lettow, E. (1972) Laparoscopic examinations in liver diseases in dogs. *Vet. Med. Rev.* 2:159–167.

Loffer, F. D., Pent, P., and Quinones, R. G. (1978) Questions and answers from the postgraduate course on the fundamentals of laparoscopy. In: *Endoscopy in Gynecology.* J. M. Phillips, ed., American Association of Gynecologic Laparoscopists, Dept. of Publications, Downey, Calif., pp. 27–38.

Rioux, J. E. (1978) An unusual complication of double-puncture laparoscopy. In: *Endoscopy in Gynecology.* J. M. Phillips, ed., American Association of Gynecologic Laparoscopists, Dept. of Publications, Downey, Calif,. pp. 76–77.

Semm, K. (1977) *Atlas of Gynecologic Laparoscopy and Hysteroscopy.* L. S. Borow, ed., W. B. Saunders, Philadelphia, pp. 6–98.

Semm, K. (1978) Gynecologic surgical interventions with the laparoscope. In: *Endoscopy in Gynecology.* J. M. Phillips, ed., American Association of Gynecologic Laparoscopists, Dept. of Publications, Downey, Calif., pp. 514–521.

Valenti, C. (1972) Endoamnioscopy and fetal biopsy:

a new technique. *Am. J. Obstet. Gynecol.* 114:561–564.

Wildt, D. E., and Seager, S. W. J. (1977) Reproduction control in the dog. *Vet. Clin. North Am.* 7:775–784.

Wildt, D. E., and Seager, S. W. J. (1978) Ovarian response in the estrual cat receiving varying dosages of HCG. *Horm. Res.* 9:130–136.

Wildt, D. E., and Seager, S. W. J. (1979) Laparoscopic determination of ovarian and uterine morphology during the reproductive cycle (of the cat). In: *Current Therapy in Theriogenology.* D. Morrow, ed., W. B. Saunders, Philadelphia (in press).

Wildt, D. E., Morcom, C. B., and Dukelow, W. R. (1975) Laparoscopic pregnancy diagnosis and uterine fluid recovery in swine. *J. Reprod. Fertil.* 44:301–304.

Wildt, D. E., Kinney, G. M., and Seager, S. W. J. (1977a) Laparoscopy for direct observation of internal organs of the domestic cat and dog. *Am. J. Vet. Res.* 38:1429–1432.

Wildt, D. E., Levinson, C. J., and Seager, S. W. J. (1977b) Laparoscopic exposure and sequential observation of the ovary of the cycling bitch. *Anat. Rec.* 189:443–449.

Wildt, D. E., Chakraborty, P. K., Panko, W. B., and

Seager, S. W. J. (1978a) Relationship of reproductive behavior, serum luteinizing hormone and time of ovulation in the bitch. *Biol. Reprod.* 18:561–570.

Wildt, D. E., Guthrie, S. C., and Seager, S. W. J. (1978b) Ovarian and behavioral cyclicity of the laboratory maintained cat. *Horm. Behav.* 10:251–257.

Wildt, D. E., Kinney, G. M., and Seager, S. W. J. (1978c) Gonadotropin induced reproductive cyclicity in the domestic cat. *Lab. Anim. Sci.* 28:301–307.

Wildt, D. E., Panko, W. B., Chakraborty, P. K., and Seager, S. W. J. (1979a) Relationship of serum estrone, estradiol-17$\beta$ and progesterone to LH, sexual behavior, and time of ovulation in the bitch. *Biol. Reprod.* 20: 648–658.

Wildt, D. E., Seager, S. W. J., and Chakraborty, P. K. (1979b) Relationship of estrous behavior, ovarian activity and serum LH and progesterone in the cat. *Biol. Reprod.* 20: Suppl. 1, 53A.

Wildt, D. E., Seager, S. W. J., Dukelow, W. R., and Chakraborty, P. K. (1979c) Ovulatory and LH response of the domestic cat. *Fed. Proc.* 38(3):1031, abstract.

# CHAPTER 4

# Laparoscopy in Monkeys and Apes*

## Richard M. Harrison, Ph.D.

## INTRODUCTION

Since the mid-1960s laparoscopy has been used extensively in nonhuman primates to examine changes on the ovaries relative to the ovulatory process. At present little data exist on the clinical applications of this procedure with respect to veterinary care of monkeys and apes. Laparoscopic techniques were first used in rhesus monkeys (Balin et al., 1966) and have since been adapted to most species commonly used in research. Recent importation restrictions of some species of monkeys have illustrated the need for conservation of nonhuman primates. Laparoscopy is a relatively atraumatic technique and is becoming increasingly important as a diagnostic and research tool to attain maximal research productivity from individual animals.

To date the majority of laparoscopic procedures performed in nonhuman primates are for the examination of the female reproductive organs in the pelvis. Fewer, but increasingly more significant numbers of examinations are conducted in males or for diagnostic purposes which may involve inspection of the upper (cranial) abdominal organs. In general, the same techniques are used whether the organs of interest are in the upper or lower abdominal regions. Certain modifications are required depending on the size of the subject, ancillary procedures to be performed, and the facilities available. Individual modifications are also made according to the laparoscopist's training and experience. This chapter details the procedures routinely used by the author to examine internal organs of large monkeys, including adult baboons, rhesus, cynomolgus and patas monkeys. These procedures have currently been used in more than 500 laparoscopic examinations, including 200 in baboons, 200 in patas monkeys, 50 in macaques, and at least 50 in other species. The author also has performed 500 laparoscopic examinations in small monkeys, including squirrel monkeys, marmosets, and infants of various species. Ancillary techniques used by others will be presented later, as will those modifications necessary for laparoscopy of the larger apes.

### Previous Laparoscopic Studies in Nonhuman Primates

In the rhesus monkey (*Macaca mulatta*), ovulations induced by human menopausal gonadotropin (HMG) and human chorionic gonadotropin (HCG) (Balin and Wan, 1969),

* The author wishes to express his appreciation to Ms. K. Reed, T. Rusca, and M. Schlenker for their assistance in the laparoscopic examinations at the Delta Primate Center. Special thanks are given to Dr. W. R. Dukelow for his assistance in learning the procedures and support through the years.

or by pregnant mares' serum gonadotropin (PMSG), HCG and prostaglandins (Batta and Brackett, 1974) have been detected by laparoscopic techniques. Bosu (1973) described a laparoscopic procedure for the examination of the ovaries in rhesus monkeys. This investigator used the technique to ascertain ovulation and to study normal ovarian steroid patterns relative to ovulation (Bosu et al., 1973). These investigators later studied the effects of postovulatory norethindrone and estrogens on reproductive hormonal patterns (Bosu and Johansson, 1974), again using laparoscopy to detect ovulation. Dierschke and Clark (1976) conducted a study to determine if frequent laparoscopy in the same animal affected normal ovarian function. A specialized "light pencil" or wand was developed that, when inserted into the abdominal cavity, provided supplemental light. By backlighting the ovary, these investigators reported that preovulatory follicles could be detected as early as day 2 or 3 of the 31 day cycle. This study was later expanded with serum luteinizing hormone (LH) and progesterone levels measured in monkeys subjected to frequent laparoscopy (Clark et al., 1978). No significant differences in the observed incidence of ovulation, length of follicular or luteal phases, or serum levels of hormones were detected in control animals compared to monkeys undergoing laparoscopy three to ten times per cycle.

Ovulation in pigtail macaques (*Macaca nemestrina*) was detected by laparoscopy and correlated with changes in vaginal cytology, body temperature, and perineal tumescence (White et al., 1973). Early detumescence and ovulation appeared to provide satisfactory correlation, with both events occurring within a 24 hour period (Blakley et al., 1977). A study of ovarian morphology in the Japanese macaque (*Macaca fuscata*) indicated that variations in follicular appearance make it difficult to precisely predict time of ovulation or estimate corpus luteum age (Nigi, 1977). This investigator reported no difficulty in determining if ovulation had occurred when careful sequential observations were made and suggested the shape of preovulatory follicles may be influenced by the location of the follicle relative to its depth from the ovarian surface.

The basic laparoscopic technique used in most nonhuman primate species today was first described in cynomolgus and squirrel monkeys (*Macaca fascicularis* and *Saimiri sciureus*, respectively) by Dukelow et al., (1971b). Using the cynomolgus monkey as a model, studies were conducted to detect changes in follicular morphology relative to ovulation (Jewett and Dukelow, 1971a, 1972a, 1973; Dukelow et al., 1972; Dukelow et al., 1971a; Rawson and Dukelow, 1973a; Dukelow, 1975), to determine cycle characteristics and gestation lengths (Jewett and Dukelow, 1971b, 1972b; Dukelow 1977), to ascertain the effects of laparoscopy on reproductive physiology (Rawson and Dukelow, 1973b; Mahone and Dukelow, 1978), and to study the effects of contraceptive agents on ovulation (Harrison et al., 1974).

Extensive laparoscopic studies have also been conducted in the squirrel monkey. The effects of megestrol acetate on ovulation when injected (Harrison and Dukelow, 1971) or administered by subcutaneous implants (Harrison et al., 1974) have been reported. The technique has been used to observe the ovarian follicular changes relative to ovulation (Harrison and Dukelow, 1974) and to detect seasonal differences in response to ovulation induction (Harrison and Dukelow, 1973; Kuehl and Dukelow, 1975). Nonfertilized ova and preimplantation blastocysts have been recovered from the squirrel monkey uterus by a laparoscopic technique (Ariga and Dukelow, 1977a,b). Laparoscopy has also been used to detect pregnancy in the squirrel monkey and to study the effects of exogenous gonadotropins on vaginal cytology, ovulation, sexual behavior, and gestation during the normal anovulatory season (Jarosz et al., 1977).

Laparoscopy has been employed as a direct technique for determining time of ovulation in baboons (*Papio anubis*) (Eddy et al., 1976). These investigators recovered ova from the reproductive tracts via laparotomy at 24, 48 or 72 hours after laparoscopically detected ovulation and were able to determine the time-course of oviductal ovum transport. A study to correlate perineal swelling with ovarian hormone levels, vaginal cytology, and ovarian follicular morphology utilized laparoscopy to detect follicular changes (Wildt *et al.*, 1977).

Although other great apes may have been subjected to laparoscopy for diagnostic studies, only the chimpanzee (*Pan troglodytes*) has undergone examinations as part of reported research efforts associated with the physiology of the great apes. Laparoscopic visualization of the ovaries in chimpanzees provided a method to accurately correlate ovulation and skin swelling detumescence (Graham *et al.*, 1973). Detailed description of successful techniques has been reported by Graham (1976) and will be described later in this chapter.

Laparoscopy provides an important tool to detect ovulation even when other less invasive techniques, such as radioimmunoassay for progesterone, are available. Reports of follicular luteinization with concomitant increases in basal body temperatures and serum progesterone levels, without ovulation, have been reported by two research groups (Marik and Hulka, 1978; Koninckx *et al.*, 1978). Even biopsies showing secretory endometrium are a reflection of luteinization and not ovulation, i.e., the release of an ovum from the follicle. Although "entrapped ova" have been described in studies involving only human subjects, similar follicles have been observed by this author in nonhuman primates that have been classified as etiopathic infertile. The follicles in these monkeys have been observed to develop and then to luteinize during periods when the monkey has mated with a fertile male (based on sperm in vaginal smear). The monkeys have shown an increase in serum progesterone levels indicative of ovulation but have not become pregnant.

## BASIC PROCEDURE FOR LAPAROSCOPY IN MONKEYS

### Equipment

The equipment used in our laboratory consists of a 5 mm in diameter, 130° laparoscope, a flexible fiber optic light cable (3 mm in diameter), and a heavy duty light projector. This projector has a 150 watt light for general diagnostic use and a 1000 watt source for photography. A 6 mm in diameter cannula with trumpet valve and pyramidal trocar are used to establish the passage for the insertion of the laparoscope into the abdominal cavity. A Verres needle is required for insufflation and is also used as a probe for organ manipulation. The gas used to insufflate the abdomen is moistened carbon dioxide ($CO_2$). If photographic documentation is desired a single lens reflex 35 mm camera with lens adapter is available. Figure 4.1 illustrates the basic instruments used for a routine examination.

Additional equipment and supplies required for the examination include clippers to remove abdominal hair, a surgical preparation solution such as Betadine, scalpel, suture, solution for sterilization of instruments, anesthesia, gauze sponges, and antibiotic powder and ointment. Other supply items, minor pieces of equipment, and accessory laparoscopic instruments required for ancillary procedures will be described in the discussion of those techniques. A table on which the animal can be restrained and then tilted in a head down supine position is required. The standard surgical table when tilted is too low to perform laparoscopy while standing and, thus, requires the examiner to sit on a low stool. Our examining table is a standard adjustable stainless steel surgical table with central drainage trough (Wahmann Manufacturing Co.). This table is 117 cm long, 61 cm wide, and 102 cm high. One end of the table can be elevated 10 to 30 cm by placing it in a wooden support (Figure 4.2). This provides an excellent working height for the laparoscopic examination and ancillary procedures.

### Preparation of Animal, Anesthesia, and Restraint

Food but not water is withheld from the animal for approximately 18 hours prior to examination. The anesthetizing drug used most extensively for large monkeys (3 kg or

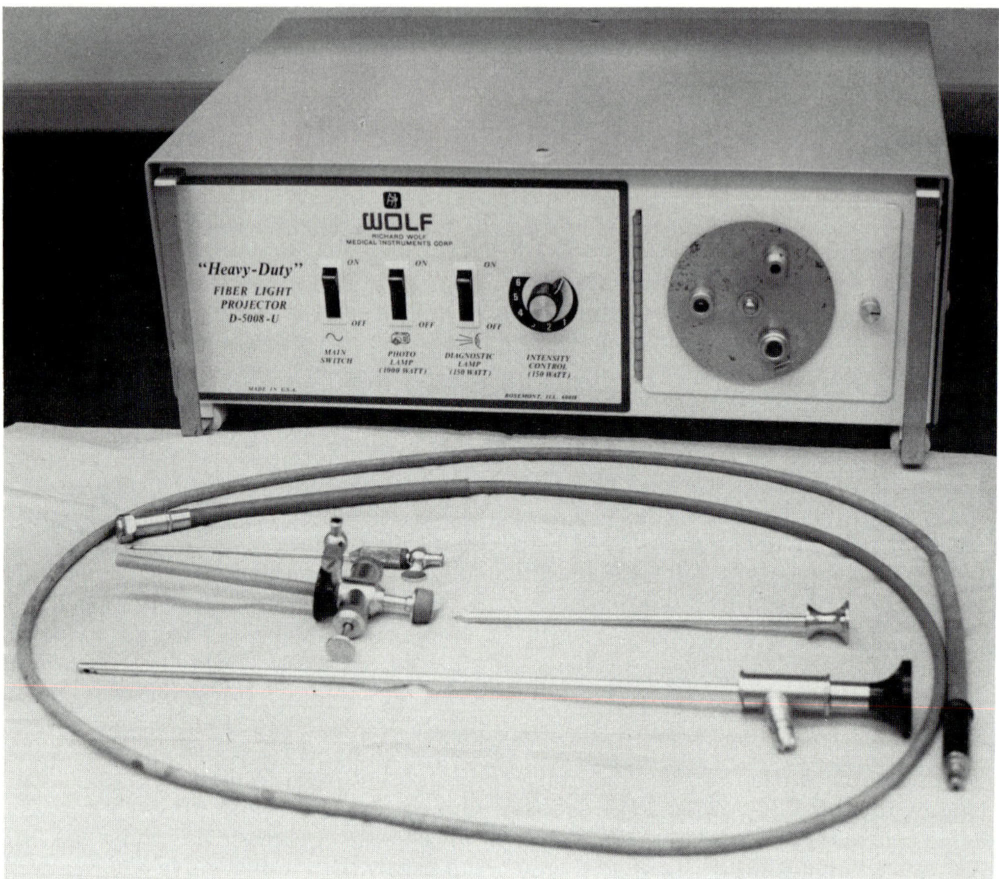


**Figure 4.1**   Basic laparoscopic instruments used for laparoscopy in monkeys and apes. Light projector has a 150 watt diagnostic lamp controlled by a rheostat and a 1000 watt lamp for photography. The flexible light cable is coiled around the 5 mm in diameter, 130° laparoscope (front), the fiberglass, trumpet valve cannula (middle-left), pyramidal trocar (right), and Verres needle (rear).

more) has been phencyclidine hydrochloride (Sernylan, BioCeutic Lab, 1 mg/kg) injected intramuscularly. A surgical plane of anesthesia is induced which is of sufficient duration (60 to 90 minutes) for laparoscopic examination and most additional procedures (i.e., collection of blood samples or vaginal smears). Since this drug is no longer commercially available the author recommends ketamine hydrochloride (Vetalar, Parke, Davis and Co., 10 mg/kg) injected intramuscularly. Compared to phencyclidine hydrochloride, animal recovery is generally more rapid (30 to 45 minutes), making ketamine hydrochloride somewhat less desirable since some procedures may require more time due to excessive fat, adhesions, distended bladder, etc. A combination of ketamine hydrochloride with acepromazine (Acepromazine maleate, Ayerst Laboratories, 10 mg/ml, ratio of 10:1) will produce a more prolonged anesthetic effect and increased muscular relaxation. As will be discussed later, gaseous anesthesia can be used to maintain the surgical plane of anesthesia but it is not generally used for routine examinations. The biological effectiveness of injected anesthesia will be more pronounced and of longer duration in any animal with impaired liver and/or kidney function since biological degradation will be prolonged.

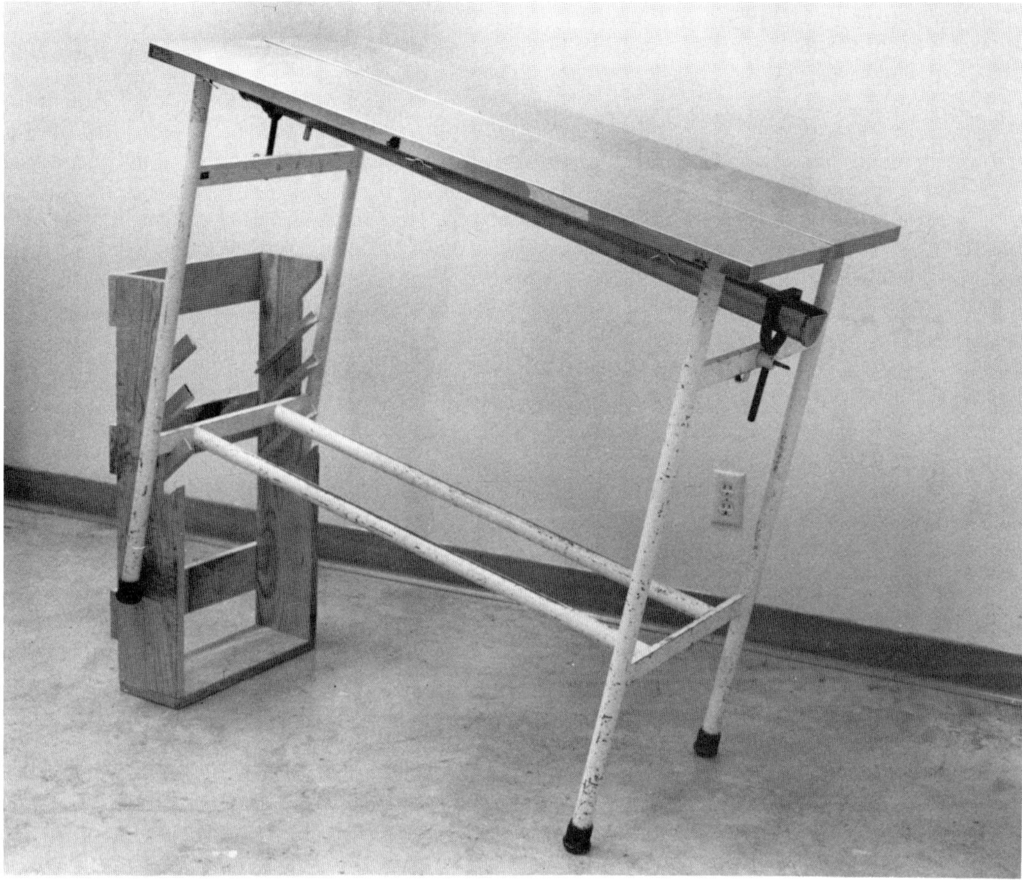

**Figure 4.2** Surgical table tilted to normal position for laparoscopic examinations. Animal's head would be at the lower (right) end and its legs would be secured by ropes. The laparoscopist can comfortably sit or stand using this type of table.

The anesthetized animal is restrained on the surgical table with ropes supporting all four limbs. The head is positioned near the end of the table, opposite the end to be elevated. No restraints are ever placed around the animal's head or neck. Surgical preparation begins with the clipping of abdominal hair from lower rib cage to pubic area, laterally to the sides. The area is then disinfected with Betadine scrub (Purdue Frederick Co.) and wiped with Betadine solution. Sterile drapes placed over the legs, chest, and to the sides assist in maintaining an aseptic area. Based on extensive experience it has not been found necessary to maintain a sterile field during most laparoscopic examinations on common laboratory primates. However, as will be discussed, sterile surgical conditions are recommended in some circumstances.

All instruments, including the laparoscope, trocar, cannula, scalpel, Verres needle, needle holder, and forceps are immersed in Amerse (Vestal Laboratories) disinfectant solution for at least 10 minutes prior to use. Other cold solutions suitable for disinfecting laparoscopes and accessory instruments are presented in Chapter 12.

### Detailed Procedure

The initial incision is made at the ventral midline in the area of the umbilicus. A 1 cm incision is made through the skin only. If serial examinations are performed at two to three day intervals, the site of incision should be changed along the midline to promote healing; in most cases after 20 or more laparoscopic examinations the total midline scar area will not exceed 5 cm.

The Verres needle is attached to the gas hose, gas is passed through to check for patency, and the needle is tested for free movement of the obturator (retractable blunt tip) before use. We use 100% $CO_2$ bubbled through a water trap as the insufflatory gas (Fig. 4.3). The water trap serves two roles by equilibrating the gas to room temperature and adding sufficient moisture to prevent any drying effect in the abdominal cavity. $CO_2$ is readily absorbed and no problems have been encountered or associated with its use. Other laboratories report using room air or 5% $CO_2$:95% air. These gases can be utilized safely, but care should be taken at the end of the examination to express as much of the insufflated gas from the abdominal cavity as possible. In human patients complaints of pain and discomfort have been related to embolisms from nonabsorbed gases. If one wishes to use room air for insufflation an insufflator can be devised using a hand bulb pump (like those used to inflate blood pressure cuffs) and an in-line glass wool filter to purify the air.

The Verres needle is inserted through the midline incision, passing through the muscle layer into the peritoneal cavity. This author holds the needle so that the blunt retractable tip (obturator) is retracted by the tissue being penetrated, exposing the sharp tip. When the peritoneal cavity is entered the obturator springs outward so that the tip is blunt and no tissue damage occurs. The abdomen is then insufflated. If an automatic insufflator is used the intraabdominal pressure gauge should read 10 to 20 mm Hg; a pressure reading in excess of 50 mm Hg indicates the Verres needle is either occluded or incorrectly positioned. If the needle tip is not in the peritoneal cavity, gas may enter the spaces between skin and muscle, as evidenced by localized distension of the skin, usually in irregular patterns. In this case the Verres needle should be removed and reinserted. If no gas pockets below the skin are observed, but the pressure reading exceeds 50 mm Hg, the gas hose should be disconnected and a syringe attached to the Verres needle. Aspiration of urine, blood, fecal material, or tissue indicates that an organ has been punctured. Corrective steps depend on the organ punctured and extent of the damage and are beyond the scope of this presentation. The novice laparoscopist exercising care should not be overly concerned since such accidents are extremely rare.

Volumes of insufflated gas vary from less than 0.5 liter in a young adult patas monkey (body weight 3 kg) to 4 to 5 liters in an adult chimpanzee (body weight 50 kg). We do not use an automatic insufflator and insufflate manually until the abdomen is firm to the touch and tympanic. The Verres needle is then removed and the table tilted to the Trendelenburg position. For most studies involving laparoscopic examination of pelvic organs in female monkeys the table is tilted 10 to 15°.

The trocar-cannula is inserted through the incision site directed toward the dorsal pelvic area (Figure 4.4). Some laparoscopists prefer passing the trocar-cannula slightly under the skin and then through the abdominal wall so that a nonalignment of insertion sites in the skin and abdominal wall exists when the instruments are removed. Our insertion technique does not provide this nonalignment and allows for a multiple tissue layer closure later. Care must be taken to insert the trocar-cannula with a steady firm movement. If the abdominal wall is penetrated too forcibly the trocar may perforate an abdominal organ; if too cautiously, the peritoneum may not be penetrated. A recognizable "pop" is usually audible when the trocar enters the cavity. The trocar should not be inserted further after it is in the peritoneal cavity. Trocar accidents are extremely rare if proper insufflation and insertion procedures are used, but can be severe if caution is not exercised. When the trocar is removed the escape of gas through the cannula can be heard, indicating that the cannula tip is within the abdominal cavity. The hose from the $CO_2$ tank is then attached to the side port of the cannula and additional gas insufflated, if required (Fig. 4.5).

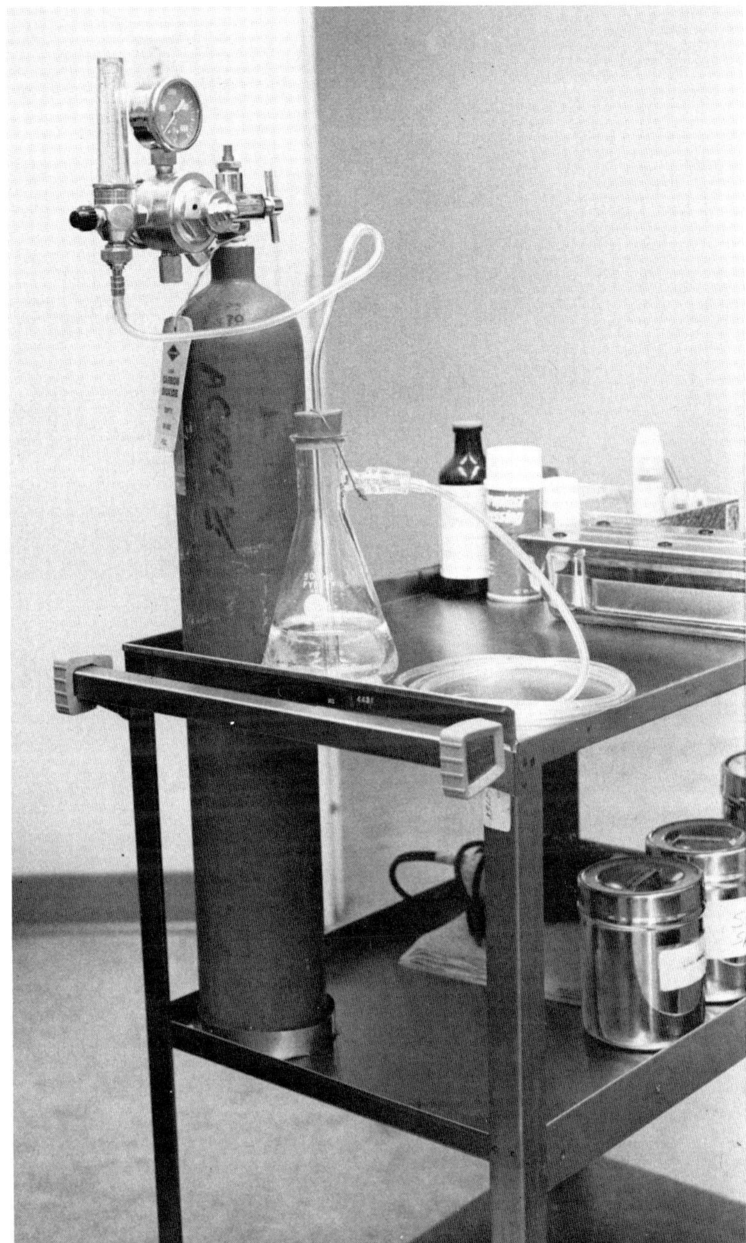

**Figure 4.3** Standard C-size $CO_2$ tank with regulator used to insufflate monkeys for laparoscopy. The gas passes through plastic and glass tubing into a stoppered, side arm flask containing sterile water; after bubbling through the water the gas passes through the side arm into plastic tubing which will be connected to the Verres needle or cannula side arm for insufflation.

The laparoscope is removed from the sterilizing solution, dried wih a sterile gauze, and inserted into the cannula. Initially, the view may be unclear; this is usually due to fogging of the terminal lens and may be avoided by rinsing the laparoscope with warm sterile water prior to insertion. The laparoscope is then attached to the light source via

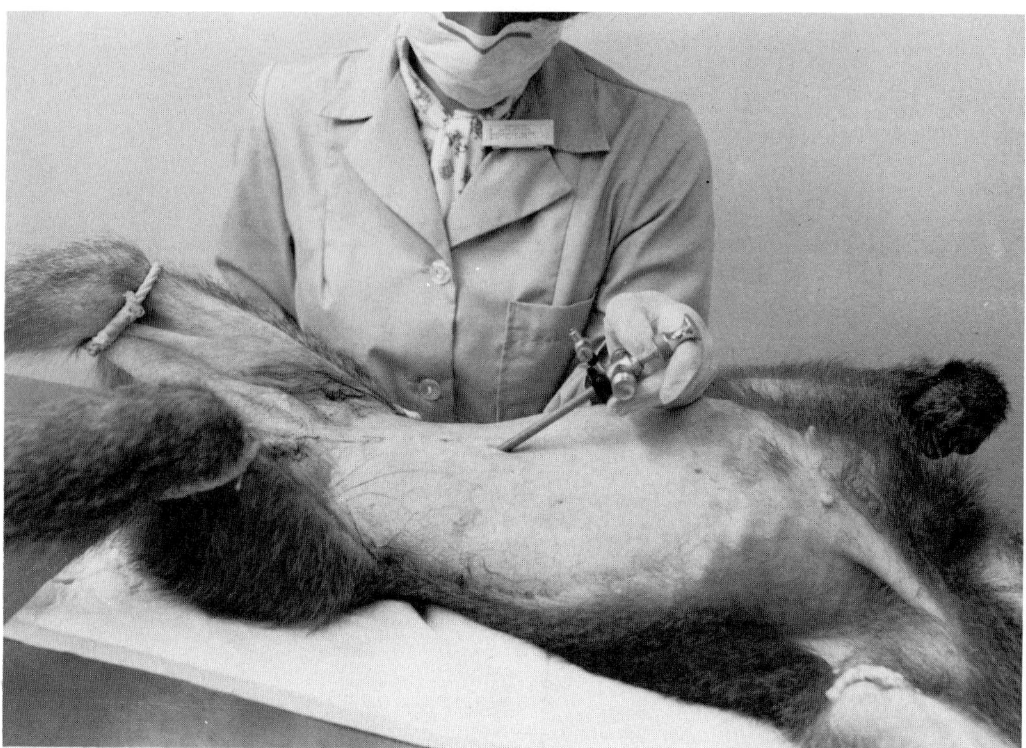

**Figure 4.4**  Cannula-trocar inserted through a 1 cm midline incision in a female baboon. The instrument was inserted at approximately a 45° angle to the table top.

the flexible light cable and the room darkened so that the abdominal wall can be transilluminated. Transillumination allows the laparoscopist to identify and avoid vasculature of the abdominal wall during the insertion of the Verres needle probe or accessory cannula. The inferior epigastric vessels are large in some species and must be avoided. The Verres needle is then reinserted in the lower right abdominal quadrant (left side if the laparoscopist is left handed) through an avascular area (Fig. 4.6). Generally, no problems are encountered from this secondary puncture. The Verres needle can be used as a manipulatory device and as a means for estimating sizes of structures visualized. The Verres needle used by the author has a diameter of 2 mm; the obturator tip is 1.5 mm in diameter; 5 mm of the tip extends beyond the cannula portion on the vent side; and the vent is 2 mm long. Knowing these dimensions, the operator is usually able to estimate sizes of internal structures. By placing the tip of the Verres needle next to a follicle, for example, one can rapidly estimate diameter and prominence of the follicle. Care must be taken that the Verres needle tip and structure measured are equidistant from the laparoscope, since magnification is considerable when the distance is reduced.

### Laparoscopic Observation of Abdominal Organs

The view through the laparoscope provides an entirely new perspective of the abdominal cavity contents. The laparoscope appears to put the observer's eye at the distal end of the instrument and not in the classic surgical overview position. Initially, the intestines and fatty tissues are generally observed. The Verres needle is used to maneuver these tissues cranially, away from the pelvis, to facilitate visualization of the

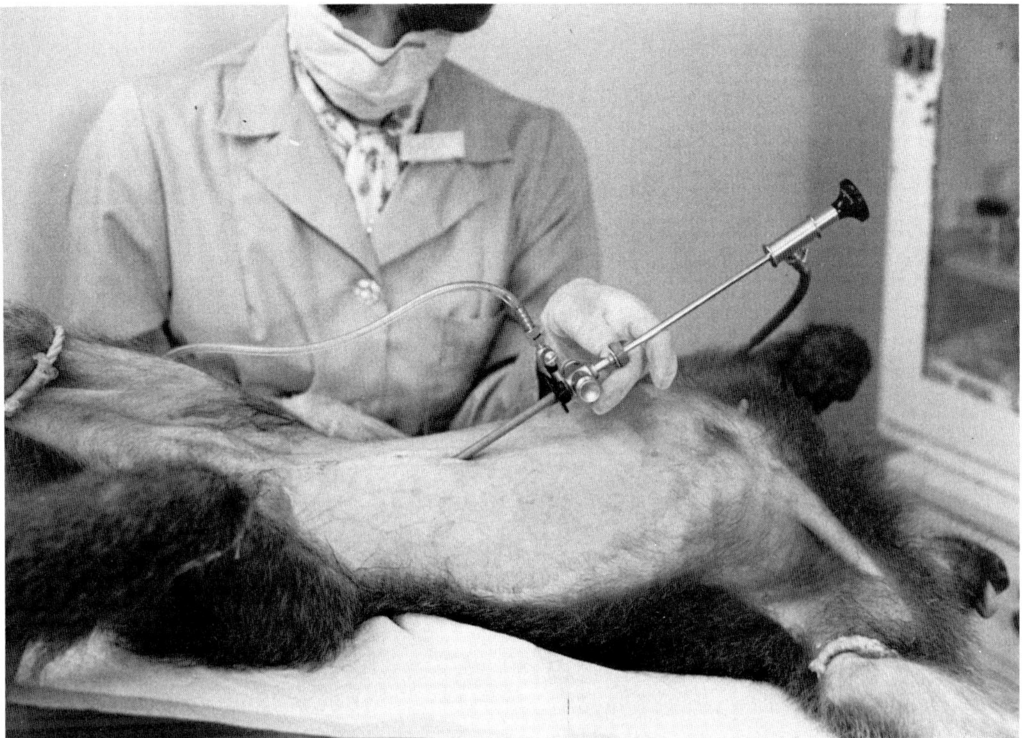

**Figure 4.5**   Trocar replaced by laparoscope with fiber optic cable attached; the tube from the $CO_2$-water trap has been attached to the cannula side arm.

reproductive organs. If the animal is in a steep Trendelenburg position these structures may already be located in this position and require no manipulation. In most subjects the bladder, uterus, and oviducts are readily identified. The ovaries frequently are caudal and dorsal to the oviducts but are easily manipulated into view using the Verres needle. The ovaries in baboons are easily rotated so all surfaces are viewed; the patas monkey's ovaries have a larger area of attachment to the mesovarium and are more difficult for the novice laparoscopist to visualize compared to those of *Papio, Macaca,* and *Saimiri.*

The bladder may be distended sufficiently with urine to obscure vision of the uterus and ovaries. If this occurs, we routinely remove the urine via a suprapubic puncture using a 50 $cm^3$ syringe and 20 gauge 38 mm (1 ½ inch) B bevel needle. The needle is attached to the syringe and inserted in a vertical position through the ventral midline 1 cm from the symphysis pubis (Fig. 4.7). (This area should be surgically prepared prior to insertion.) The needle can usually be visualized internally using the laparoscope and guided into and through the bladder wall, taking care to avoid large vessels. The syringe plunger is then withdrawn and urine aspirated. If more than 50 $cm^3$ of urine is removed, the syringe is disconnected and emptied. The needle remains *in situ* until sufficient urine has been removed to facilitate viewing. Baboons and patas monkeys frequently require the aspiration of 100 to 150 $cm^3$ of urine. (Since this urine is sterile it is suitable for various tests in clinical situations.) We find this technique to be easier and more rapid than urethral catheterization. However, either procedure is suitable; the method of choice should depend on the expertise of the investigator.

The laparoscopist should learn to recognize normal and pathologic changes in the pelvic organs. Blanched areas may appear on the nonpregnant uterus (*Color Atlas,* Pl.

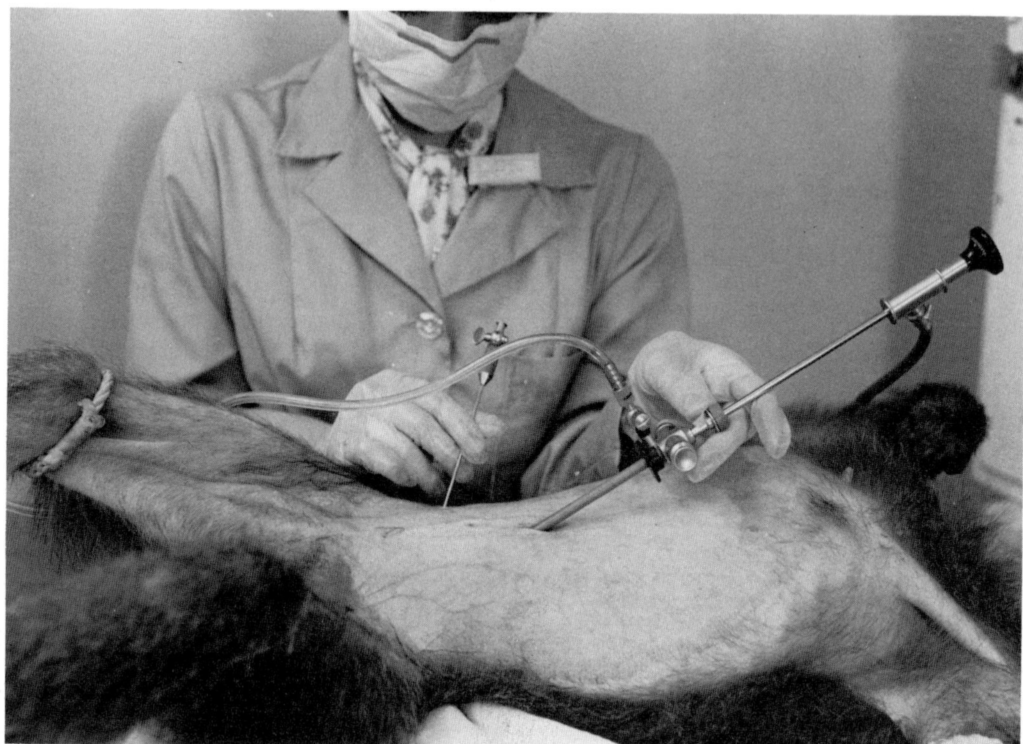

**Figure 4.6**   Verres needle inserted in lower right abdominal quadrant following transillumination of ventral abdominal wall to select an avascular area.

3, Fig. 3); ovaries may appear as pale pink featureless oval structures (Pl. 3, Fig. 4) or with numerous dark luteal scars (Pl. 3, Fig. 5). As ovulation approaches follicles initially appear as translucent areas of generalized swelling, then later may become fluid-filled in appearance with surface vascularization (Pl. 3, Fig. 6). Immediately before ovulation the follicle may become cloudy and appear to contain intrafollicular hemorrhage. The follicle at this time usually is more spherical (Pl. 3, Fig. 7) than soon after ovulation, when it usually appears less rounded and hemorrhagic (Pl. 3, Fig. 8), and becomes pale red as luteinization occurs (Pl. 4, Fig. 1). In most monkeys, by five to seven days after ovulation the follicle appears as a cratered orange colored structure (Pl. 4, Fig. 2). By six weeks the corpus luteum in the nonpregnant monkey has regressed and appears only as a pale yellow scar (Pl. 4, Fig. 3). Plate 4, Figure 4 illustrates how the Verres needle supporting the ovary provides a means to estimate size of the follicle; the needle is 2 mm in diameter.

Sequential changes in the follicle vary between animals, species, and individual cycles. In some animals extensive luteinization occurs rapidly, in others the corpus remains hemorrhagic for several days. Initially, luteinization usually appears as orange colored tissue around the base of the follicle; within two to three days the entire follicle appears orange to yellow in coloration. As the corpus luteum ages it will sequentially become more yellow, pale to a yellow-white, and eventually turn to a white structure, the corpus albicans. The period of time postovulation in which an identifiable structure can be laparoscopically detected is extremely variable, but usually exceeds 10 weeks.

Uterine appearance is related to the stage of the reproductive cycle. Uterine tissue is more vascular in the luteal (postovulation) stage and if touched with the Verres needle appears flaccid. The gravid uterus is quite hyperemic and extreme caution should be

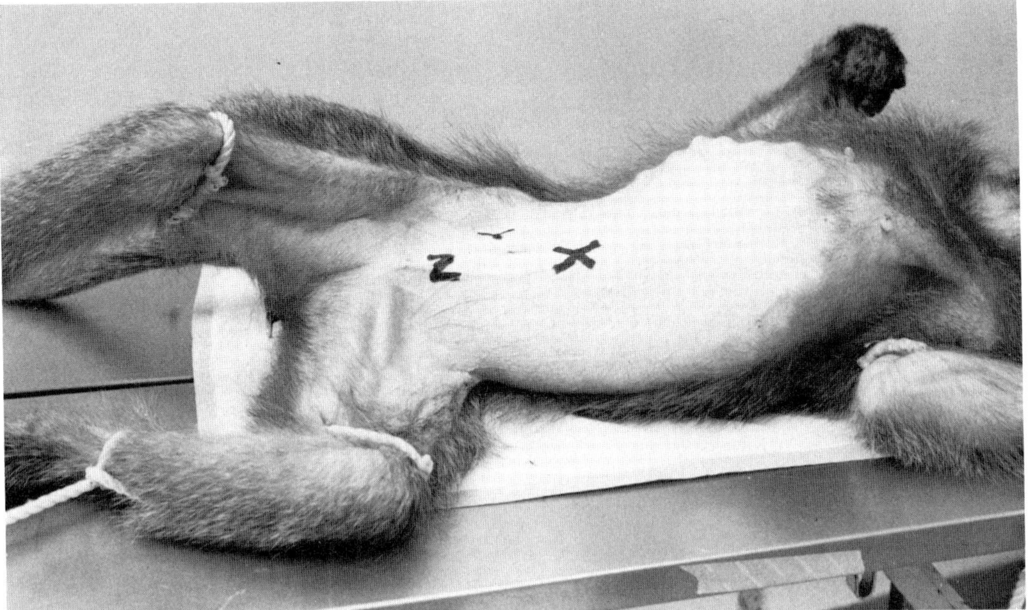


**Figure 4.7** Baboon with abdominal area clipped prior to surgical scrub. Note sites marked: X, area for midline incision for primary insertion; Y, area for insertion of secondary cannula or Verres needle used as an ancillary probe; Z, midline area 1 cm cranial to symphysis pubis where suprapubic puncture is performed to aspirate urine from the bladder, if necessary.

exercised to avoid inducing uterine hemorrhage when examining a pregnant animal. The oviducts are pale pink tubes and the fimbriae usually appear as pink lacy structures. Cysts on the ovaries and oviducts should be noted, if present, as well as any adhesions that may be attached to these organs. The bladder is usually bluish in color with prominent vessels and the intestines are greyish white. Fatty tissue in the omentum and around the reproductive organs is yellow and in an obese monkey makes it difficult to locate the reproductive organs. Increasing the degree of table tilt to allow greater shift of internal tissues may assist in the laparoscopic examination of such animals.

The experienced laparoscopist is able to judge reproductive cyclicity, including time of ovulation, with some reliability, by serial observations of the ovaries. Vascular patterns on the peritoneal surface of the uterus can assist in detecting the location of the placenta, and, in some monkeys, morphologic changes in the uterus can be used to detect pregnancy as early as 16 to 20 days postmating. Laparoscopy in combination with a smaller endoscope, such as the Needlescope[R] (Dyonics, Inc.) has been used in our laboratory for the examination of the conceptus *in utero* (fetoscopy) during the first two-thirds of pregnancy. Basically the procedure involves laparoscopic visualization of the ventral surface of the uterus, insertion of the small trocar-cannula through the abdominal wall, and then under laparoscopic guidance, through the uterine wall. Caution to avoid vessels on the uterine surface must be exercised. The trocar is removed and the small endoscope inserted. Visualization is not as satisfactory as with the larger laparoscope, but is adequate for fetal sexing, subcutaneous injections, and obtaining fetal tissue and blood. The procedure has a higher morbidity rate than most other laparoscopic procedures. Amnionic fluid loss from the puncture site appears to be minimal.

Examination of the organs located in the upper (cranial) half of the abdominal cavity can be made through the same midline infraumbilical puncture site as previously described. The author inserts the trocar-cannula directed caudally towards the pelvis, replaces the trocar with the laparoscope, and then rotates the instrument laterally until the laparoscope is pointed cranially toward the upper abdomen. If a table is used that can be tilted side to side as well as end to end, the animal being examined can be positioned so that the investigator can see the diaphragm, greater curvature of the stomach, portions of the spleen and left kidney (Pl. 4, Fig. 5), liver, gallbladder (Pl. 4, Fig. 6), the intestines, urinary bladder, uterus, oviducts, ovaries, and anterior peritoneal wall. The seminal vesicles and abdominal portions of the spermatic cords (vas deferens and testicular vessels) can be observed in males. The laparoscope can be used to assist the veterinarian in the diagnosis of diseases involving the organs of the pelvic and abdominal cavities.

Biopsy of various organs can be performed under laparoscopic guidance and intraabdominal hemorrhage suppressed by laparoscopic electrocoagulation. The author has had limited experience in these areas and recommends the discussion provided by Dr. Wildt in Chapter 3.

### Laparoscopic Photography

In most monkeys the bladder, uterus, oviducts, and ovaries can be observed in a single field of vision (Pl. 3, Fig. 3). As the laparoscope is moved closer, the total area visualized is reduced but the target tissue viewed is magnified. For example, at extreme closeness a follicle 5 mm in diameter will fill the field of vision. In trying to document the observations by photography the laparoscopist will learn that his eye can accommodate to low level light much better than the camera. The beginner at laparoscopic photography can expect to waste some film before learning to judge the most suitable light and distance required for good photographs. The best results have been achieved in our laboratory using high speed color film (ASA 400 for slides and for prints) with a shutter speed of ⅛ to 1/30 second. At the slower shutter speeds the breathing movements of the animal must be considered, since movement during photographic exposure will cause blurring. A written record should be maintained on each photograph taken, including structure photographed, shutter speed, and film type used. If a projection unit is used that does not have a high intensity bulb for photography (1000 watts) one can still obtain high quality photographs in small primate species. Using 150 watts of projected light, a 5 mm laparoscope, and film of the speed mentioned above, the author has obtained excellent photographs of the ovarian morphology in squirrel monkeys (Harrison and Dukelow, 1974). An interesting study was also undertaken to determine if infrared film could provide a means to detect minute details in ovarian follicular morphology (Jewett and Dukelow, 1972c). The technique did appear to provide greater clarity but additional efforts have not been reported.

### Termination of Examination and Postoperative Care

At the end of the examination the Verres needle is removed first to allow the puncture site to be laparoscopically examined on the innerperitoneal side. The telescope is then slowly removed and the valve of the cannula left open so that the insufflated gas can be evacuated. The cannula is also removed slowly from the abdominal cavity to avoid extracting omentum through the puncture site. The latter rarely occurs and omentum can be easily returned into the abdomen by gentle probing with the Verres needle or a similar blunted instrument.

We routinely close the midline incision with 3-0 chromic suture on an atraumatic cutting edge ¾ circle needle. Usually one suture is placed in the peritoneum-muscle layer and then nitrofurazone (Eaton Veterinary Laboratories) is sprinkled into the site.

Skin closure is accomplished with one to three interrupted stitches and the entire sutured area is covered with Furacin ointment (Eaton Veterinary Laboratories). The lateral secondary puncture wound of the Verres needle is routinely not closed but is covered with ointment. In the event that the animal is pregnant, one skin suture is inserted in the secondary site primarily as a precautionary measure. No prophylactic antibiotic injections are administered unless indicated by some clinical diagnosis or ancillary procedure. Using these postoperative techniques only two monkeys have developed minor staphylococcal wound infections in over 1000 laparoscopic procedures. Only one monkey required antibiotic treatment (three injections of 150,000 units of Flo-Cillin, Bristol Laboratories, at 48 hour intervals).

## Modification of Techniques for Use in Large and Small Primates

If the nonhuman primates to be examined are not of the size described above (3 to 15 kg) some modifications in laparoscopy procedure are recommended.

### SMALL PRIMATE LAPAROSCOPY

Small primates, such as adult squirrel monkeys or marmosets, or infant macaques in the 500 gm to 2 kg body weight range, can be laparoscopically examined with no technical problems.

Anesthesia can be induced using sodium pentobarbitol (Nembutal, Abbot Laboratories, 10 mg/kg) injected intraperitoneally. Surgical preparation is as described above but the examination may be facilitated by using a restraint table of the adjustable stage type placed on a suitable counter or table (Dukelow and Ariga, 1976) (Fig. 4.8); (Dierschke and Clark, 1976) (Figs. 4.9 and 4.10). In the larger animals, insufflation through a Verres needle precedes the insertion of the trocar-cannula. But the distance between the anterior abdominal wall and the underlying organs in these insufflated animals is 4 to 5 cm, a sufficient distance to prevent organ damage due to trocar puncture. In a smaller monkey, such as a 600 gm squirrel monkey, even after insufflation the organs are only 1 to 2 cm below the muscle layer and the possibility of organ perforation is increased. In these smaller animals it is best to incline the animal's body head down on the table tilted at a 30 to 45° angle prior to any insertion. The skin and muscle layer are then lifted, either manually or with towel clips, and the trocar-cannula inserted through the incision, under the skin, and then dorsally through the abdominal wall. A pneumoperitoneum is then produced through the midline cannula, the laparoscope is inserted, and the procedure continues as described above. With this insertion technique one or two sutures in the skin layer are usually sufficient for incision repair since there is nonalignment of puncture sites through the skin, muscle, and peritoneum.

### LAPAROSCOPY IN APES

The technique of laparoscopy in chimpanzees, as described by Graham (1976), is similar to that described earlier for large monkeys, with certain more elaborate alterations in technique. Some of these modifications are necessary in these more expensive and valuable primates to provide minimal risk to the animal. Preanesthesia is induced with ketamine hydrochloride (10 to 20 mg/kg, i.m.) and concomitant atropine (atropine sulfate, W. A. Butler, 0.4 mg, i.m.). An endotracheal tube is passed and inhalation anesthesia maintained with 1 to 2% halothane, 60% nitrous oxide and 40% oxygen. The abdomen, vagina, and perineum are cleansed and a urethral catheter is used to empty the bladder. An intravenous drip of lactated Ringer's solution is administered throughout the procedure. The chimpanzee is positioned on the table so that the rump is even with the end of the table. A cervical cuff (Fig. 4.11) is inserted and, if necessary, held by

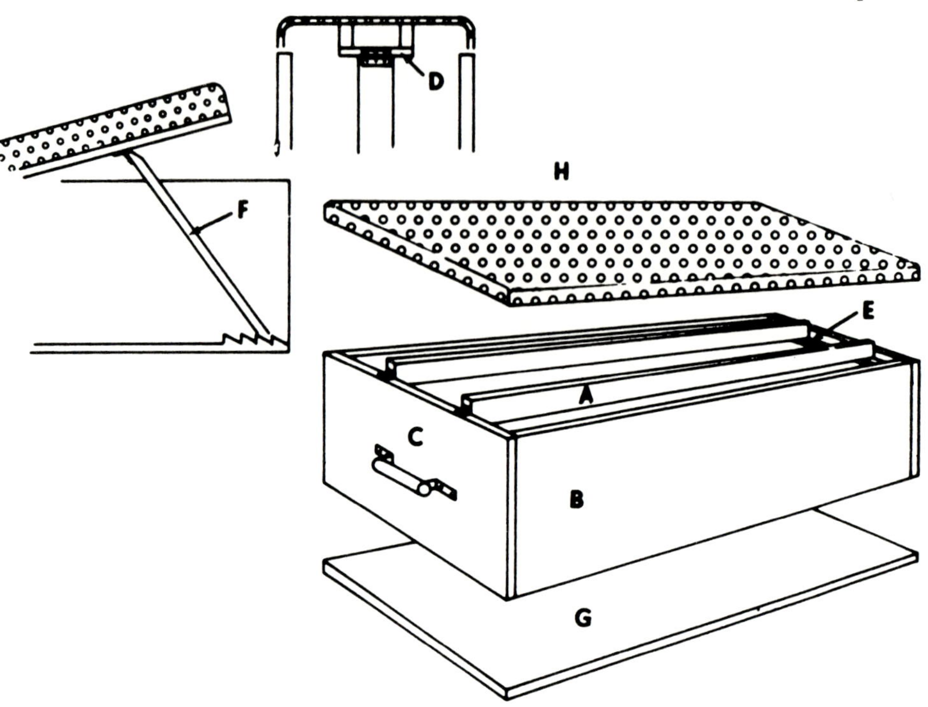



**Figure 4.8**  Variable angle laparoscopy stage. Identification of pieces, their quantity ( ), and size in cm: **A**, (2), 66.9 × 4.1 × 8.9; **B**, (2), 66.9 × 23.8 × 1.6; **C**, (2), 33.0 × 23.8 × 1.6; **D**, (1), 67.3 × 24.1 × 1.6; **E**, (1), 25.4 × 1.6 × 2.5; **F**, (1), 38.1 × 12.7 × 1.6; **G**, (1), 36.2 × 72.4 × 0.6; **H**, (1), perforated stainless steel shaped to fit. **H** is screwed to **A**'s which are hinged to frontpiece **C** and rest on brace **E**. **D** is attached to lower side of **A**'s about 17 cm from free ends. **F** is hinged to **D** and by bracing it in various positions controls tilt of stage. Stage can be placed on surgical table, counter top, etc. (Reproduced with permission from W. R. Dukelow and S. Ariga, *Journal of Medical Primatology* 5:82–99, 1976.)

slight suction. The cervical cuff can be moved during the examination to aid the laparoscopist in locating the uterus. The patient is draped and a sterile field maintained. Instruments are sterilized by gas or wet sterilization. The table is tilted so that the animal is in a steep Trendelenburg position prior to any surgical intervention. Insufflation is accomplished using the Verres needle inserted through the infraumbilical incision. Because of the greater field of view, a 10 mm in diameter laparoscope is usually used in these larger animals but the smaller 5 mm and 8 mm instruments will also provide adequate visualization. Inexplicably, adhesion formation (usually bowel to peritoneum) is not uncommon even in chimpanzees unoperated on previously; such adhesions may cause viewing problems. Compared to smaller primates, the reproductive organs are not as easily identified and visualized in these larger sized species. Consequently, an ancillary grasping forceps inserted through a secondary cannula in the lower abdominal quadrant is usually required to assist in manipulating the organs. Postoperative treatment and care are similar to that described earlier.

### General Technical Considerations

Certain considerations must be made by the operator using laparoscopic techniques in nonhuman primates. The size of the animals to be used and the planned frequency

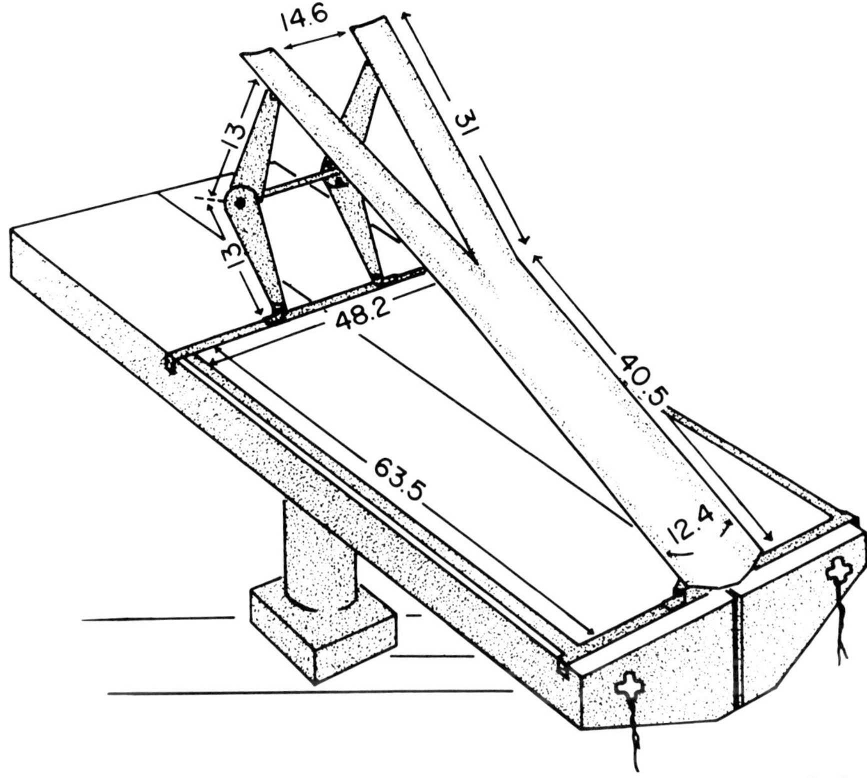



**Figure 4.9**  Diagram of tilt rack. All dimensions are in cm. It is constructed of stainless steel and brass and is usually mounted to a standard surgical table. The rear legs of the monkey are secured to the split ends of the rack and the front legs tied by ropes at the opposite end. (Reproduced with permission from D. J. Dierschke and J. R. Clark, *Journal of Medical Primatology* 5:100–110, 1976.)

of examinations should be considered prior to the purchase of a specific laparoscopic telescope. If the animals to be used are generally small (3 kg or less), or if repeated examinations are to be performed in a larger monkey, then the 5 mm in diameter laparoscope is the instrument of choice. If the subject is larger, 25 kg or more, or if laparoscopic examinations will be infrequently performed in individual animals, then an 8 or 10 mm laparoscope may be preferred. The larger instruments provide more light for photography, television, or video recording and are also available with operative channels for single puncture, ancillary procedures. If only a single laparoscope is to be purchased the author recommends the 5 mm instrument because of its overall versatility.

The direction of view through a laparoscope usually varies from 180° (straight ahead) to 160°, or 130° (see Chapter 2). In the author's experience the 180° instrument allows more rapid orientation for the novice laparoscopist. However, the 130° instrument has an extended tip that can assist the lens from being obscured or contaminated by body tissue. Regardless of instrument type the operator may discover the view obscured due to lens fogging. There are three basic causes of fogging other than instrument failure due to damage: (1) tissue has contaminated the distal lens; (2) temperature difference between the laparoscope tip and the abdominal cavity; and (3) eyepiece fogging due to the operator's breath on the eyepiece. This last problem is especially common if the examiner is wearing a surgical mask which directs exhalatory air towards the eyes. In the first and last instances the problem is solved by wiping the fogged lens with a sterile gauze. The temperature problem can be prevented by placing the instrument in warm sterile water prior to insertion.

Some technical aspects of laparoscopy vary between investigators and even between primate species. Although some laparoscopists prefer a steep Trendelenburg position, ~45°, others prefer the subject tilted only slightly, 10 to 15°. The steep position may induce respiratory problems if the procedure is prolonged, and especially if 100% $CO_2$ is used for insufflation. (Pressure on the diaphragm decreases respiratory effectiveness and large quantities of absorbed $CO_2$ can induce hyperventilation.) Under such circumstances vital signs should be monitored. One may also consider the advantages of an automatic insufflation unit. This equipment is quite valuable in clinical situations in which a sterile field must be maintained. Conversely, a standard $CO_2$ tank with regulator, connected to a flask containing water, is more economical and works satisfactorily when an assistant is present to release $CO_2$ as needed.

The degree of sterility maintained during a laparoscopic examination and the use of prophylactic antibiotics also varies with the individual laparoscopist. If only a single set of instruments is available and multiple daily examinations are performed, gas sterili-

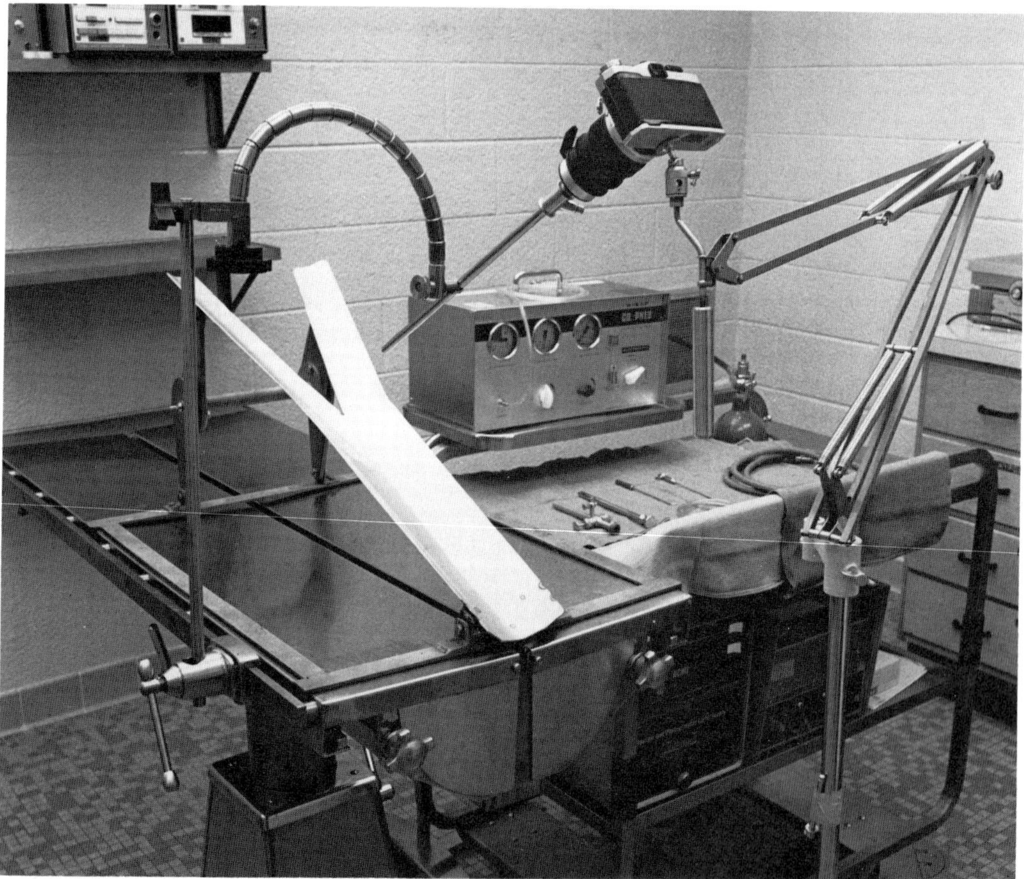

**Figure 4.10** Equipment for laparoscopy in monkeys. Tilt rack is attached to a standard surgical table, camera and telescope held by Siegler flexbar holder/positioner, automatic insufflator and cart in background. (Reproduced with permission of D. J. Dierschke and J. R. Clark, *Journal of Medical Primatology* 5:100–110, 1976.)

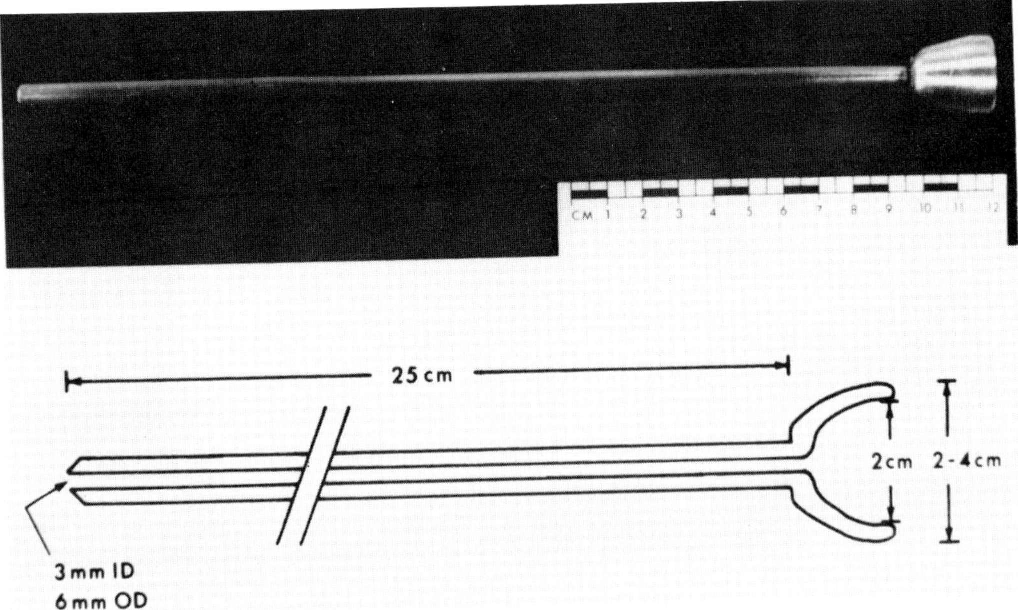


**Figure 4.11** Cervical cuff, showing details of construction. Cuff is made of stainless steel and fits over the ectocervix; it is rarely necessary to retain it by suction. (Reproduced with permission from C. E. Graham, *Journal of Medical Primatology* 5:111–123, 1976.)

zation is not feasible and antibiotics may be considered as an important supplement to liquid instrument sterilization. Certain species of primates may be quite expensive or the research design may dictate prolonged use. In such cases more precaution and emphasis on elaborate sterile techniques are required. In a clinical, nonhuman primate veterinary practice, or when the examination is performed in a rare or endangered species, then sterile surgical conditions are recommended for laparoscopy. An assistant is essential when the procedure is to be performed under sterile conditions or when the animal being examined is suspected of having an infectious condition. The assistant makes the connections to the light and gas sources so that the laparoscopist is not contaminated by these areas.

Most laparoscopists find it convenient to have a mobile cart containing the instrumentarium. The cart requires a restraint appparatus for the compressed gas tank and a space for the light source, instrument sterilization pan, and miscellaneous supplies (i.e., drugs, gloves, syringes, etc.). A standard laboratory cart with an opening cut in the top shelf, of sufficient size to pass a size "C" gas tank, serves quite well. A collar welded to the second shelf below the opening supports the tank. A heavy duty light projector, because of its size and weight, should be placed on the bottom shelf (Fig. 4.12). Specialized endoscopy carts are commercially available (See Chapter 12).

When recording observations the operator should be consistent in using descriptive terminology of the internal organs. Terms such as blanched, red, anterior, lower, etc., have subjective meanings. For example, an ovary may be "under," "behind," "below," or "posterior" to the bladder and be in the same location in all four instances. Use of terms such as ventral-dorsal, medial-lateral, anterior-posterior as medically defined should be adhered to as much as possible. Even then, professionals in the veterinary medical field do not define terms in the same manner as those in the human medical field. Physicians refer to upper and anterior abdominal surfaces, whereas veterinarians refer to the same as cranial and ventral surfaces.

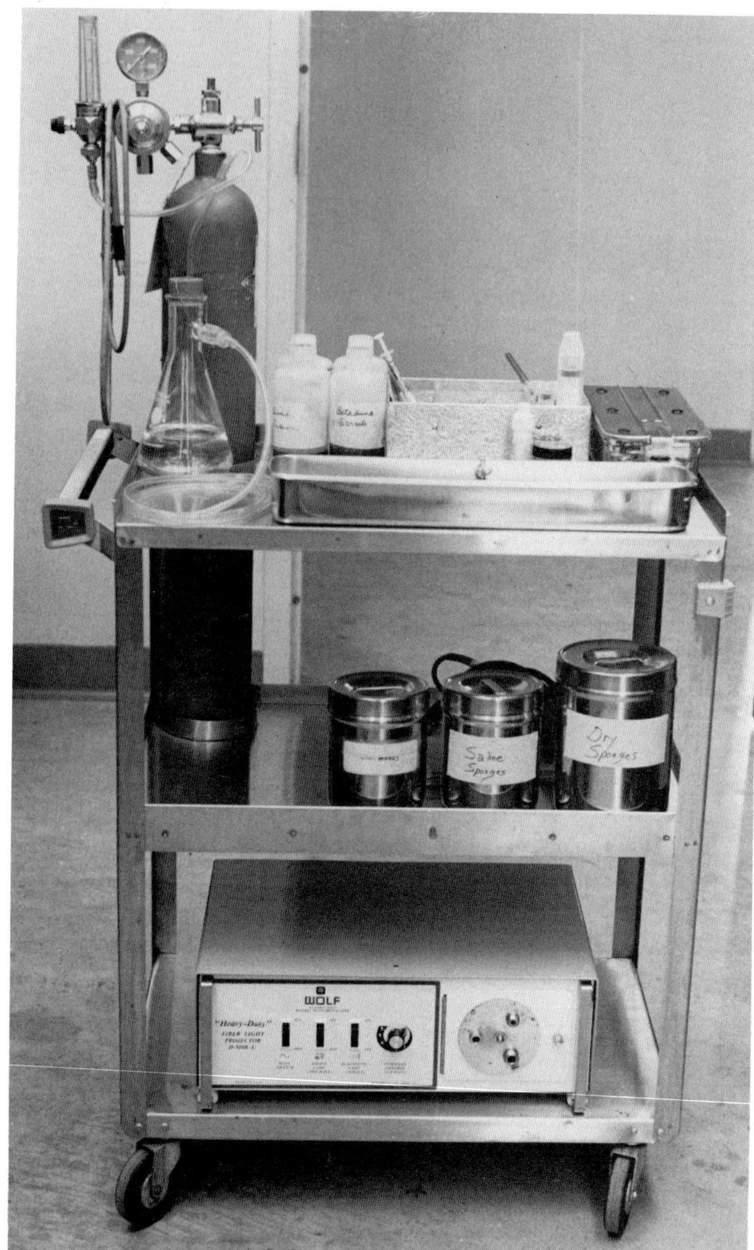

**Figure 4.12**  Standard laboratory cart modified for use as a laparoscopy cart. Upper shelf holds instrument trays for soaking laparoscope, cannula, trocar, Verres needles and other ancillary instruments; squeeze bottles with disinfectant solutions; tray with sutures, needles, tubes, and antibiotic preparations; and water trap connected to $CO_2$ tank. Second shelf usually contains boxes with surgical gloves, masks, clippers, and containers with alcohol, saline, and dry sponges.

The ovary is not fixed in place *in situ* and the laparoscopist must manipulate it to a standard orientation so that medial edges are not considered to be anterior or lateral at a different examination. In describing the location of structures on the ovaries it is usually advisable to note relationships to other structures, such as luteal scars, vessels, etc. Some organs (i.e., liver, small intestines) have specific nomenclature for various anatomical regions which should be used when recording observations. The novice laparoscopist may find it difficult to identify such areas initially even if familiar with abdominal anatomy from the surgeon's standard viewpoint. Colors are difficult to describe and may appear to change if the light source is altered. For example, yellow and pink colors fade when the photographic 1000 watt lamp is used compared to the diagnostic 150 watt lamp.

The ancillary procedures available to the laparoscopist depend on his dexterity, experience, and the type of accessory laparoscopic equipment available. Some reported procedures in monkeys include follicular aspiration and intrafollicular injection (Dukelow and Ariga, 1976; Rawson and Dukelow, 1978), topical application of compounds to the surface of the ovary (Rawson, 1975), uterine flushing (Ariga and Dukelow, 1977a), oviductal deposition of ova or solutions (Dukelow and Ariga, 1976), and lysis of adhesions (Graham, 1976). (See Chapter 5 for details of these procedures.) Procedures that are routinely performed in humans and can be adapted for use in nonhuman primates include tubal occlusion with clips (Hulka and Omran, 1972), tubal ligation with suture (Clarke, 1972), and aspiration of fluid from the cul-de-sac, ovarian cysts and hydrosalpinges (Siegler and Garret, 1970).

The organs that can be visualized and the extent to which they can be examined will depend on species, animal, size, amount of internal fat, previous surgical procedures, and the dexterity of the laparoscopist. The laparoscopic procedures are relatively atraumatic to the subjects; more than 20 examinations in individual patas monkeys during a two year period have not affected their reproductive efficiency. Some baboons were examined daily for five days and as frequently as 10 times in a 32 day cycle with no changes in cyclic parameters.

Only two deaths in approximately 1000 laparoscopic examinations have been in any way associated with the procedure. Both deaths occurred in baboons; one was due to an anesthesia reaction prior to the examination; the second was caused by massive hemorrhage when the inferior vena cava was cut by a pyramidal trocar. The second accident occurred while the laparoscopist was instructing a technician in the technique and was due to failure of the beginner to recognize that the trocar had completely entered the abdominal cavity. The only contraindication to primate laparoscopy, as discovered by the author, is prior abdominal surgery. Extensive lymph node dissections and splenectomies in patas monkey females, as part of other research projects, have resulted in the formation of large vascular adhesions that make it impossible to laparoscopically visualize the abdominal organs in these monkeys.

Laparoscopy is a valuable tool for both research and diagnostic purposes. Its usefulness in veterinary medicine involving nonhuman primates will certainly be further explored in the future.


### References

Ariga, S., and Dukelow, W. R. (1977a) Nonsurgical (laparoscopic) uterine flushing and egg recovery technique in the squirrel monkey (*Saimiri sciureus*). *Primates* 18:452–457.

Ariga, S., and Dukelow, W. R. (1977b) Recovery of preimplantation blastocysts in the squirrel monkey by a laparoscopic technique. *Fertil. Steril.* 28:577–580.

Balin, H., Wan, L. S., and Israel, S. L. (1966) Recent advances in pelvic endoscopy. *Obstet. Gynecol.* 27:30–43.

Balin, H., and Wan, L. S. (1969) A study of induction of ovulation in *Macaca mulatta*. *J. Reprod. Med.* 2:273–284.

Batta, S. K., and Brackett, B. G. (1974) Ovulation induction in rhesus monkey by treatment with gonadotropins and prostaglandins. *Prostaglandins* 6:45–54.

Blakley, G. A., Blaine, C. R., and Morton, W. R. (1977) Correlation of perineal detumescence and ovulation in the pigtail macaque. (*Macaca nemestrina*). *Lab. Anim. Sci.* 27:352–355.

Bosu, W. T. K. (1973) Laparoscopic technique for the examination of the ovaries in the rhesus monkey. *J. Med. Primatol.* 2:124–129.

Bosu, W. T. K., Johansson, E. D. B., and Gemzell, C. (1973) Ovarian steroid patterns in peripheral plasma during the menstrual cycle in the rhesus monkey. *Folia Primatol.* 19:218–234.

Bosu, W. T. K., and Johansson, E. D. B. (1974) Effects

of postovulatory norethindrone and estrogens on the plasma levels of estrogen and progesterone in rhesus monkeys. *Contraception* 9:357–367.

Clark, J. R., Dierschke, D. J., and Wolf, R. C. (1978) Hormonal regulation of ovarian folliculogenesis in rhesus monkeys: 1. Concentration of serum luteinizing hormone and progesterone during laparoscopy and patterns of follicular development during successive menstrual cycles. *Biol. Reprod.* 17:779–783.

Clarke, H. C. (1972) Laparoscopy—new instruments for suturing and ligation. *Fertil. Steril.* 23:274–277.

Dierschke, D. J., and Clark, J. R. (1976) Laparoscopy in *Macaca mulatta*: Specialized equipment employed and initial observations. *J. Med. Primatol.* 5:100–110.

Dukelow, W. R. (1975) The morphology of follicular development and ovulation in nonhuman primates. *J. Reprod. Fertil.* (Suppl.) 22:23–51.

Dukelow, W. R. (1977) Ovulatory cycle characteristics in *Macaca fascicularis. J. Med. Primatol.* 6:33–42.

Dukelow, W. R., and Ariga, S. (1976) Laparoscopic technique for biomedical research. *J. Med. Primatol.* 5:82–99.

Dukelow, W. R., Harrison, R. M., Jewett, D. A., and Johnson, M. P. (1971a) Follicular morphology and ovulation induction in the nonhuman primate. In: *Fertility and Sterility, Proceeding of the 7th World Congress Oct. 17–25, 1971.* T. Hasegawa, ed., Excerpta Medica, Amsterdam, pp. 593–595.

Dukelow, W. R., Jarosz, S. J., Jewett, D. A., and Harrison, R. M. (1971b) Laparoscopic examination of ovaries in goats and primates. *Lab. Anim. Sci.* 21:594–597.

Dukelow, W. R., Harrison, R. M., Rawson, J. M. R., and Johnson, M. P. (1972) Natural and artificial control of ovulation in nonhuman primates. In: *Medical Primatology, 1972, Part 1.* E. I. Goldsmith and J. Moor-Jankowski, eds., Karger, Basel, pp. 232–236.

Eddy, C. A., Turner, T., Kraemer, D. C., and Pauerstein, C. J. (1976) Pattern and duration of ovum transport in the baboon. *Obstet. Gynecol.* 47:658–664.

Graham, C. E. (1976) Technique of laparoscopy in the chimpanzee. *J. Med. Primatol.* 5:111–123.

Graham, C. E., Keeling, M., Chapman, C., Cummins, L. B., and Haynie, J. (1973) Method of endoscopy in the chimpanzee: Relations of ovarian anatomy, endometrial histology and sexual swelling. *Am. J. Phys. Anthropol.* 38:211–216.

Harrison, R. M., and Dukelow, W. R. (1971) Megestrol acetate: Its effect on the inhibition of ovulation in squirrel monkeys. *J. Reprod. Fertil.* 25:99–101.

Harrison, R. M., and Dukelow, W. R. (1973) Seasonal adaptation of laboratory maintained squirrel monkeys. *J. Med. Primatol.* 2:277–283.

Harrison, R. M., and Dukelow, W. R. (1974) Morpho-

logical changes in the *Saimiri sciureus* ovarian follicles as detected by laparoscopy. *Primates* 15:305–309.

Harrison, R. M., Rawson, J. M. R., and Dukelow, W. R. (1974) Megestrol acetate: II. Effects on ovulation in nonhuman primates as determined by laparoscopy. *Fertil. Steril.* 25:51–56.

Hulka, J. F., and Omran, K. F. (1972) Comparative tubal occlusion: Rigid and spring-loaded clips. *Fertil. Steril.* 23:633–639.

Jarosz, S. J., Kuehl, T. J., and Dukelow, W. R. (1977) Vaginal cytology, induced ovulation and gestation in the squirrel monkey (*Saimiri sciureus*). *Biol. Reprod.* 16:97–103.

Jewett, D. A., and Dukelow, W. R. (1971a) Follicular morphology in *Macaca fascicularis. Folia Primatol.* 16:216–220.

Jewett, D. A., and Dukelow, W. R. (1971b) Laparoscopy and precise mating techniques to determine gestation length in *Macaca fascicularis. Lab. Prim. Newsl.* 10:16–17.

Jewett, D. A., and Dukelow, W. R. (1972a) Serial observations of follicular morphology near ovulation in *Macaca fascicularis. J. Reprod. Fertil.* 31:287–290.

Jewett, D. A., and Dukelow, W. R. (1972b) Cyclicity and gestation length of *Macaca fascicularis. Primates* 13:327–330.

Jewett, D. A., and Dukelow, W. R. (1972c) Infrared photo-laparographic techniques for ovulation studies in primates. *J. Med. Primatol.* 7:223–227.

Jewett, D. A., and Dukelow, W. R. (1973) Follicular observation and laparoscopic aspiration techniques in *Macaca fascicularis. J. Med. Primatol.* 2:108–113.

Koninckx, P. R., Heyns, W. J., Corvelyn, P. A., and Brosens, I. A. (1978) Delayed onset of luteinization as a cause of infertility. *Fertil. Steril.* 29:266–269.

Kuehl, T. J., and Dukelow, W. R. (1975) Ovulation induction during the anovulatory season in *Saimiri sciureus. J. Med. Primatol.* 4:23–31.

Mahone, J. P., and Dukelow, W. R. (1978) Reproductive performance in *Macaca fascicularis* following repeated laparoscopy. *J. Med. Primatol.* 7:185–188.

Marik, J., and Hulka, J. (1978) Luteinized unruptured follicle syndrome: A subtle case of infertility. *Fertil. Steril.* 29:270–274.

Nigi, H. (1977) Laparoscopic observations of ovaries before and after ovulation in the Japanese monkey (*Macaca fuscata*). *Primates* 18:243–259.

Rawson, J. M. R. (1975) Physiological and biochemical parameters of gonadotropin-induced ovulation in the nonhuman primate. Ph.D. thesis, Michigan State University, East Lansing.

Rawson, J. M. R., and Dukelow, W. R. (1973a) Observation of ovulation in *Macaca fascicularis. J. Reprod. Fertil.* 34:187–190.

Rawson, J. M. R., and Dukelow, W. R. (1973b) Effect

of laparoscopy and anesthesia on ovulation, conception, gestation, and lactation in a *Macaca fascicularis*. *Lab. Prim. Newsl.* 12:4–5.

Rawson, J. M. R., and Dukelow, W. R. (1978) Effects of intrafollicular administration of gonadotropins in two species of nonhuman primates using laparoscopy. *J. Med. Primatol.* 7:223–227.

Siegler, A. M., and Garret, M. (1970) Ancillary techniques with laparoscopy. *Fertil. Steril.* 21:763–773.

White, R. J., Blaine, C. R., and Blakley, G. A. (1973) Detecting ovulation in *Macaca nemestrina* by correlation of vaginal cytology, body temperature, and perineal tumescence with laparoscopy. *Am. J. Phys. Anthropol.* 38:189–194.

Wildt, D. E., Doyle, L. L., Stone, S. C., and Harrison, R. M. (1977) Correlation of perineal swelling with serum ovarian hormone levels, vaginal cytology, and ovarian follicular development during the baboon reproductive cycle. *Primates* 18:261–270.

# CHAPTER 5

# Laparoscopy in Small Animals and Ancillary Techniques*

## W. Richard Dukelow, Ph.D.

## INTRODUCTION

The advantages of laparoscopy techniques over invasive surgical procedures (i.e., laparotomy) for observing the internal abdominal organs have been described by other authors in this volume. The advantages of having complete laparoscopic visualization of the abdominal cavity for observational or diagnostic purposes are obvious. Yet, for all its simplicity, the ultimate application of laparoscopic techniques to research lies in its modification and adaptation to particular scientific procedures. The limits of such modifications exist only in the limitations of ingenuity and resourcefulness of the laparoscopist. Procedures thought to be impossible several years ago are now commonplace and new expertise and equipment are being developed at an ever expanding rate to accommodate the technology of modern science.

The present chapter examines laparoscopic application to rather standard research procedures in many biomedical fields, including repeated observations, recovery of body fluids, administration of compounds, and recovery of tissues. Since the author's expertise lies in the area of reproductive physiology, this field will be used as an exemplary mode, but the ingenious reader will readily see application to a variety of physiological fields.

Similarly, it is necessary to select particular research models for demonstration and, in this chapter, these represent the species most extensively studied in the author's laboratory. Brief reference will be made to efforts conducted in some of the more common laboratory animals in which no published reports have been made concerning the use of laparascopy for clinical or research purposes. Again, the reader is reminded

* The techniques described in this chapter have been utilized in the author's laboratory during the past ten years and are the result of original studies by a large number of individuals whose ability and friendship are cherished by the author. For these pioneering efforts special appreciation is expressed to Drs. R. M. Harrison, D. A. Jewett, D. E. Wildt, J. M. R. Rawson, T. J. Kuehl, C. B. Morcom, J. P. Mahone, S. Fujimoto, S. J. Jarosz, and S. Ariga. Without their skills, the techniques reported here would not have been possible. Research partially reported in this chapter was supported by the National Foundation-March of Dimes and the National Institutes of Health.

that development of a single technique in one species is usually rather readily adapted to other species. The basic laparoscopic observational procedures used in the author's laboratory have been previously reported for primates (Dukelow et al., 1971; Jewett and Dukelow, 1973; Dukelow and Ariga, 1976; Dukelow, 1978), rabbit (Fujimoto et al., 1974), goats and sheep (Dukelow et al., 1971; Snyder and Dukelow, 1974), and swine (Wildt et al., 1973; Wildt et al., 1975).

## Instrumentation

A wide variety of suitable laparoscopic equipment is available from the several manufacturers in this field. The primary choice relates only to the size of the laparoscope relative to the size of the animal being examined. The choice of a 130, 160, or 180° laparoscope, pyramidal or conical pointed trocar, and the type of insufflation instrumentation is largely one of personal preference by the laparoscopist. In all of the work described in this paper the following equipment, manufactured by Richard Wolf GMBH (Knittlingen, West Germany) was used: 5 mm in diameter pediatric laparoscopic telescope; trocar sleeve with piston valve, 6 mm in diameter; Verres needle; manipulatory prove with centimeter markings (for use with large domestic animals); 5.5 mm in diameter fiber optic cable; and the 4000 model light generator (for standard laparoscopy) or the flash generator, proximal type (no. 5005) when photography was desired. Photography in our laboratory has involved 35 mm cameras (Exacta, Canon, and Olympus) fitted with the 95 mm adapter made by Richard Wolf Medical Instruments Corporation. The photographic procedures have been previously described (Dukelow et al., 1971).

## ANCILLARY PROCEDURES

### Laparoscopic Injection and Aspiration from the Follicle

The procedure for follicular aspiration in most species is identical to that used with laparotomy with the exception that the aspirating needle is passed through the skin and abdominal wall and guided to the ovary under laparoscopic visualization. In nonhuman primate species we have used a 25 gauge needle (⅝ inch long) passed through the skin and abdominal wall at a point 2 to 3 cm lateral and caudal to the laparoscopic entry point. With the bevel side down, the needle is then gently inserted into the follicle and a slight suction applied with a 1 ml tuberculin syringe. Normally about 0.1 ml of appropriate medium is contained in the syringe prior to aspiration. A more complex system for follicular aspiration, eliminating the need for aspiration into the medium, has been described by Jewett and Dukelow (1973), but the simple syringe aspiration procedure has been successfully used in a wide variety of primates, laboratory and domestic animals. Similar laparoscopic systems, employing catch reservoirs for recovery of human oocytes, have been described by Steptoe and Edwards (1970) and Morgenstern and Soupart (1972).

Certain experiments may necessitate the injection of various experimental substances into the follicle and traditionally this is performed using midventral laparotomy and injection with a microsyringe. This procedure can be adapted to laparoscopic procedures by the insertion of a 32 gauge needle through a 24 gauge needle-cannula inserted through the lower abdominal wall. The 32 gauge needle can be attached to a Micrometer syringe (Gilmont Instruments, Inc.) and, under laparoscopic visualization, the needle is inserted at the base of the follicle. Generally, only vesicular follicles (i.e., showing surface vascular patterns and antrum development) are used and caution must be exercised to avoid penetration of the vascular supply to the follicles. Injections can be made in 1 $\mu$l volumes without damage to the physical integrity of the follicle (Rawson and Dukelow, 1978). As with follicle aspiration, this technique can be adapted, by varying needle sizes, to many laboratory and domestic experimental animals.

## Laparoscopic Deposition of Substances into the Oviduct

Techniques have been developed in the squirrel monkey (*Saimiri sciureus*) for the laparoscopic deposition of test substances and fertilized ova directly into the ampullar region of the oviduct. Using this procedure (anesthesia: 16 mg sodium pentobarbital, injected intraperitoneally to 600 to 800 gm animals) the ovaries are first located laparoscopically utilizing an accessory manipulatory probe (generally a Verres needle) 2 to 3 cm lateral and caudal to the laparoscopic point of entry. The accessory probe is then withdrawn and replaced with a Hartman alligator forceps.

The forceps are then used to manipulate the fimbria so that the opening of the ampulla is visible through the laparoscope (Fig. 5.1). The substance (or embryos) to be deposited is contained in a volume of 1 to 3 $\mu$l within a micropipette (Micro/pettor A, Scientific Manufacturing Industries). The micropipette is inserted through an accessory

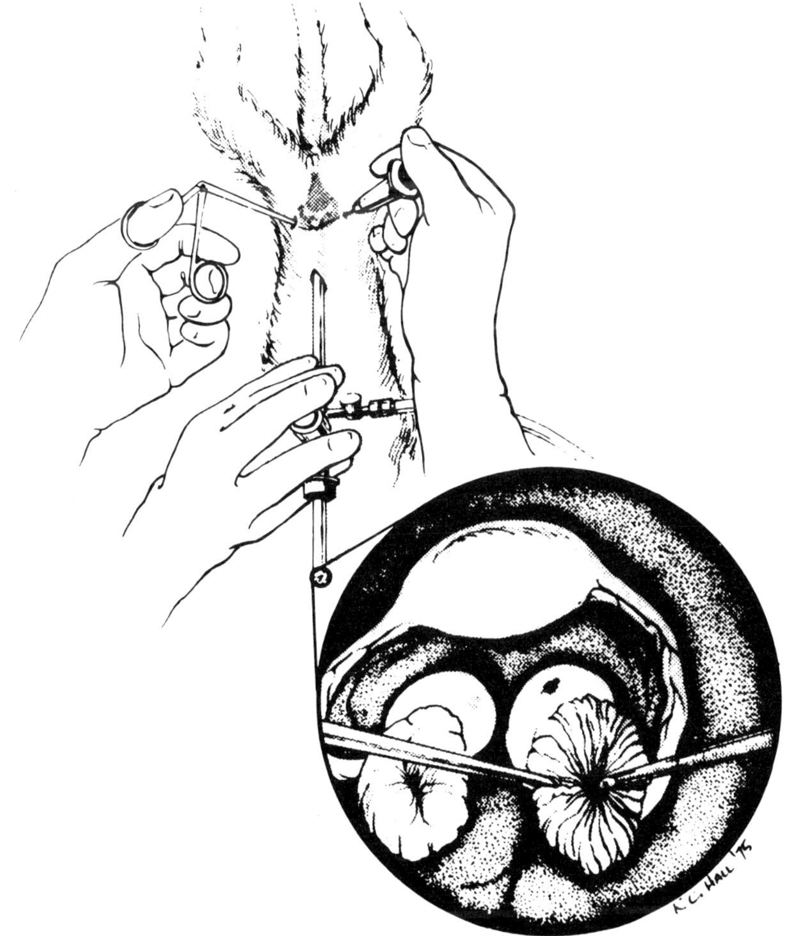

**Figure 5.1**  Diagrammatic representation of the technique for laparoscopic oviductal transfer in the squirrel monkey. (Reproduced wih permission from *Journal of Medical Primatology* 5:82–99, 1976.)

probe puncture site ipsilateral to the oviduct to be entered. Under laparoscopic visualization the micropipette is then inserted into the ampulla (steadied by the alligator forceps) and the plunger depressed. The micropipette must be withdrawn slowly to prevent reverse suction within the oviduct. Similarly, the plunger of the micropipette must remain depressed until the instrument has been withdrawn. When testing the efficacy of this transfer with a 0.05% solution of trypan blue dye, no leakage from the oviduct has been observed with 3 $\mu$l deposition or less, even when penetration of the oviduct was as little as 1 mm. With greater volumes (4 to 5 $\mu$l) leakage has been observed.

In larger animals similar procedures have been used. Efforts to reduce the volume of previously frozen semen required for artificial insemination in swine has resulted in some technical studies on oviductal insemination of semen using the laparoscope (Morcom and Dukelow, unpublished data). The basic laparoscopic procedure has been previously described for swine ovarian visualization (Wildt *et al.*, 1973). For the insemination procedure the bladder is catheterized to facilitate location and manipulation of the oviduct. Using the laparoscope the reproductive tract is identified and the laparoscopic grasping forceps are inserted and used to grasp the oviduct near the tubal-uterine junction. A 22 gauge, 3.5 inch spinal needle is then directed into the fimbrial end of the oviduct and 2 to 4 ml of extended semen is deposited. The procedure is then repeated with the opposite oviduct. This procedure obviously requires a great degree of laparoscopic skill. In preliminary studies our laboratory has achieved two pregnancies in seven attempts. Live offspring have been born following gestation of normal duration.

## Laparoscopic Recovery of Uterine Fluid and Blastocysts

Laparoscopic techniques have been employed in both swine and nonhuman primates to recover uterine fluid samples. In the case of swine (Wildt *et al.*, 1975), after visualization of the reproductive tract, an accessory trocar-cannula is inserted laterally from the midline through the abdominal wall. The trocar is then removed and laparoscopic grasping forceps are inserted. The uterine horn is grasped with the forceps and held in position while a 15 gauge needle, three inches long, is inserted through the skin and abdominal wall at a site anterior to the point of cannulation. After insertion of the needle through the wall of the uterine horn, polyethylene tubing (PE 90, Clay Adams Co.) with the terminal end sealed and small perforations along 4 cm of its length is inserted through the needle and into the uterine lumen (Fig. 5.2). The cannulation needle can then be withdrawn and the cannula left in the uterine horn. Sterile saline (6 to 10 ml) is then injected through the tubing and immediately aspirated. Recovery rates of aspirate are normally between 30 and 50%. Little or no bleeding occurs and no incidence of uterine infection has been observed.

In primates, uterine fluid (and blastocysts) can be recovered by flushing sterile saline through the uterus and collecting the fluid via a cervical catheter. This technique has been developed for use in the squirrel monkey and requires a preliminary ovulation induction regimen if ova or blastocysts are required. The induction regimen is illustrated in Figure 5.3. Ovulation is detected laparoscopically by examination of the ovaries within 24 hours of the exogenous administration of the ovulatory dose of human chorionic gonadotropin (HCG). Uterine flushing is performed four to seven days after the HCG injection.

After initial observation through the laparoscope, urine is removed from the bladder by suprapubic puncture (see chapter 4, *Laparoscopy in Monkeys and Apes*). The manipulatory probe (a Verres needle) is removed and a Hartman alligator forceps inserted as described earlier. The uterine ligament is grasped with the forceps to steady the uterus during flushing (Fig. 5.4). A 25 gauge, ⅝ inch needle, with a 3 ml syringe attached, is inserted through the lower abdominal wall, the fundus of the uterus, and into the uterine lumen. Warmed physiological saline or normal electrolyte solution is then flushed gently and slowly through the uterus. The fluid is recovered through a

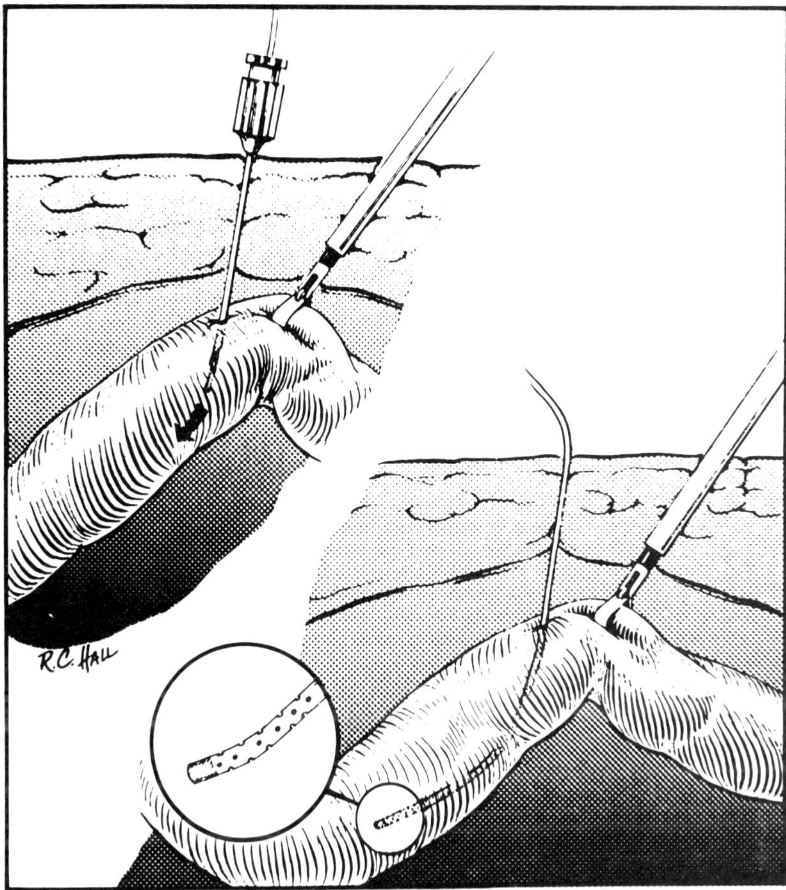

**Figure 5.2**   Diagram (left) of the uterus of a female pig being grasped with the forceps and the insertion of a 15 gauge needle. Diagram (right) showing the needle removed, leaving only the polyethylene tubing *in utero*. (Reproduced with permission of Wildt *et al., Journal of Reproduction and Fertility* 44:301–304, 1975.)

polyethylene catheter (PE 200, Clay Adams Co.) attached to a Pasteur pipette. The large end of the pipette is placed in the vagina and caps over the external os of the cervix. A hollow glass slide or similar device can be used to contain the flushed fluid for later examination for ova or blastocysts. A fluid recovery rate of 70 to 90% is normally found (Ariga and Dukelow, 1977a, b). A photo of a 93 hour old recovered blastocyst from a squirrel monkey is shown in Figure 5.5.

### Laparoscopic Topical Application of Materials

The basic laparoscopic technique also can be utilized to apply test compounds or treatments directed to selected organs of the body. In this laboratory this technique has been used to study the effects of various gonadotropins and ovulation inducing compounds on the ovarian surface.

To apply the substances a 2 mm disk is made from either no. 42 filter paper (Whatman Co.) or Gelfoam (Upjohn Co.). A simple way of making these is by using an ear punch such as is used in identifying laboratory animals. These disks are then saturated with the test solution and, using a 3 mm grasping forceps (Richard Wolf Medical Instruments

# Schedule for Uterine Flushing
# in Saimiri sciureus

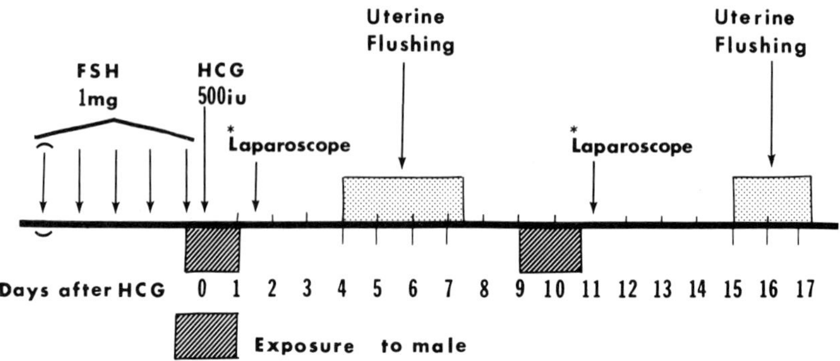


**Figure 5.3**   Schedule for uterine flushing in *Saimiri sciureus*.

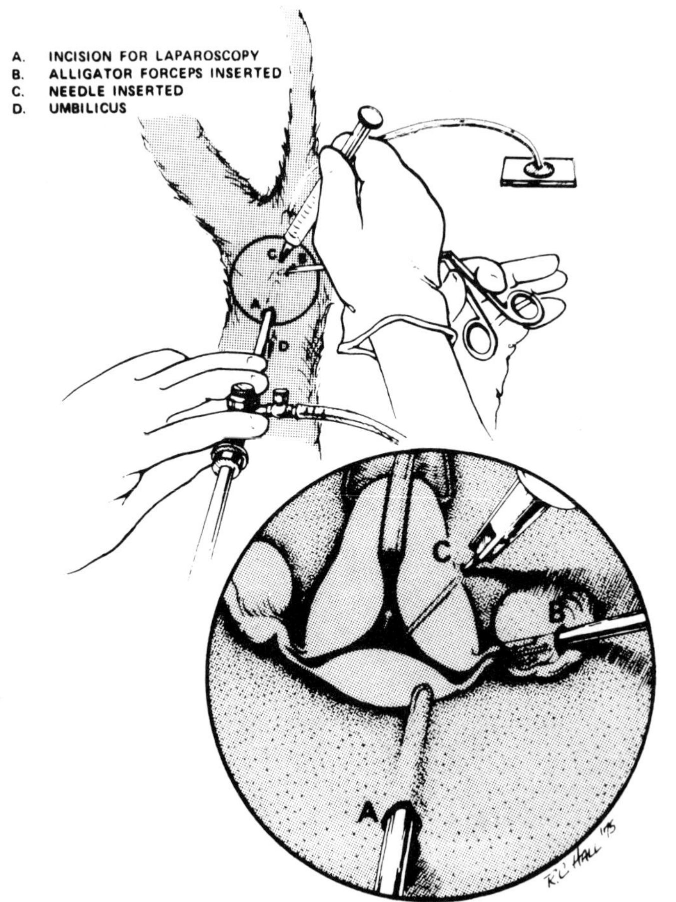


**Figure 5.4**   Diagrammatic presentation of uterine flushing technique used in the squirrel monkey. (Reproduced with permission from *Journal of Medical Primatology* 5:82–99, 1976.)

# Blastocyst (ĖFA 93—109hours)

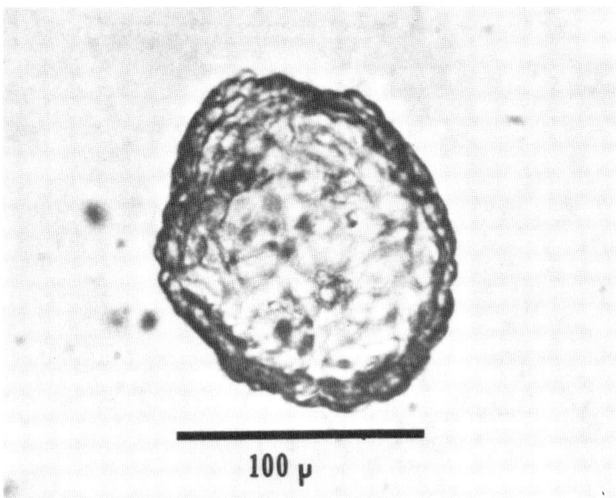


**EFA   Estimated Fertilization Age**

**Figure 5.5**   Recovered five day blastocyst from *Saimiri sciureus*. Estimated fertilization age, 93 to 109 hours.

Corp.) under laparoscopic visualization, the disks are placed on the surface of the organ to be studied. In our own studies such disks placed on the ovarian surface remain adhered to the ovary for at least two hours and can easily be removed with the same grasping forceps.

### Extensive Laparoscopy and Reproductive Studies

Prior to using the ancillary procedures described above one may be concerned that extensive use of such procedures may influence reproductive parameters and affect the reproductive potential of the animals. This section examines the extensive use of laparoscopy in nonhuman primates and its effects on the reproductive status of these animals.

The use of laparotomy for abdominal visualization is generally limited to four or five procedures, due to adhesion formation, and these are generally not possible at intervals of less than 24 hours. Laparoscopy, on the other hand, has been carried out in several species over extended time periods or extensively for short time periods.

In nonhuman primates, particularly the menstruating macaque species in which effects of surgical stress can be measured by subsequent variation in cycle length, several colonies of animals have been subjected to extensive laparoscopic procedures. The earliest report of such extensive studies involved a single, regularly cycling cynomolgus macaque (*M. fascicularis*) that was exposed daily to a fertile male, anesthetized (0.15 mg phencyclidine hydrochloride), and bled by venipuncture. The mating, anesthesia and venipuncture were continued for 33 days (Rawson and Dukelow, 1973). During this high stress period of intensive manipulation the animal was also laparoscopically examined twice, on days 7 and 10. The animal ovulated and conceived on day 16 of the cycle (day 3 of anesthesia and venipuncture) and showed implantation bleeding 18 days later. Laparoscopy was performed again during the seventh week of gestation and pregnancy continued. On day 169 of gestation a normal female infant was delivered. Following parturition, the adult female was laparoscopically examined at 6,

10, 14, 16, and 22 weeks to detect resumption of ovarian activity. No deleterious effect of the procedure on lactation was noted and the infant was weaned at 24 weeks of age with a normal body weight of 840 gm. Twenty-one days after separation from the infant regular menstruation began. Ovulation was confirmed at laparoscopy on day 16 after weaning and a subsequent menses was observed on day 27. A complete history of the procedures and reproductive activities of this female is illustrated in Figure 5.6.

Other investigators have studied the effect of repeated laparoscopic examinations (6.4 ± 0.3 per cycle, mean ± S.D.) on cycle length in the rhesus monkey (*M. mulatta*). The mean cycle length prior to, during, and subsequent to laparoscopic examination was found to be 28.9 ± 0.6, 27.5 ± 0.6, and 28.9 ± 0.8 days respectively (Dierschke and Clark, 1976). Similarly, in the author's laboratory with a mean of 2.3 laparoscopic observations per cycle in cynomolgus macaques, the mean cycle length for 252 cycles was 30.6 ± 5.0 (S.E.). This value was no different than the control animals (not subjected to laparoscopic examination) with 334 cycles which averaged 29.4 ± 11.1 days (Dukelow, 1977).

Intensive studies over a short time interval have been conducted for investigation of follicular morphology just prior to ovulation in the cynomolgus macaque (Jewett and Dukelow, 1972). Six animals were subjected to laparoscopic examination at approximately hourly intervals for an eight to nine hour period without ill effect and without blocking ovulation.

The reproductive performance of 16 cynomolgus macaques, subjected to various numbers of laparoscopic examinations ranging from 31 to 82 each, was reported by Mahone and Dukelow (1978). Eight of the 16 became pregnant and of these eight, the number of laparoscopic examinations prior to pregnancy ranged from 38 to 67. The authors concluded that, although extensive laparoscopy did produce occasional abdominal adhesions, the animals' ability to become pregnant and to deliver normal, healthy young was not inhibited.

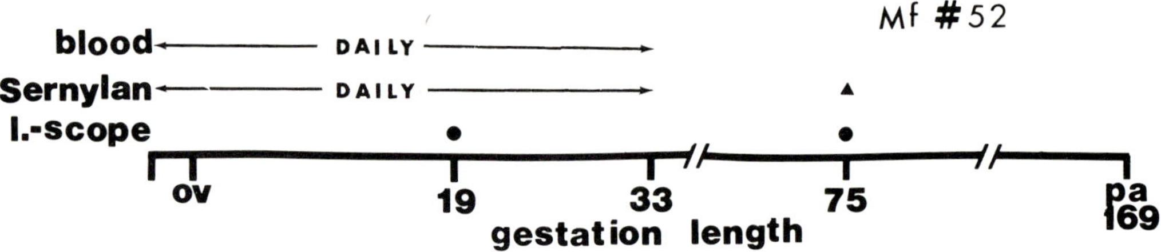


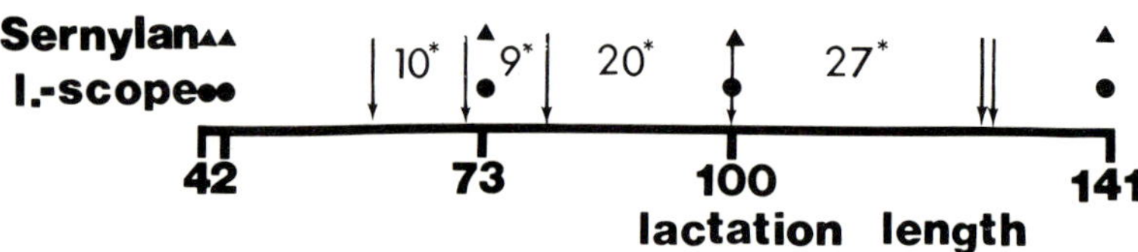


**Figure 5.6**  Summary of procedures carried out during gestation and lactation in *M. fascicularis* female no. 52. Triangles indicate day of administration of the anesthesia, phencyclidine hydrochloride.

# SMALL ANIMAL TECHNIQUES

## Special Techniques Applicable to Small Laboratory Rodents

It was earlier stated that the application of laparoscopic techniques is limited only by the ingenuity of the laparoscopist and this, indeed, applies to the laparoscopy of small laboratory rodents. In our laboratory limited laparoscopic examinations for the observation of uterine and ovarian changes have been carried out on mice, rats, mink, *tylomys*, and *ototylomys* (the latter two are wild Mexican rodents). Anesthesia was induced either by ether inhalation or sodium pentobarbital injected intraperitoneally. Alternative anesthetic regimens for most small laboratory species can also be found in a recent textbook (Harkness and Wagner, 1977). All laparoscopy was with the 5 mm, in diameter, pediatric laparoscope previously described; however, the size of this instrument is approaching the maximum size (especially with mice). For routine laparoscopy the author suggests that the smaller 1.7 to 2.7 mm, in diameter, laparoscopes might be preferable. No problems, however, were encountered when using the 5 mm laparoscope in these small animals.

All of these species have an ovarian bursa (periovarian sac) around the ovary that precludes direct observation of the ovarian surface. However, manipulation of the ovary within the sac allows reasonable observations of the ovary through the membrane. Observation of the uterine horn shortly after implantation (days 6 to 9 in the rodents listed) allows easy counting of the embryos and emphasizes the value of laparoscopy for studies of early embryonic mortality. To accomplish this the laparoscopist locates the bifurcation of the uterine horns and moves the laparoscope along the length of the horn towards the ovary. He then repeats the procedure on the opposite uterine horn. Such a procedure does not interfere with pregnancy. In one mouse, for example, laparoscopically examined at midpregnancy and found to have 16 implanted embryos, delivery was normal at term with the birth of the full complement of offspring.

Completion of the laparoscopic procedure in laboratory rodents, with suturing, is identical to that described for other species.

## Laparoscopy in the Rabbit

Special considerations are necessary in the rabbit. Because of the flaccid nature of the abdomen it is more difficult to laparoscopically examine than most other laboratory or domestic animals. Maintenance of an adequate level of abdominal insufflation is difficult unless a commercial insufflator is used and, additionally, there is a tendency for the organ being examined, such as the ovary, to sink within the abdominal contents and make examination impossible. Accordingly, a technique has been developed by Fujimoto *et al.* (1974), which allows suspension of the ovary from a suture passed through the abdominal wall. The rabbit is initially anesthetized with sodium pentobarbital (20 to 25 mg/kg body weight, injected intravenously), and the laparoscope inserted in the standard manner used with other species. After locating the ovary using the laparoscope and a manipulatory probe (usually the Verres needle) a large curved needle with attached 3-0 suture is threaded through the abdominal wall, around or through the ovarian ligament, and back through the wall where the ends are loosely tied or clamped with a needle holder (Fig. 5.7). A similar procedure is repeated for the second ovary. Manual elevation of the external portion of the sutures makes observation of the ovaries a simple procedure. At the completion of the examination, the sutures are merely withdrawn through the abdominal wall.

A very similar technique has been used in ovulation studies in the guinea pig (Dr. J. M. R. Rawson, personal communication). The animal was anesthetized with sodium pentobarbital (28 to 35 mg/kg, intraperitoneally) and the 5 mm, 180° laparoscope

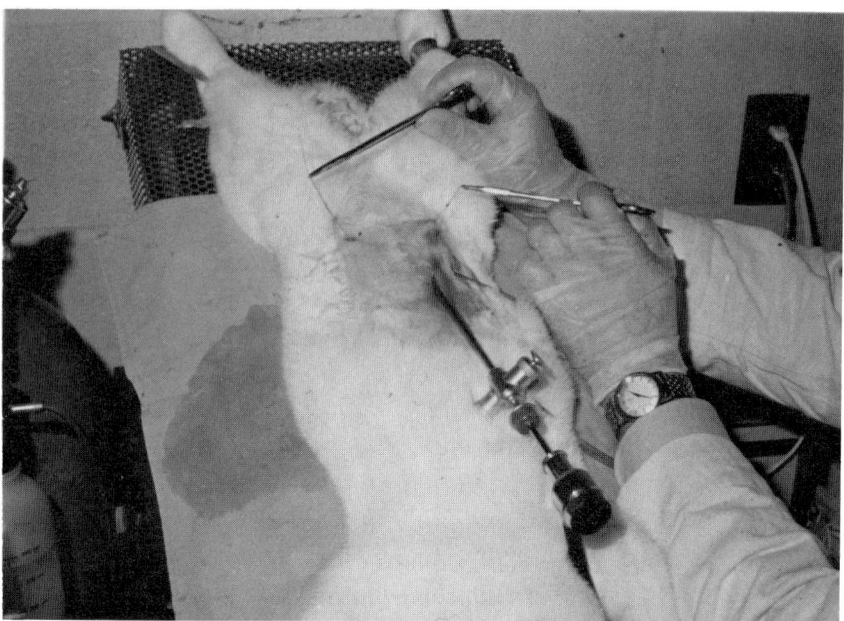

**Figure 5.7**  Elevation of the external portion of sutures laparoscopically placed around the ovarian ligaments to facilitate suspension and observation of the ovaries in a rabbit. (Reproduced with permission of Fujimoto *et al.*, *Journal of Reprod. Fertil.* 38:97–103, 1974.)

inserted through a midventral approach. The transabdominal suturing technique was used to elevate and facilitate visualization of the ovaries of this species also.

## CONCLUSIONS

Most of the examples provided in this chapter are those utilized experimentally in the laboratory of the author. Rather than serving as a complete listing of available research techniques for laparoscopists, they serve only as examples of types of problems which can be faced and solved with skilled laparoscopy. If the listing of these few simple procedures serves to stimulate the imagination of laparoscopists to develop more intricate and advanced approaches to the solution of research and clinical problems, then the function of this chapter will have been served.

**References**

Ariga, S., and Dukelow, W. R. (1977a) Nonsurgical (laparoscopic) uterine flushing and egg recovery technique in the squirrel monkey (*Saimiri sciureus*). *Primates* 18:453–457.

Ariga, S., and Dukelow, W. R. (1977b) Recovery of preimplantation blastocysts in the squirrel monkey by a laparoscopic technique. *Fertil. Steril.* 28:577–580.

Dierschke, D. J., and Clark, J. R. (1976) Laparoscopy in *Macaca mulatta*: Specialized equipment employed and initial observations. *J. Med. Primatol.* 5:100–110.

Dukelow, W. R. (1977) Ovulatory cycle characteristics in *Macaca fascicularis*. *J. Med. Primatol.* 6:33–42.

Dukelow, W. R. (1978) Laparoscopic research techniques in mammalian embryology. In: *Methods in Mammalian Reproduction*. J. C. Daniel, ed., Academic Press, New York, pp. 437–460.

Dukelow, W. R., and Ariga, S. (1976) Laparoscopic techniques for biomedical research. *J. Med. Primatol.* 5:82–99.

Dukelow, W. R., Jarosz, S. J., Jewett, D. A., and Harrison, R. M. (1971) Laparoscopic examination of the ovaries in goats and primates. *Lab. Anim. Sci.* 21:594–597.

Fujimoto, S., Rawson, J. M. R., and Dukelow, W. R.

(1974) Hormonal influences on the time of ovulation in the rabbit as determined by laparoscopy. *J. Reprod. Fertil.* 38:97–103.

Harkness, J. E., and Wagner, J. E. (1977) *The Biology and Medicine of Rabbits and Rodents.* Lea and Febiger, Philadelphia, pp. 46–52.

Jewett, D. A., and Dukelow, W. R. (1972) Serial observations of follicular morphology near ovulation in *Macaca fascicularis. J. Reprod. Fertil.* 31:287–290.

Jewett, D. A., and Dukelow, W. R. (1973) Follicular observation and laparoscopic aspiration techniques in *Macaca fascicularis. J. Med. Primatol.* 2: 108–113.

Mahone, J. P., and Dukelow, W. R. (1978) Reproductive performance in *Macaca fascicularis* following repeated laparoscopy. *J. Med. Primatol.* 7:185–188.

Morgenstern, L. L., and Soupart, P. (1972) Oocyte recovery from the human ovary. *Fertil. Steril.* 23: 751–758.

Rawson, J. M. R., and Dukelow, W. R. (1973) Effect of laparoscopy and anesthesia on ovulation, conception, gestation, and lactation in a *Macaca fascicu-laris. Lab. Prim. Newsl.* 12:4–5.

Rawson, J. M. R., and Dukelow, W. R. (1978) Effects of intrafollicular administration of gonadotropins in two species of nonhuman primates using laparoscopy. *J. Med. Primatol.* 7:223–227.

Snyder, D. A., and Dukelow, W. R. (1974) Laparoscopic studies of ovulation, pregnancy diagnosis, and follicle aspiration in sheep. *Theriogenology* 2: 143–148.

Steptoe, P. C., and Edwards, R. G. (1970) Laparoscopic recovery of preovulatory human oocytes after priming of ovaries with gonadotropins. *Lancet* 4: 683–689.

Wildt, D. E., Fujimoto, S., Spencer, J. L., and Dukelow, W. R. (1973) Direct ovarian observation in the pig by means of laparoscopy. *J. Reprod. Fertil.* 35:541–543.

Wildt, D. E., Morcom, C. B., and Dukelow, W. R. (1975) Laparoscopic pregnancy diagnosis and uterine fluid recovery in swine. *J. Reprod. Fertil.* 44: 301–304.

# CHAPTER 6

# Laparoscopy in the Sheep and Goat*

Karl H. Seeger, Dr. Med. Vet., and
Peter R. Klatt, Dr. Med. Vet.

## INTRODUCTION

Numerous research investigations have required exploration and examination of the abdominal contents of the sheep and goat. Because these species are common and relatively inexpensive, it has been feasible to conduct a number of novel approaches of viewing into the peritoneal cavity.

Many of these methods have involved standard laparotomy or minilaparotomy (Hulet and Foote, 1968) procedures or the use of a chronic peritoneal fistula in conjunction with endoscope insertion (Lamond and Holmes, 1965; Dierschke and Hyatt, 1969; Boyd and Ducker, 1975). In the latter procedure, an indwelling rubber, Silastic, or Plexiglas cannula was placed in the paralumbar fossa region and used as a channel to insert a laparoscope. The theory behind such a technique was sound since the animal could be examined without inducing a surgical plane of anesthesia. However, a number of problems were encountered, including granuloma formation over the implanted fistula and peritonitis. In addition, because of the cannula location in the paralumbar fossa, some difficulty was reported in locating and visualizing specific organs.

In 1968, the first report on laparoscopy in sheep, using the ventral trocar-cannula approach and refined fiber optic systems was published (Roberts, 1968). In the following year, Thimonier and Mauleon (1969) using similar methodology reported the usefulness of laparoscopy to study estrous behavior-ovarian pituitary relationships in the ewe. Several years later, a doctoral thesis, subsequently published, utilized laparoscopy effectively to investigate estrual-ovarian activity in Texel sheep (Muurling, 1971, 1972). In this same year, laparoscopy was reported as a safe and reliable means of diagnosing pregnancy and estimating fetal numbers in this species (Phillippo et al., 1971). More recent endoscopic investigations in sheep have been concerned with analysis of various anesthetic regimens (Boyd and Ducker, 1973); detailing procedures and describing ovarian morphology (Seeger, 1973); utilizing ancillary techniques for collecting ova for subsequent in vitro culture (Snyder and Dukelow, 1974); and simply determining ovulation rate (Bindon et al., 1979; Quirke et al., 1979).

* The authors wish to thank Michael Ochs and Gert Reinhardt for their technical assistance and Sabine Müller for typing the manuscript.

The authors are aware of only two reports on laparoscopy in goats (Dukelow *et al.*, 1971; Jarosz *et al.*, 1971). These investigators, using techniques similar to that used in sheep, characterized the reproductive ovarian cycle of the African Pygmy and Toggenburg goat.

The present chapter outlines the authors' recommendations for performing laparoscopy in sheep. Unless otherwise specifically discussed, all advised procedures are equally effective in goats.

## LAPAROSCOPIC TECHNIQUE

### Animals, Anesthesia, and Restraint

In 1972, our laboratory began using laparoscopy in a study designed to induce estrous behavior and ovarian activity in anestrous ewes using gonadotropin releasing hormone (GnRH). Laparoscopy was employed as a safe means of confirming ovarian follicle development and ovulation. A total of 176 sheep were utilized, from six months to seven years of age and from 20 to greater than 50 kg in body weight. A wide variety of breeds were represented, including Merino, German black face, Texel, Heidschnucken, East Friesian dairy and mixed breeds. No males were examined. The following recommendations are based on our experiences with these animals.

When performing laparoscopy in a relatively large animal such as the sheep, the number of personnel available is a critical factor. If only a single animal is to be examined, a minimum of two, the operator and assistant, are required. In a setting necessitating a number of laparoscopies, it is recommended to have available the laparoscopist and, in addition, two assistants, preferably three. One of these individuals should be a skilled technician familiar with general anesthesia, insufflation, record keeping, and photolaparoscopy procedures. The remaining two assistants can cooperate in the physical handling and restraint of each animal, thereby allowing the laparoscopist to maintain a reasonable degree of cleanliness. This teamwork approach has been very effective in the authors' laboratory, allowing routine examinations of the reproductive organs to require 10 minutes or less per animal.

Food is withheld from animals for 24 hours prior to conducting laparoscopy. Withholding water is unnecessary. The operator may be more comfortable with catheterizing the bladder before the operation. However, little danger exists in puncturing the bladder. In 619 laparoscopies, only one animal suffered such an accident.

Laparoscopy in sheep can be performed using one or a combination of anesthetics. Our laboratory generally utilizes sodium pentobarbital (Narcoren, JFFA-Merieux or Halatal Solution, Jen-Sal Laboratories.) injected intravenously via the jugular vein at a dosage of 20 mg/kg body weight. Two-thirds of the estimated total dose is injected rapidly, the last third sequentially and slowly until a surgical plane of anesthesia is achieved. The major physical indicator of this state is corneal reflex. Drug injection is stopped coincidentally with the loss of this reflex. A surgical plane of anesthesia is maintained with this drug regimen for approximately 30 minutes. As a supporting measure, a local spray anesthetic (ethylchlorine, $C_2H_5Cl$, Chemisches Werk) is administered to the proposed incision sites. Injectable anesthetics (lidocaine, xylocaine) work equally well for this purpose.

The dosage of pentobarbital can be reduced by pretreating the sheep with a tranquilizing drug. Snyder and Dukelow (1974) injected 250 to 350 mg of promazine hydrochloride (Sparine, Wyeth Laboratories.) intramuscularly, waited five to ten minutes and noted that only 9 to 10 mg of pentobarbital/kg of body weight were required to induce anesthesia suitable for laparoscopy. Ether or halothane (Fluothane, Ayerst Laboratories) inhalation through a face mask breathing apparatus can also be used as needed to maintain anesthesia.

The most efficacious approach for laparoscopic insertion in sheep and goats is in the ventral inguinal region. One of the essentials for successful laparoscopy is the proper positioning and restraint of the animal to achieve optimum access to this anatomical area. A standard surgical table with tilting apparatus is satisfactory, as well as various types of self constructed sheep cradles similar to that first described by Hulet and Foote (1968), and later by Blockey (1972). A very simple restraint device can be devised by binding together two short ladders into a V shape. Our laboratory uses a restraint apparatus modified from that of Hulet and Foote (1968) and constructed of metal and canvas (Fig. 6.1). The anesthetized animal is tied head-down in a dorsal recumbent position on the table sloped at a 45° angle. If food has been withheld for 15 to 24 hours,

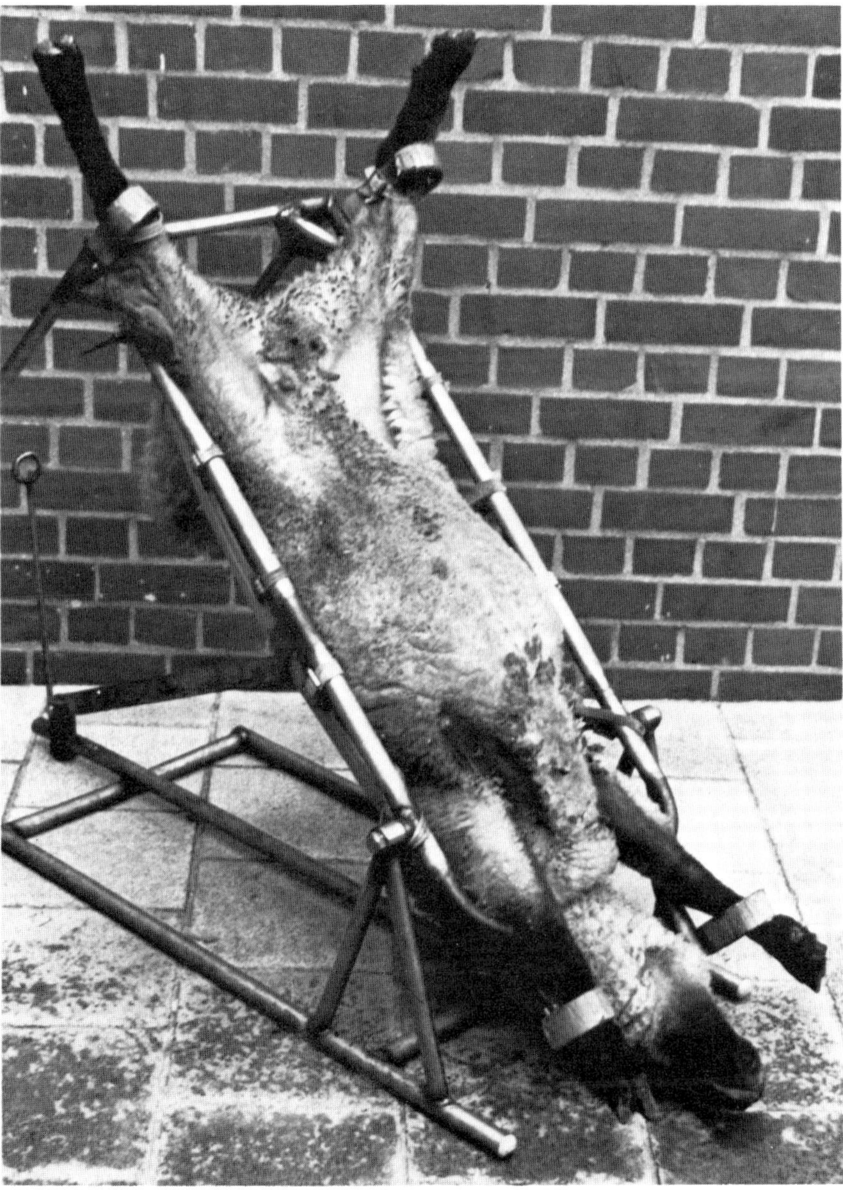

**Figure 6.1** Anesthetized sheep positioned in cradle prior to surgical preparation.

this position will allow the gut and omentum majus to move cranially and lessen the danger of trocar-cannula insertion.

## Equipment

The essential instruments required for laparoscopy in the sheep and goat include the conical tip trocar, spherical cannula with valve and gas inlet, and laparoscope. The laparoscope used in our laboratory consists of a telescope, 1 cm in diameter, 30 cm in length, with a 130° field of view (Richard Wolf GMBH, Knittlingen, West Germany). The corresponding trocar-cannula for this laparoscope is 1.1 cm in diameter. A smaller diameter (5 mm, 130°) laparoscope has been used successfully in sheep (Snyder and Dukelow, 1974) and goats (Dukelow *et al.*, 1971; Jarosz *et al.*, 1971).

The light source used in our facility consists of an illumination generator (Richard Wolf GMBH, Knittlingen, West Germany) containing a halogen bulb (150 watts) for diagnostic observations and an electronic flash system for photolaparoscopy. Both diagnostic and photo illumination is transferred from the light source to the laparoscope through a glass fiber cable, 180 cm in length and 3.5 mm in diameter. Some accessory manipulation is generally required using a manipulatory probe or forceps inserted through a secondary cannula. We utilize an 11 mm secondary cannula similar to the one used for laparoscope insertion; however, the 6 mm cannula described by Snyder and Dukelow (1974) works equally well. Insufflation of the peritoneal cavity is accomplished using an automatic insufflating device which allows the operator to maintain a constant intraabdominal pressure and air space. Although convenient, this commercial apparatus is not an absolute necessity for sheep laparoscopy. The laparoscopist can also create a pneumoperitoneum using a hand pump (Fig. 6.2) with bacteria tight filter to force air through the insufflating needle and into the abdominal cavity. Although a standard Verres needle device can be used to pass the gas through the abdominal wall, the operator can also employ an ordinary pointed cannula of about 10 cm in length with an inner diameter of 0.4 mm. Carbon dioxide, nitrous oxide or air have all been utilized to produce pneumoperitoneum in sheep. No physiologic differences have been discerned among animals insufflated with these three gases. Our laboratory utilizes air or $CO_2$ in air—the latter has also been used with satisfactory results in goats (Dukelow *et al.*, 1971; Jarosz *et al.*, 1971).

Documentation of observations has been performed using a single lens reflex camera and a 95 mm lens adapter (Elbaflex 1000, Richard Wolf GMBH, Knittlingen, West Germany). Other cameras with various lens adapters can also be used effectively. Photographs in goats have been obtained using a 35 mm Canon TL camera and laparoscopic adapter (Jarosz *et al.*, 1971).

Several routine surgical instruments are required, including a scalpel and forceps. In the event that internal trauma or hemorrhage is diagnosed or occurs as a result of inappropriate laparoscopic techniques, a sterile surgical pack should be available for laparotomy. Incision sites are repaired with Michel clamps or absorbable suture. The former require removal approximately 10 days after examination.

## Equipment and Surgical Preparation

In our research program, a sterile field has not been maintained during laparoscopic examination of ewes. An attempt is made to keep the immediate surgical site, the laparoscopic instruments, and the operator's hands as uncontaminated as possible. Such an approach has not resulted in postoperative infections. In the event that laparoscopy is used clinically in this species, the authors recommend that no uncertain precautions be taken, and if the surgeon feels uncomfortable with our procedure, that standard measures for maintaining sterility be employed.

Surgical and laparoscopic instruments are sterilized in ethylene oxide or alternatively

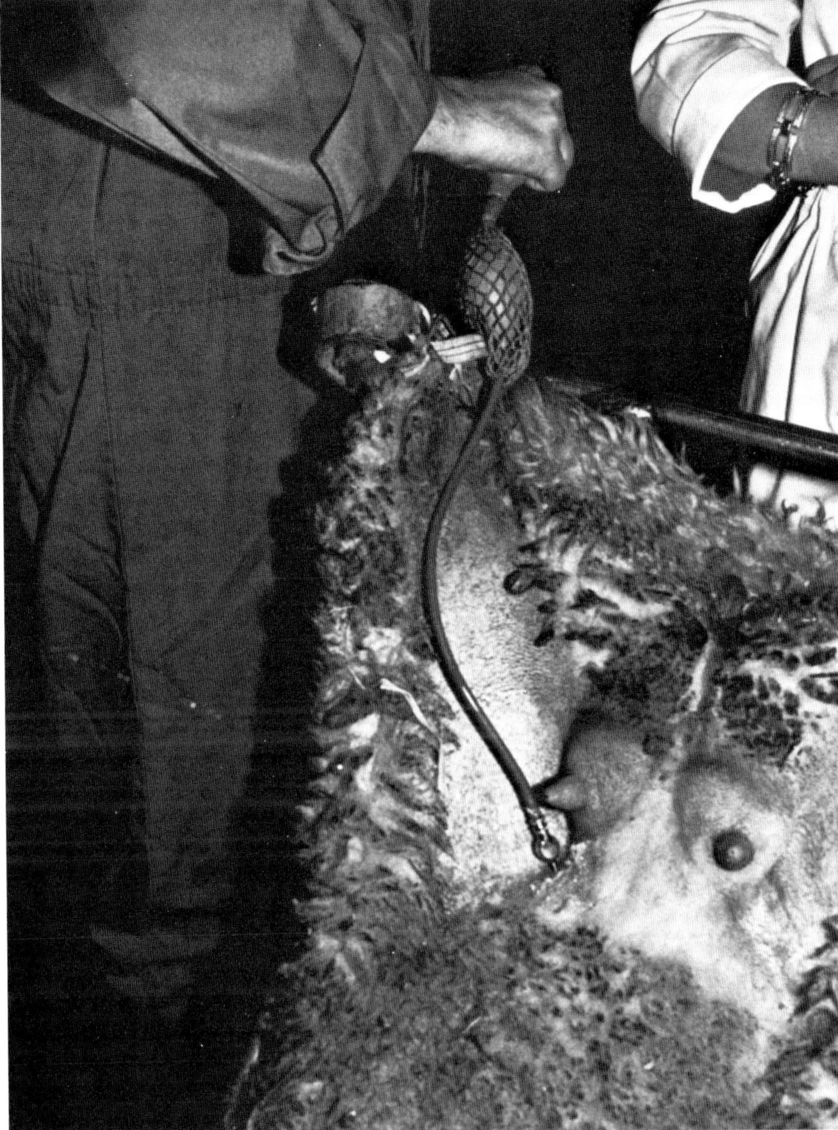

**Figure 6.2**   The hand pump used to insufflate the ewe with room air. The insufflatory needle is inserted lateral to the midline.

immersed in a germicidal solution recommended by the equipment manufacturer. The instruments are cleaned thoroughly between examinations by wiping with sterile gauze soaked in 70% ethanol. Following induction of anesthesia and restraint of the sheep, the posterior abdominal region in the area of the pubis is surgically prepared. An area approximately 12 to 15 cm in length and located in the vicinity of and cranial to the mammary gland is clipped or manually depilated of wool (Fig. 6.3). This preparation is extended approximately 10 cm to each side of the midline. This inguinal region of woolless skin is then disinfected by scrubbing with 90% ethanol or benzalkonium chloride (Zephiran, Winthrop Laboratories). The specific sites for insertion of the trocar-cannula(e) are more thoroughly cleansed by the application of povidone iodine (Beta-

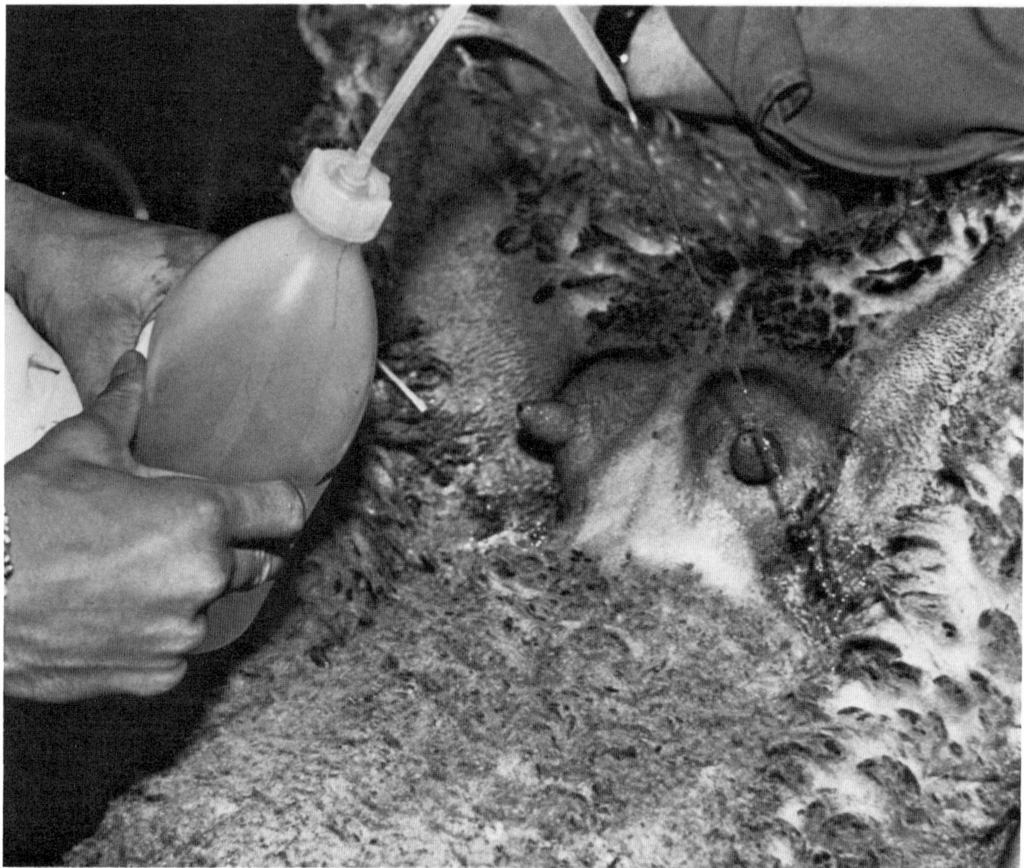

**Figure 6.3** The posterior abdominal region is surgically prepared by clipping or depilating and then applying ethanol.

dine, Purdue Frederick Co.) or Lugol's solution (20 gm potassium iodide, 1 gm iodine in 300 ml of distilled water).

### Insufflation and Laparoscope Insertion

The pneumoperitoneum is created prior to the insertion of the laparoscope. In our laboratory, to avoid internal contact with the inserted laparoscope or forceps, the insufflatory cannula (or Verres needle) is placed 4 to 6 cm to the left of the midline (Fig. 6.2). Normally, a small volume of gas exists in the peritoneal cavity. Before insufflating, a syringe is attached to the inserted cannula and an attempt made to aspirate air from the cavity. Successful suction of abdominal air gives the operator reasonable confidence that the cannula is properly in place and not located within the bowel. The bulb pump (Fig. 6.2) or hose from the pneumoperitoneum apparatus is then attached to the insufflatory cannula and the pneumoperitoneum established. For an average adult 30 kg ewe approximately 4 to 6 liters of gas are required or until the abdominal wall becomes slightly distended. Insufflation volume may vary considerably due to rumen size and positioning.

When the rumen constitutes a large portion of the abdominal cavity, such as in the sheep and goat, the site of the trocar-cannula insertion is critical. In addition, one must consider that major vasculature for draining the mammary gland exists in the inguinal region of these species. The optimum location for intromission of this instrument is approximately 2 cm cranial to the mammary gland (Fig. 6.4). Compared to other species, this site for the laparoscope is at an extremely caudal location, but necessary to avoid false placement of the trocar-cannula into the rumen. The skin incision can be made on the midline or within a 4 cm range to either side of this location. The authors prefer to insert the laparoscopic trocar-cannula slightly to the left of the midline. This allows the accessory trocar-cannula to be placed closely and immediately adjacent to the right of the midline. Such a procedure facilitates simultaneous observation-manipulation.

The trocar-cannula assembly is inserted in a horizontal, dorsomedial direction. The trocar is removed, the laparoscope immediately inserted, and the examination initiated. With the animal in the Trendelenburg position, the operator can generally immediately observe a portion of the urinary bladder, uterus, gut, and sometimes ovaries.

### Insertion and Use of Accessory Instruments

To perform precise examination of specific organs in the sheep and goat, it is almost always necessary to utilize a manipulatory forceps. The corresponding trocar-cannula for this device is inserted on the opposite side of the ventral midline from the laparoscope (Fig. 6.4). This positioning allows support of the endoscope and convenient

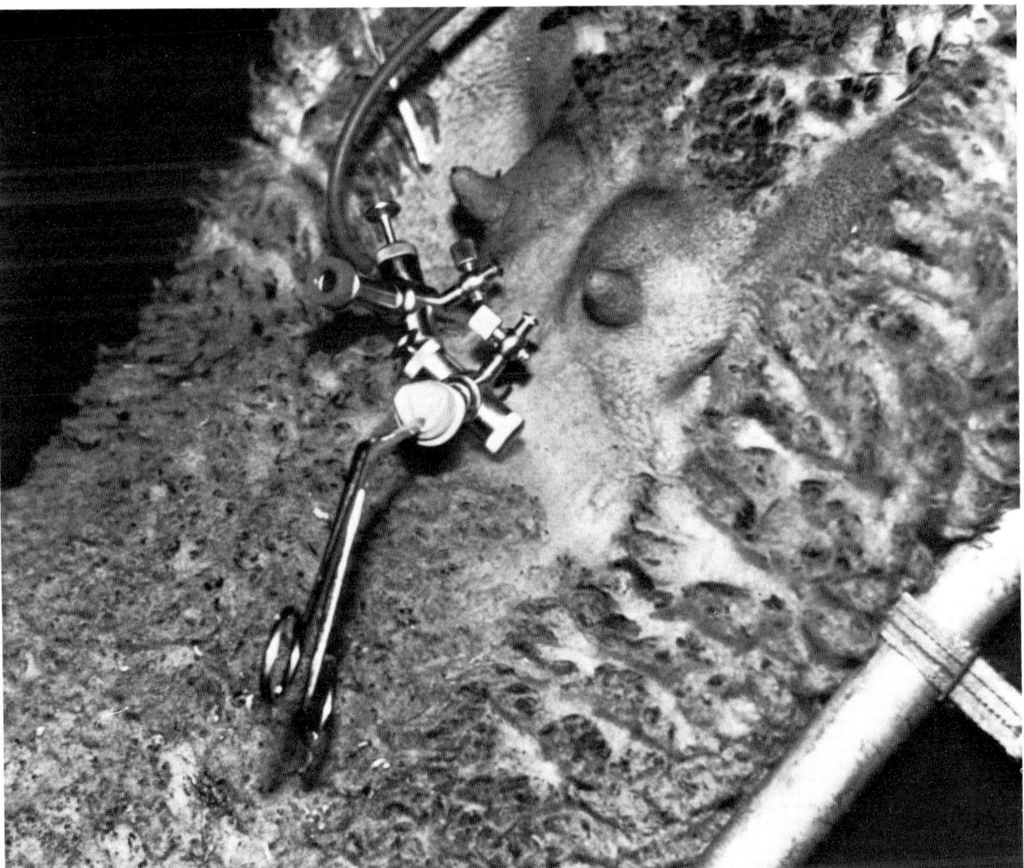

**Figure 6.4** Anatomical sites for insertion of the laparoscopic cannula (upper) and accessory cannula (lower). A rubber diaphragm is placed over the end of the latter device to inhibit insufflatory loss when using a small diameter manipulatory forceps.

manipulation of the ancillary forceps. As previously indicated, our laboratory does not have available a standard accessory trocar-cannula unit for forceps insertion. Instead, we have adapted an 11 mm standard endoscopic cannula for forceps use. After insertion, a rubber diaphragm (from a rubber surgical glove) is fitted over the entrance of the cannula and then the forceps are inserted through the diaphragm. The latter allows the forceps to be used in the oversized cannula without loss of insufflation (Figs. 6.4 and 6.5).

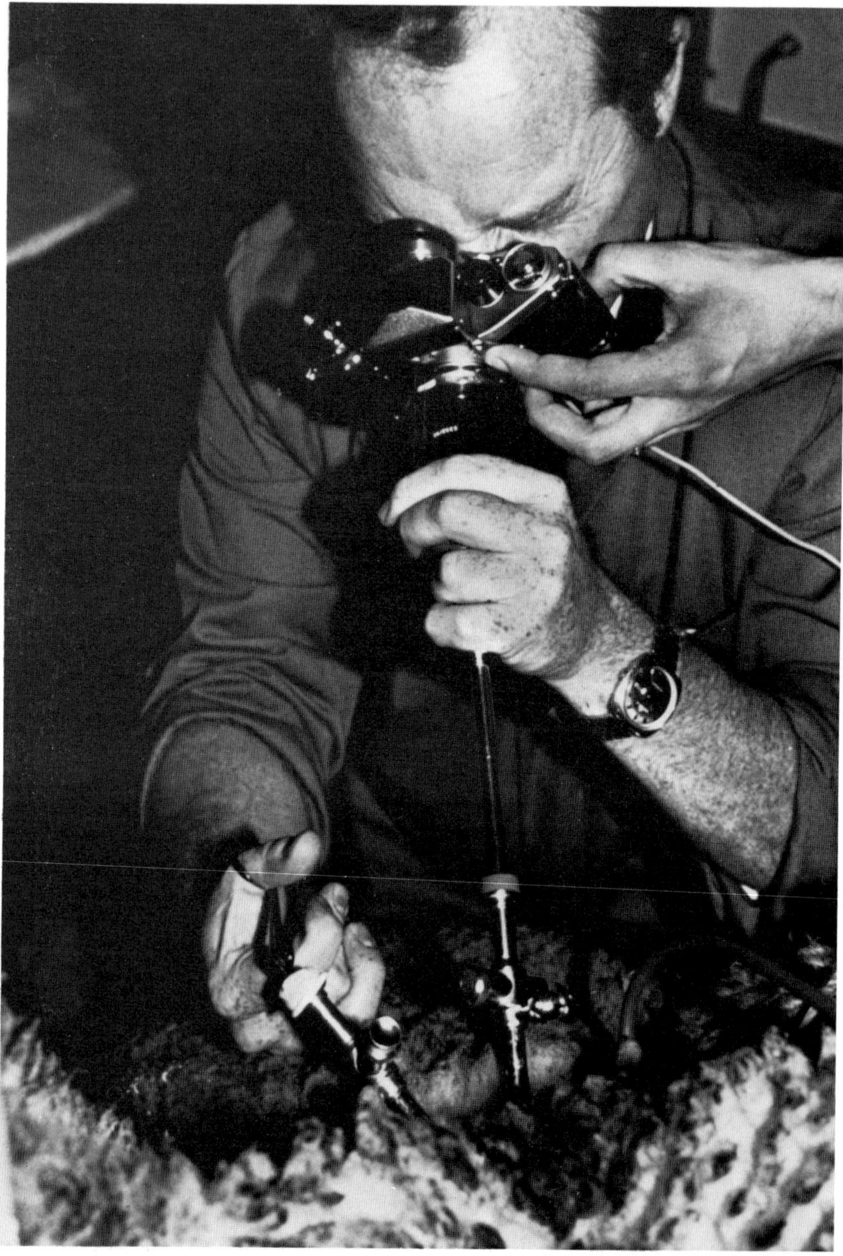

**Figure 6.5**  Photolaparoscopy in the sheep. An assistant aids in controlling the camera.

## CAPABILITIES OF LAPAROSCOPY IN THE SHEEP

### General Visualization

The beginner will require some time to develop the skills to allow the simultaneous coordination of the accessory instrument with the visual field. With an internal forceps for maneuvering organs, the laparoscopist can now make a more complete diagnostic examination of the bladder and reproductive tract. In females, the uterine body, bifurcation, both uterine horns, oviducts, fimbrae, and ovaries can be observed. In the nonpregnant ewe, the use of accessory forceps or an elongated tactile probe allows the operator to "roll" the uterus to examine the dorsal aspect. Ovarian observation is best accomplished by using the forceps to grasp the uterine ligament or mesosalpinx and elevate the ovary and ovarian blood supply into view. With the animal in the Trendelenburg position, a considerable portion of the lower gastrointestinal tract is observable, including the small intestine and colon. The transparency of the latter tissue allows the operator to observe feces within the colon. The accessory forceps can be used to grasp and maneuver the small intestine for more thorough investigation.

In the event that the operator is interested in visualizing the organs of the cranial peritoneal cavity, he may consider adapting the paralumbar fossa approach, similar to that described in this text for the cow and horse. Our laboratory has had limited experience with such a technique, but because of the ease of restraint and passive temperament of most sheep, this approach can be successful. Methodology is similar to that described for the cow (Seeger, 1977). The animal is restrained in a standing position, local anesthetic applied to the right paralumbar fossa area, and the trocar-cannula inserted through a skin incision in the fossa. Following insertion of the laparoscope into the peritoneal cavity, the telescope is directed cranially to view the liver. This paralumbar approach is less effective than midventral insertion for evaluating uterine and ovarian anatomy.

Our laboratory has made no attempt at examining other ovine organs (i.e., pancreas, gallbladder, kidney) or implementing standard biopsy procedures; it is reasonable to assume that if the organ is visible, little additional diligence is required to obtain tissue samples.

### Laparoscopy for Diagnoses, Surgery, and Reproductive Study

Beyond reproductive study, little information is available on the usefulness of laparoscopy for diagnosis or surgical alteration in ovine veterinary medicine. We have utilized laparoscopy successfully as a simple and efficient means of diagnosing or confirming cases of vesiculitis caused by urinary calculi. Both subtle and dramatic alterations in the morphology of the gut as viewed through the endoscope have been reliable indicators of gastrointestinal tissue inflammation.

By far, the most extensive use of laparoscopy in the sheep and goat has been for reproductive study. It is the only means to sequentially monitor ovarian activity in individual animals, since most ewes cannot withstand multiple laparotomies because of extensive adhesion formation and the possibility of peritonitis. In addition, laparoscopy is a much more rapid procedure than laparotomy. Following laparoscope insertion, examination of both ovaries and uterine horns is generally completed in 10 minutes. In our laboratory, this technique has been a useful tool to investigate the role of ovarian function in the control of the reproductive cycle and to diagnose pregnancy. A series of laparoscopic photographs illustrates the normal expected alterations in ovarian morphology throughout the estrous cycle of the sheep (*Color Atlas*, Pl. 4, Figs. 7 and 8; Pl. 5, Figs. 1 to 7). Corresponding peripheral plasma concentrations of progesterone (as determined by radioimmunoassay) for each stage of the cycle for individual females are also provided in each figure description. In contrast to studying natural cyclic ovarian activity, Snyder and Dukelow (1974) used laparoscopy to evaluate the effect of various gonadotropin regimens on ovarian function in ewes. More recently, laparoscopy has been used to assess ovarian activity to aid in comparing the relationship of ovulation rate and serum hormone levels in various sheep breeds (Quirke *et al.*, 1979) and to determine the effect of a prostaglandin analogue on corpus luteum (CL) function (Bindon *et al.*, 1979).

Phillippo *et al.* (1971) first demonstrated the feasibility of using laparoscopy to detect early pregnancy in the ewe. Diagnosis was based on the size and form of the CL and the degree of distention and vasculature of the uterus. A positive diagnosis could be made as early as the 17th day after mating. Pregnancy was correctly diagnosed in 90.5% of the ewes and nonpregnancy in 91.5% of the animals. The number of lambs carried was correctly estimated from the number of CL in 20 out of 24 ewes. Snyder and Dukelow (1974) also studied the efficacy of laparoscopy to confirm early pregnancy. These investigators also claimed that pregnancy could be detected as early as 15 to 17 days after estrus due to the failure of the CL to visibly regress. We have observed that by day 25 of pregnancy, the uterus shows distinct distension and a variation in color from rosy pink to a grayish blue. At this early period of gestation, the uterine horns take on a segmented appearance (Pl. 5, Fig. 8; Pl. 6, Fig. 1) and the uterine epithelium becomes infiltrated by numerous large diameter vascular patterns. Neither our laboratory nor others have reported any adverse effects of laparoscopy on embryo viability or gestation length.

The pregnant sheep has served as an important animal model for the testing of fetoscopic procedures currently being used in clinical human medicine. The possible implications of fetoscopy in animal research and clinical veterinary medicine have been discussed in a previous chapter (see Chapter 3). In recent years, fetoscopy has become a potential alternative to other prenatal evaluation techniques, including amniocentesis. Some of these early studies have utilized the sheep because it is inexpensive, easily obtained, and anatomically possesses a sizable uterus with often a single conceptus.

Pregnant ewes between 85 and 95 days of gestation (term, 140 days) have been used (Morris *et al.*, 1976). In this study a percutaneous approach was used with a 2.7 mm in diameter endoscope inserted directly through the abdominal wall and into the gravid uterus. Excellent visualization of the fetus and particularly the fetoplacental circulation was reported. More recently, these investigators reported an improved technique in which the ewe was initially subjected to laparoscopy to preselect an avascular uterine site for insertion of the fetoscope (Morris *et al.*, 1977). Under direct visualization by laparoscopy, the operator guided the fetoscopic trocar-cannula unit to the uterine surface and observed its insertion. Use of the laparoscope in conjunction with the fetoscopy procedure provided several advantages. The brilliant illumination of the laparoscope allowed the detection of large, convoluted plexes of veins transversing the surface myometrium of the uterus (these were generally not noted at laparotomy). In addition, the quantity of light provided through the laparoscope when placed in close opposition to the uterine wall, transilluminated the relatively thin myometrial wall and allowed identification of underlying individual placental caruncles (characteristic of the ovine). Both of these observations apparently permitted the laparoscopist to insert the fetoscopic trocar-cannula while avoiding these vascular and placental areas. Fetoscopy was performed randomly throughout gestation with some ewes subjected to two to four such examinations. The fetus and associated blood supply apparently could be clearly visualized. The authors reported a 23.6% abortion rate in ewes in which the fetus had been directly examined endoscopically.

Ovine laparoscopy has been conducted successfully for the collection of ovarian oocytes for subsequent *in vitro* culture (Snyder and Dukelow, 1974). In this study, the ovary containing visible follicles was held stationary with ancillary laparoscopic forceps. An 18 gauge cannula was inserted at the midline at the cranial border of the mammary gland. A 23 gauge, 11 cm needle was inserted through the cannula, visually directed to the ovarian surface, and used to puncture the follicle wall. A syringe containing 2.5 ml of sterile saline was attached to the needle hub and used to aspirate the follicular contents. Ova were recovered from 28% of the follicles. This particular technique has tremendous potential as a means of supplying viable ova for *in vitro* fertilization studies.

## Termination of the Examination and Postoperative Care

The laparoscopy examination is terminated by cautiously removing the laparoscope and forceps from each respective cannula. With the valves opened on the cannulae, the gas can be evacuated from the cavity by manually pressing the abdominal wall dorsally. The cannulae are removed from the peritoneal cavity and the two puncture sites closed with Michel clamps or suture. It is unnecessary to repair the site at which the insufflation cannula is inserted.

Following closure of the incision sites, the anesthetized animal is closely monitored during the recovery phase. The sheep should be placed on straw within view of the laparoscopy team. Animals anesthetized with pentobarbital will attempt to stand approximately 30 minutes after examination and are moving rather normally 60 minutes postsurgery. As with most ruminants, bloating may develop after anesthesia. To prevent this occurrence, the sheep should be positioned with the head and neck extended away from the thorax.

In field or certain research circumstances, the setting often does not permit laparoscopy to be performed under sterile surgical conditions conducive to avoiding infections. In addition, one of the main advantages of laparoscopy for the researcher is the simplicity and speed with which an abdominal cavity examination can be made. When a number of animals are to be examined, normally the most time consuming role is played by the assistants who must anesthetize, restrain, and surgically prepare each ewe.

Under such circumstances, to avoid infection problems, the laparoscopist should be concerned with two critical actions. First, it is imperative to thoroughly clean the instruments between examinations, particularly the laparoscope, trocar-cannula, and accessory forceps. The ethanol decontamination procedure described previously is sufficient to maintain relatively disinfected instrumentation. Second, the laparoscopist should not be involved in the preparation of the animals. The operator should recall that to properly restrain and surgically prepare the animal highly contaminated anatomical areas of the sheep cannot be avoided (i.e., legs, anal and vaginal areas, inguinal region). Consequently, if possible, the operator should concern himself only with handling the endoscopic instruments, supervising the adequate surgical preparation of the operation site, and conducting the laparoscopic observations. Minimally, the laparoscopist should disinfect the hands and wear and change sterile surgical gloves after each individual examination. As a means of postoperative prophylaxis, a broad spectrum antibiotic or a combination of antibiotic drugs that cover the range of gram-positive and gram-negative bacteria should be administered intramuscularly.

## General Results, Complications, and Contraindications

Previous researchers who have desired frequent laparoscopy for the sheep have advocated the use of an indwelling cannula (Lamond and Holmes, 1965; Dierschke and Hyatt, 1969; Boyd and Ducker, 1975). The problems with this chronic fistula technique have been discussed earlier in the chapter. The indwelling cannula may be helpful in the event that laparoscopy is required at 24 hour intervals or less; however, further study is required to assure that such a chronic implant does not adversely disturb certain physiologic events, including ovulation. In our experiments, laparoscopy by means of a midventral approach is generally performed at 48 hour intervals which is not contraindicated. As many as 10 ovarian examinations within a single animal's 18 day cycle have been conducted without consequence. Snyder and Dukelow (1974) reported a similar frequency of examinations and a total of 170 laparoscopies in 19 ewes. In our experiments, 619 examinations were performed with one ewe subjected to 17 laparoscopies. Several other animals underwent 10 to 12 such examinations. During the course of the study, five sheep died as a result of anesthetic accident.

It is possible during insertion of the laparoscopic trocar-cannula to additionally penetrate the rumen, small intestine, or colon. This generally occurs only in unfasted animals. If digested or fecal material is not laparoscopically observed to escape into the peritoneal cavity, it is sufficient to remove the instruments and simply administer a high dosage of antibiotic (one million units of penicillin-streptomycin). Infection does not usually occur. However, if the animal is exhibiting diarrhea, which inevitably results in fecal contamination of the abdominal cavity, postoperative complications can occur. In our study, one animal died as a result of trocar penetration of the intestine. This individual was noted to have diarrhea; laparoscopic observation of the intestinal site immediately after puncture confirmed the escape of ingesta into the peritoneal cavity. If this problem occurs, the operator should immediately perform laparotomy to repair the intestinal perforation and then treat the animal intensively with antibiotics.

Another complication is adhesion development attributable to the laparoscopy procedures. Although obviously fewer in number and extent than that observed following laparotomy, nevertheless, adhesions do form following repeated examination. Sheep with extensive adhesion development are very difficult, if not impossible, to laparoscopically examine.

Insertion of the trocar-cannula at a site too far cranially will result in the laparoscope being located on the anterior side of the omental net. This is indicated when the operator has no clear view of the organs and instead observes only fatty-whitish appearing surroundings. This may be corrected by retracting the telescope and cannula until the ends of each approach the ventral abdominal wall. The assembly should then be directed caudally against the ventral wall to escape the omentum. The use of accessory forceps to manipulate the omentum from the terminal viewing lens of the endoscope may also be helpful.

Due to anatomical location of widespread vasculature in the ventral abdominal wall, it is possible to inadvertently sever a vessel during insertion of the trocar-cannula. This occurrence can be frustrating and sometimes serious if hemorrhage is extensive. Blood will generally flow down the barrel of the telescope, clotting, and hindering visualization from the terminal lens. The cannula-laparoscope assembly should be removed from the peritoneal cavity, the puncture site repaired, and the laparoscope reinserted at an adjacent (usually caudal and lateral) avascular location. Extensive continued hemorrhage may necessitate additional surgery to ligate the severed vessel.

Possible side effects of the laparoscopy procedure on reproduction may exist. Previous research has indicated that anesthetics, including sodium pentobarbital, halothane, ether, and morphine can prevent or delay ovulation in small laboratory animals (Whitehead and Ruf, 1973; Chappel and Barraclough, 1976; Packman and Rothchild, 1976). These drugs have been shown to specifically act by altering the pituitary release of preovulatory gonadotropins, FSH and LH. The authors are unaware of similar evidence for this adverse effect occurring in sheep anesthetized with pentobarbital. In addition, laparoscopy has not been shown to disturb reproductive cyclicity of this species (Thimonier and Mauleon, 1969; Seeger, 1973). It is possible that the operation and particularly aggressive manipulation of the uteroovarian anatomy could conceivably alter reproductive function. It would be interesting to investigate the effect of laparoscopic manipulation on the conveyance of the luteolysin prostaglandin $F_{2\alpha}$ from the uterine mucosa to the corpus luteum, or the effect of vigorous laparoscopy on serum concentrations of reproductive hormones. It has recently been demonstrated that laparoscopy performed at 48 hour intervals during proestrus and estrus has no effect on serum concentrations of LH, estradiol-17$\beta$, and progesterone in the female dog (see Chapter 3). Similar study deserves investigation in other species, including the sheep.

## Laparoscopic Photography and Records

A major advantage of laparoscopy for the researcher is that observations can be easily documented by photography (Fig. 6.5). Illumination provided by our electronic flash system simulates daylight, hence, daylight films are used to produce realistic colors. Excellent results have been obtained using Kodachrome II (ASA 25). Color slide film is recommended which later can be converted to color or black and white prints.

Photographic results vary with the type of instrumentation used. The above described film used with a different size laparoscope or illumination source may not produce quality photographs. No commercial information on the intensity of our electronic flash system is available. This particular light generator does produce three photographic light intensities. The ovary with distinct, prominent structures such as CL can be photographed with any of the flash intensities. Inactive ovaries or ovaries containing follicles are more successfully photographed with the lowest intensity. In this case, brighter illumination can result in pictures with a blanched, or "washed out" appearance or poor contrast. The photolaparoscopist should also remember that the variation in photograph quality is often more a result of variation in the distance between the terminal lens of the endoscope and the target organ than due to absolute intensity of the light generator.

We have had no experience with photographic documentation using illumination sources with only the 150 watt diagnostic lamp. Jarosz *et al.* (1971) had success with photographing the ovary of the goat using a 5 mm in diameter, 130° laparoscope and a 150 watt diagnostic lamp.

It should be stressed that it is of extreme importance to keep records of photographs as well as written explanations of observations. The operator should not rely on memory with respect to observations or photographic records. A simple method of identifying photographs consists of giving each roll of film an identification number. After loading the film, the camera is used to photograph a sheet of paper containing the identification number, the animal number to be examined, the date and the particular experimental protocol. Similar sheets are photographed between animal examinations. Although this requires considerable film, the expense is secondary compared to the elimination of confusion upon return of the processed film.

## CONCLUSIONS

The sheep, because of its ready availability and minor expense, will continue to play a valuable role in various physiologic experimentations. As in most other comparatively large domestic animals, laparoscopy, to date, has not been utilized to its fullest in terms of surgical or research usefulness. Our results and others have indicated the effectiveness of laparoscopy for general observation of the reproductive organs, bladder, and portions of the gastrointestinal tract. Certainly, further investigations will be conducted in the near future to ascertain the full potential of laparoscopy in this species.

**References**

Bindon, B. M., Blanc, M. R., Pelletier, J., Terqui, M., and Thimonier, J. (1979) Periovulatory gonadotrophin and ovarian steroid patterns in sheep of breeds with differing fecundity. *J. Reprod. Fertil.* 55:15–25.

Blockey, M. A. deB., Englund, I. K. J., and Cumming, I. A. (1972) A modified surgical cradle for mass laparotomy of ewes. *Aust. Vet. J.* 48:564–566.

Boyd, J. S., and Ducker, M. J. (1973) A method of examining the cyclic changes occurring in the sheep ovary using endoscopy. *Vet. Rec.* 93:40–43.

Boyd, J. S., and Ducker, M. J. (1975) A preliminary

report on the use of a chronic peritoneal fistula for endoscopic examination of ovine ovarian activity. *Vet. Rec.* 96:78–81.

Chappel, S. C., and Barraclough, C. A. (1976) The effects of sodium pentobarbital or ether anesthesia on spontaneous and electrochemically-induced gonadotropin release. *Proc. Soc. Exp. Biol. Med.* 153: 1–6.

Dierschke, D. J., and Hyatt, J. L. (1969) Peritoneoscopy via a chronically implanted cannula to observe ovarian activity in ewes. *J. Anim. Sci.* 28:645–649.

Dukelow, W. R., Jarosz, S. J., Jewett, D. A., and Harrison, R. M. (1971) Laparoscopic examination of the ovaries in goats and primates. *Lab. Anim. Sci.* 21:594–597.

Hulet, C. V., and Foote, W. C. (1968) A rapid technique for observing the reproductive tract of living ewes. *J. Anim. Sci.* 27:142–145.

Jarosz, S. J., Deans, R. J., and Dukelow, W. R. (1971) The reproductive cycle of the African Pygmy and Toggenburg goat. *J. Reprod. Fertil.* 24:119–123.

Lamond, D. R., and Holmes, J. H. G. (1965) Suitable endoscope and laparotomy techniques for ovarian activity in the cow. *Aust. Vet. J.* 41:324–328.

Morris, J. A., Davidson, E. C., Maidman, J. C., Arce, J. J., Brown, J. E., and Frazer, R. (1976) Sampling the fetoplacental circulation. I. The pregnant ovine. *Am. J. Obstet. Gynecol.* 125:1121–1124.

Morris, J. A., Davidson, E. C., Maidman, J. C., Arce, J. J., Brown, J. E., and Frazer, R. (1977) Sampling the fetoplacental circulation. II. Combined laparoscopy-fetoscopy in the pregnant ovine. *Am. J. Obstet. Gynecol.* 128:279–286.

Muurling, F. (1971) Oestrische en ovariële aktiviteit bij Texelse schapen in Nederland (Oestrual and ovarian activity in Texel sheep in the Netherlands).

Dissertation Rijksuniversiteit Utrecht.

Muurling, F. (1972) Oestrische en ovariële aktiviteit bij Texelse schapen in Nederland (Oestrual and ovarian activity in Texel sheep in the Netherlands). *Tijdschr. Diergeneeskd.* 97:401–407.

Packman, P. M., and Rothchild, J. A. (1976) Morphine inhibition of ovulation: Reversal by naloxone. *Endocrinology* 99:7–10.

Phillippo, M., Swapp, G. H., Robinson, J. J., and Gill, J. C. (1971) The diagnosis of pregnancy and estimation of fetal numbers in sheep by laparoscopy. *J. Reprod. Fertil.* 27:129–132.

Quirke, J. F., Hanrahan, J. P., and Gosling, J. P. (1979) Plasma progesterone levels throughout the estrous cycle and release of LH at estrus in sheep with different ovulation rates. *J. Reprod. Fertil.* 55:37–44.

Roberts, E. M. (1968) Endoscopy of the reproductive tract of the ewe. *Proc. Aust. Soc. Anim. Prod.* 7: 192–194.

Seeger, K. (1973) Die Laparoskopie, eine Technik zur Routineuntersuchung des Genitaltrakts beim Schaf. *Tieraerztl. Prax.* 1:295–299.

Seeger, K. (1977) Laparoscopic investigation of the bovine ovary. *Vet. Med. Small Anim. Clin.* 72:1037–1044.

Snyder, D. A., and Dukelow, W. R. (1974) Laparoscopic studies of ovulation, pregnancy diagnosis, and follicle aspiration in sheep. *Theriogenology* 2: 143–148.

Thimonier, J., and Mauleon, P. (1969) Variations saisonnières du comportement d'oestrus et des activités ovariennes et hypophysaires chez les ovins. *Ann. Biol. Anim., Biochim. Biophys.* 9:233–250.

Whitehead, S., and Ruf, K. B. (1973) The effects of halothane on ovulation in the rat. *Experientia* 29: 880–881.

# CHAPTER 7

# Laparoscopy in the Pig*

## David E. Wildt, Ph.D.

### INTRODUCTION

Laparoscopy has been used in the pig for reproductive research studies (Wildt *et al.*, 1973; Wildt *et al.*, 1975). Fortunately, it is not often necessary to subject pigs to anesthesia and laparotomy for clinical diagnoses. Nevertheless, laparoscopy can be utilized safely and effectively in most sizes of pigs whenever it is necessary to examine or sample organs of the peritoneal cavity. The basic technique of laparoscopy in the pig is quite similar to that described in the previous chapter for the sheep. Modifications are necessary in terms of anesthesia and the site of laparoscope insertion.

### LAPAROSCOPIC TECHNIQUE

#### Animals, Anesthesia, and Restraint

Techniques reported in this chapter are based on research investigations involving 64 pre- or postpuberal gilts ranging from 5 to 12 months of age and 82 to 145 kg in body weight. All animals were of the Yorkshire, Hampshire, or Yorkshire-Hampshire crossbred type and maintained under standard dietary and housing conditions. The smaller the pig, the easier it is to perform the endoscopic examination. However, depending on proper anesthetization and restraint, variations in age, size, and breed of pig do not appear to limit the overall effectiveness of laparoscopy in this species.

#### *PREEXAMINATION PREPARATION OF ANIMALS*

Withholding food and water immediately prior to the operation is not an absolute prerequisite for the pig, particularly when the examination is limited to the reproductive tract. The anesthetized pig rarely vomits and, with proper abdominal insufflation, even a distended gut does not interfere markedly with observation of the reproductive organs. As a rule, feed is withheld the day of the laparoscopy if the reproductive tract is to be

* This work was conducted at the Endocrine Research Unit, Michigan State University. The author acknowledges the support of this laboratory's director, Dr. W. Richard Dukelow, and the assistance of colleagues, Drs. C. B. Morcom and J. L. Spencer.

examined and for 24 hours if a gastrointestinal, hepatic, or splenic examination is scheduled. Water is always provided *ad libitum*. Catheterization of the bladder is not performed. The problem of a distended bladder inhibiting laparoscopic visualization is solved using the superpubic puncture procedure described in Chapters 3 and 4.

Because of difficulty in handling and due to the large animal size, laparoscopy in the pig generally requires the laparoscopist and at least one assistant. If a series of animals require laparoscopy, the procedure is greatly facilitated by the presence of the operator and two assistants. This number of personnel is generally required to adequately record results, induce anesthesia, monitor animal recovery, and maintain a relatively aseptic operational field.

## ANESTHESIA

Laparoscopy in the pig is performed with the animal in a surgical plane of anesthesia. The author has made several unsuccessful attempts to subject gilts to laparoscopy using tranquilization and a paralumbar approach (similar to that described for the cow and horse). General anesthesia and midventral insertion of the laparoscope appear to be, by far, the superior technique for this species. The use of gaseous anesthesia administered in a rebreathing system is undoubtedly the safest and most satisfactory form of general anesthesia in swine (Jennings, 1971). Intravenous injection for induction of anesthesia is difficult due to the sparsity of superficial veins and the temperament of the species. Virtually the only peripheral vasculature that can be used for intravenous injection is that of the ear or the anterior vena cava. The former can be observed readily but is of small caliber and not suitable for injections of large volumes of fluids. This approach is often frustrated by the pig shaking its head when attempts are made to inject into the ear vein. The author has had success administering the anesthetic drug via the anterior vena cava. Initial restraint of the pig is accomplished using a nose snare and the anterior vena cava is located by inserting a 7 cm, 18 gauge needle in the vicinity of the junction of the first rib and sternum. The drug most frequently used has been sodium pentobarbital (Halatal Solution, Jen-Sal Laboratories, 65 mg/ml) which has been used either as the initial induction agent or for producing the surgical plane of anesthesia. For the latter purpose, sodium pentobarbital at a variable dosage of 10 to 32 mg/kg body weight is required. Unmated gilts require significantly more of this drug/kg body weight than pregnant gilts to achieve similar planes of surgical anesthesia. A surgical plane for the pig is generally judged by the observation of slow, regular respiration, slight palpebral reflex, and a relaxed musculature and jaw.

Pentobarbital is a poor analgesic, and relatively high doses must be administered before pain perception is inhibited. This drug has a marked depressant effect on the medullary respiratory centers and the high dose required to achieve a plane of surgical anesthesia conducive to laparoscopy approaches the lethal dose capable of eliciting respiratory failure. Consequently, operators using sodium pentobarbital should have access to respiratory stimulants such as pentylenetetrazol (Am-Pent, Jen-Sal Laboratories) or doxapram hydrochloride (Dopram-V, A. H. Robins Co.) for intravenous administration.

The dose level of sodium pentobarbital used is directly proportional to the rate at which it is administered. In general, injections of this drug are administered in 10 ml increments. The first unit produces basal narcosis and usually allows the pig to be restrained in a dorsal-supine position. If a surgical plane of anesthesia is to be induced and maintained with gas, this basal narcotic state allows the snout of the pig to be masked for inhalation anesthesia. If pentobarbital alone is to be utilized, additional units of this drug are administered at approximately five minute intervals until the proper plane of anesthesia is achieved (Fig 7.1). The pig generally remains totally immobilized for 30 to 50 minutes. Recovery occurs in two to five hours and no adverse effects have been observed resulting from three times weekly sodium pentobarbital administration.

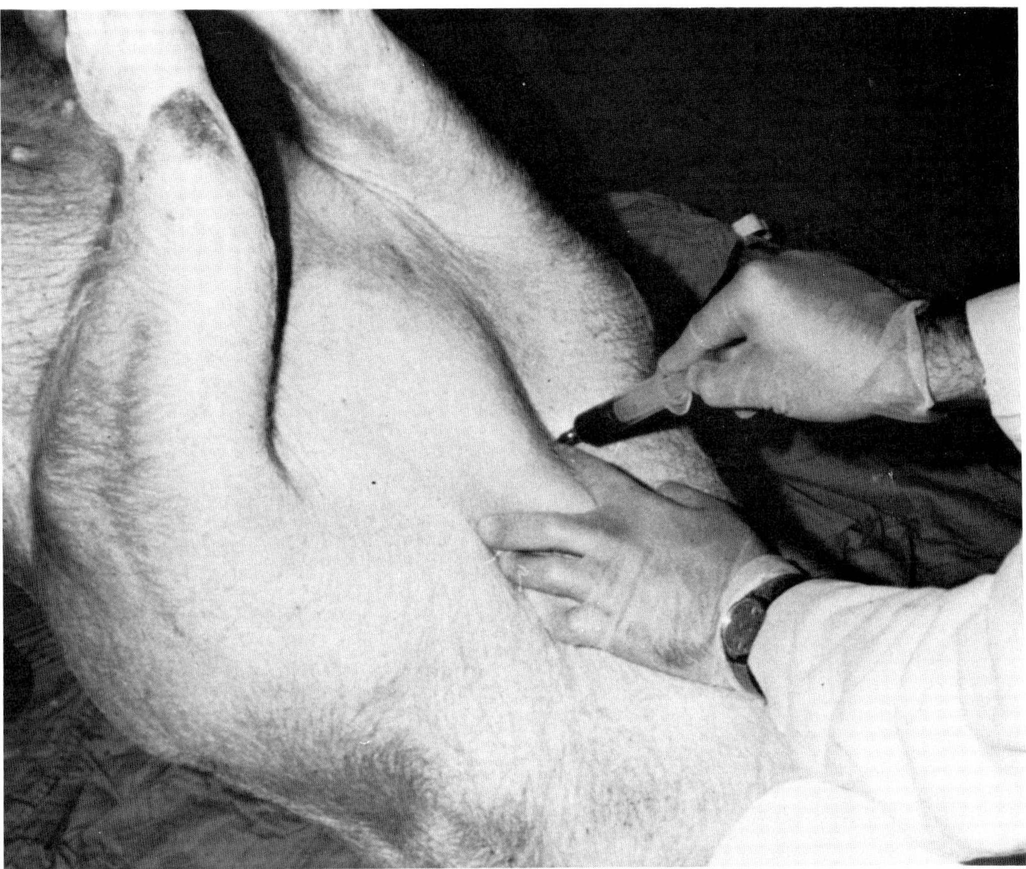

**Figure 7.1**   Administration of the anesthetic drug intravenously into the anterior vena cava.

Thiopental sodium is also reported as an excellent drug for inducing anesthesia in swine (Jennings, 1971). The recommended dosage given as a 5 or 10% solution is 29 mg/kg for small pigs and 24 mg/kg for large pigs adminstered via the ear vein or anterior vena cava. There is also at least one report concerning the use of ketamine hydrochloride (Ketaset, Bristol Laboratories) administered intramuscularly for immobilizing pigs (Rossoff, 1974). The high recommended dosage (29 mg/kg), however, would likely make the routine use of this drug economically unfeasible. Ketaset for inducing swine anesthesia should likely be considered as a last resort in the event that previous attempts at intravenous injections of barbiturates have been unsuccessful.

Fortunately, the shape of the snout of the pig is quite conducive to the fitting of a face mask. Safe and satisfactory anesthesia can be maintained in pigs using this method and no endotracheal intubation. Halothane is an excellent inhalation anesthetic agent for swine. Recently, Morcom and Dukelow (unpublished data) have reported excellent anesthetic results for pig laparoscopy using sodium pentobarbital injected intravenously as the inducing agent and a combination of halothane (Fluothane, Ayerst Laboratories) and nitrous oxide as the maintenance anesthetic.

## RESTRAINT

The anesthetized pig is restrained on its back on a standard surgical table with tilt capacity. As in other species, the target organ to be viewed dictates the positioning of the table. For insertion of instruments and observation of the caudal abdominal cavity contents, the table is angled to the Trendelenburg position. To observe the cranial portion of the peritoneal cavity following laparoscope placement, the table is returned to a flat, 180° plane. In examinations in which only the reproductive organs are to be viewed, the animal can be placed head down on a simply constructed, sloped (30°) trough table (Fig. 7.2). The table is modified from that described by Hulet and Foote (1968) and Jarosz et al. (1971). The animal is supported in this position primarily by a leather strap encompassing the neck and attached to the anterior portion of the table (Fig. 7.3). The hind legs are bound loosely, allowing the greatest proportion of weight to be supported by the neck strap.

## Equipment

### LAPAROSCOPE AND TROCAR-CANNULA ASSEMBLY

The endoscope used in these studies consisted of a 5 mm in diameter, 130° laparoscope, 20 cm in length (Richard Wolf Medical Instruments Corp.). The pig, however, is readily adaptable to a variety of rigid laparoscopes of standard lengths and from 5 to 10 mm in diameter. For easy organ identification, examination, and photographic documentation in adult swine, a laparoscope of 8 to 10 mm in diameter is preferable. The desired angle of the direction of view of the endoscope is based on the operator's experience and personal preferences (see Chapter 3).

The trocar-cannula assembly must correspond to the diameter of the laparoscopic telescope. Either the pyramidal or conical tip trocar is satisfactory. It is advantageous that the cannula contain a trumpet or clip valve and side arm sleeve to assist in producing and maintaining a pneumoperitoneum.

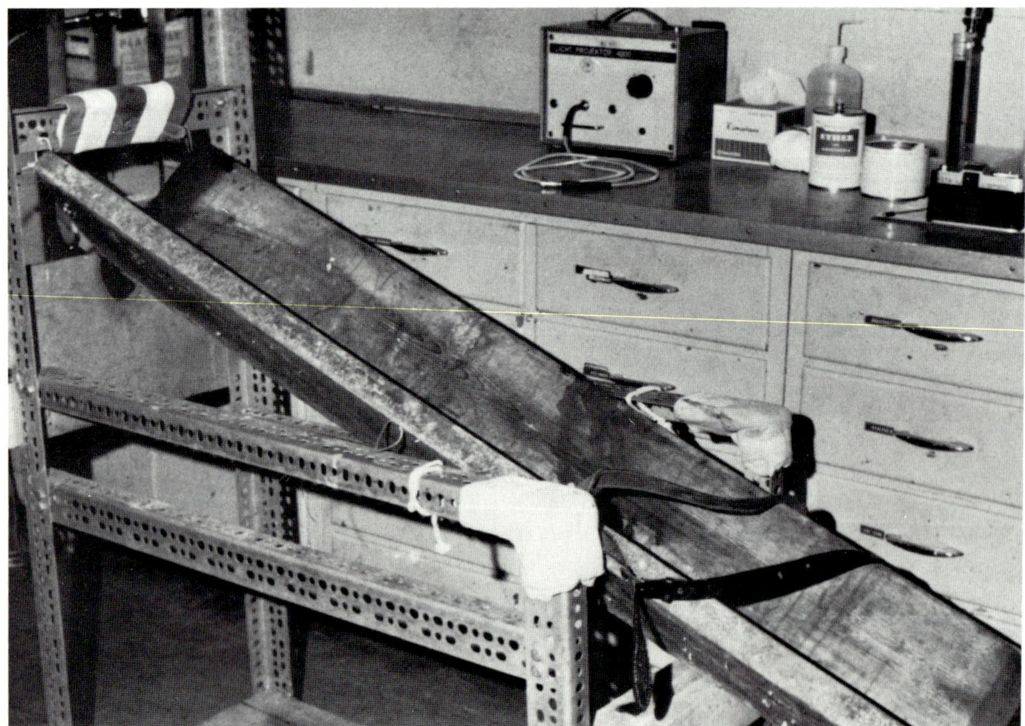

**Figure 7.2**   A self constructed, sloped trough table suitable for pig laparoscopy.

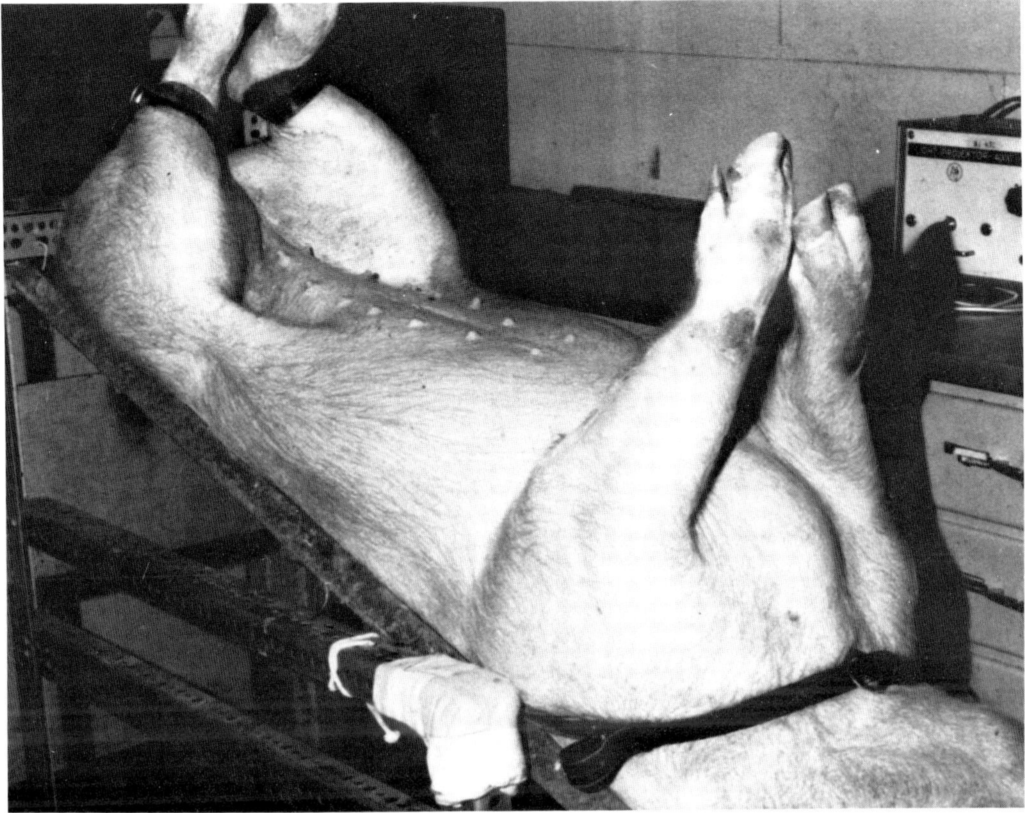

**Figure 7.3**  The pig supported in the Trendelenburg position. Most of the animal weight is supported by the encompassing neck strap.

## ILLUMINATION SOURCE AND PNEUMOPERITONEUM INSTRUMENTATION

Since most pig laparoscopy is associated with research investigation, a light source and cable capable of providing illumination adequate for photographic documentation should be utilized. These devices are discussed in detail in Chapter 12. The most inexpensive sources contain a single 150 watt lamp which allows diagnostic examination but inadequate illumination for quality photography of the internal organs of the pig.

The creation of a pneumoperitoneum is a prerequisite for satisfactory laparoscopic visualization in this species. Although convenient, a commercial pneumoperitoneum apparatus is probably an unnecessary expense for those operators performing only swine laparoscopy. A suitable alternative is to simply insufflate the animal directly from a commercial tank containing either 100% carbon dioxide ($CO_2$) or 5% $CO_2$ in air. When using this technique, the precautions outlined in Chapter 3 should be considered closely. Insufflation prior to laparoscope insertion requires a Verres needle, approximately 150 mm in length.

## SURGICAL AND ACCESSORY LAPAROSCOPIC INSTRUMENTS

A scalpel and blade, thumb forceps, needle holder, and suture (3-0 Dexon absorbable suture, American Cyanamid Co.) are required. Due to the elongated anatomy of the uterine horns and the vast length and coiled position of the small and large intestines, a secondary forceps or probe is frequently required for manipulation (the Verres needle used for this function in the dog, cat, and monkey is of insufficient length in the adult pig). An ancillary probe (5 mm in diameter, 29 cm in length) is produced by at least one manufacturer (Richard Wolf Medical Instruments Corp.) which is of adequate size for use in swine. This tactile probe is graduated with centimeter markings, which allows intraabdominal measurement and, as will be described, can be inserted directly through the abdominal wall or through an accessory 6 mm in diameter cannula. As an alternative method, an accessory forceps can be inserted through the secondary cannula and used for internal manipulation. Any of a variety of forceps are practical in this species. Maximum versatility is achieved by the use of a combination forceps, such as the Palmer forceps (see Chapter 3, Fig. 3.9) which allows manipulation and the added potential of biopsy and electrocoagulation.

The author is unaware of any one camera being superior for laparoscopic photography in the pig. The operator should consider utilizing camera, film types, and techniques successfully used in the dog and cat (see Chapter 3) or nonhuman primate (see Chapter 4).

### Surgical Preparation

In research investigations, the laparoscopic examinations have not been performed using sterile techniques. The pig does not appear to be predisposed to the development of infections following such minor invasive surgery as laparoscopy. Laparoscopic instruments are disinfected by brief (10 to 20 minutes) immersion in benzalkonium chloride (Zephiran, Winthrop Laboratories) or chlorhexidine (Nolvasan-S, Fort Dodge Laboratories, Inc.). If necessary, the caudal portion of the ventral region is clipped of hair. This area is scrubbed either with benzalkonium chloride or a povidone-iodine solution (Betadine, Purdue Frederick Co.). The laparoscopist should wear sterile surgical gloves during the examination.

### Insufflation, Instrument Insertion, and Termination of the Operation

A pneumoperitoneum is necessary to adequately observe internal organs of the pig. However, if the small 5 mm in diameter laparoscope is scheduled for use, insufflation does *not* necessarily have to be performed *before* inserting the corresponding laparoscopic trocar-cannula. Avoiding preinsufflation eliminates the danger of false placement of gas between the skin and peritoneum or into bowel or bladder. Little chance of perforating internal organs exists when using the 6 mm in diameter trocar-cannula assembly in a pig that is not insufflated.

The experienced operator using a greater diameter endoscope and corresponding cannula unit may prefer preinsertion insufflation. Following surgical preparation of the ventral abdominal region, the Verres needle is inserted through the abdominal wall at a site on the midline, 2 to 4 cm caudal to the umbilicus depending on animal size (see Chapter 3 on the mechanics and insertion of this device). The hose from the gas source is attached and gas passed into the cavity. Generally 2 to 4 liters of gas are required; insufflation continues until the ventral abdominal wall appears slightly distended. The Verres needle may then be removed from the peritoneal cavity.

The site of the trocar-cannula insertion is on the midline in the vicinity of the umbilicus. For examination of the reproductive organs, the skin incision is made 2 to 8 cm caudal to the umbilicus (Fig. 7.4); for observation of the anterior abdominal contents, the incision is made at the umbilicus or within 6 cm cranial to this site. The length of the incision depends on the diameter of the trocar-cannula assembly used. As a rule, the length of the incision should generally be extended 0.5 to 1.0 cm longer than the diameter of the trocar-cannula assembly. The latter is then passed subdermally about 2 cm and then directed dorsally at a 60° angle through the musculature of the abdominal wall (Fig 7.5). Because of the relatively thick subdermal fat and muscular wall in this

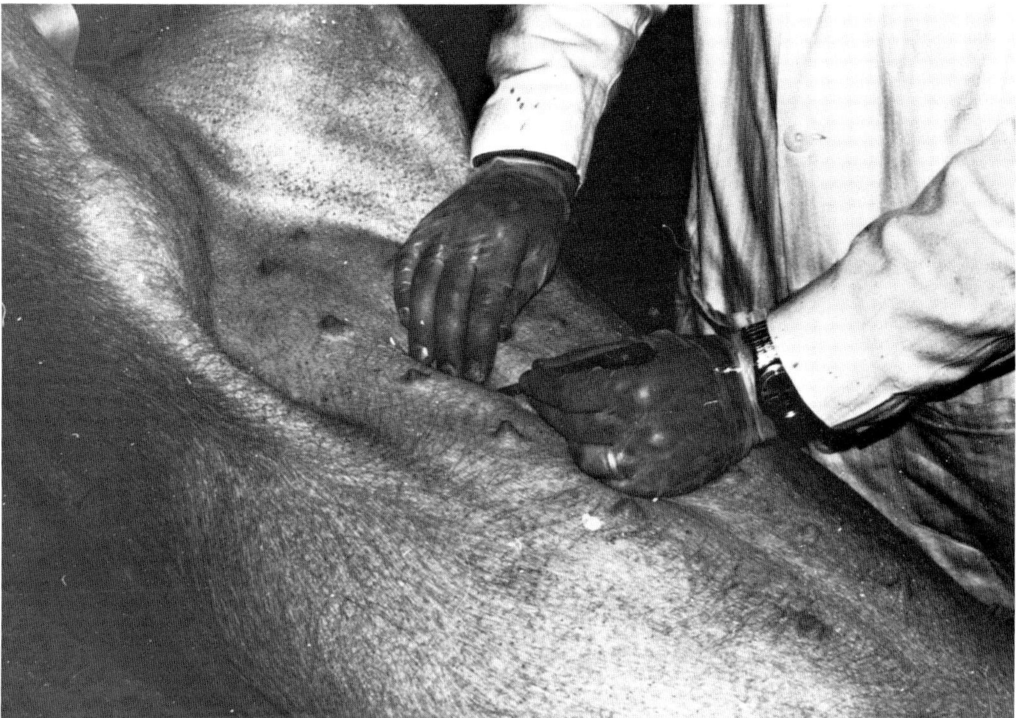

**Figure 7.4** The skin incision through which the laparoscopic trocar-cannula unit is inserted is made 2 to 8 cm caudal to the umbilicus.

species, this insertion procedure allows natural closure of the incision after examination and alleviates concern of possible herniation.

The trocar is removed and the laparoscope is introduced through the cannula (Fig. 7.6). Additional insufflation is sometimes required during the examination and this can be accomplished by attaching the gas hose directly to the sleeve of the midline cannula (Fig. 7.6). The operator should immediately scan the abdominal cavity to ensure against possible complications due to the insertion technique (i.e., hemorrhage or perforated bowel).

The laparoscopist then determines the necessity of ancillary manipulatory instruments. In reproductive studies involving internal maneuvering of the uterus and ovaries, a secondary 0.5 cm skin incision is made 4 cm caudal and 10 cm lateral to the midline incision. The tactile probe does not require intromission through a previously inserted cannula. This instrument can simply be thrust through the muscle and peritoneal layers (Fig 7.7). Manipulation (Fig. 7.8) of this probe is considerably more flexible and versatile when this direct technique is utilized. Because of the thick abdominal wall, insertion through the accessory cannula actually restricts the maneuvering capabilities of this probe. The accessory trocar-cannula is used for the insertion of an ancillary grasping, biopsy, or cautery forceps (Fig. 7.9). Both the tactile probe and accessory trocar-cannula are inserted by holding each device at a 70 to 80° angle to the plane of the body with the tip of the probe or trocar pointed at a 45° angle to the animal's ventral midline.

At the end of the examination, all instruments are withdrawn with the exception of the midline cannula which is used to assist in the evacuation of the pneumoperitoneum. Using a 1 cm skin incision and the described subdermal insertion technique, suturing the puncture site is unnecessary. If a larger diameter trocar-cannula unit is used, 1 to 3 sutures are placed in the skin layer only. An antibacterial ointment or powder is applied

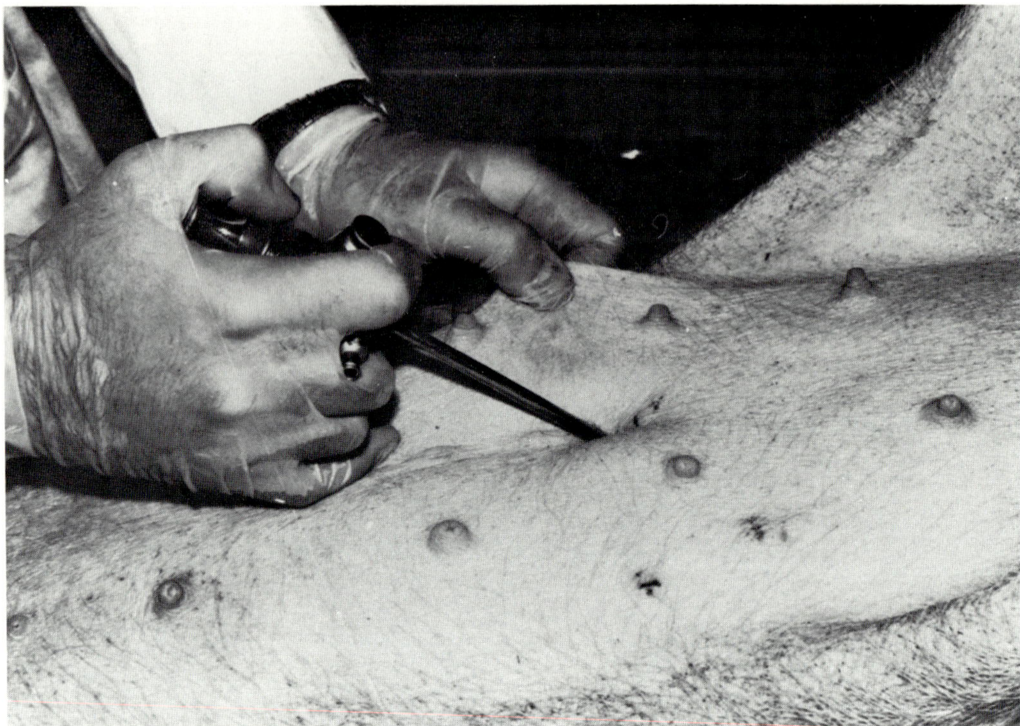

**Figure 7.5**   Insertion of the trocar-cannula assembly. The abdominal wall is supported with the operator's free hand.

to the incision site(s) and a penicillin-streptomycin solution (600,000 units penicillin, 750 mg streptomycin) is administered intramuscularly as a prophylactic measure. The pig is transferred to suitable quarters for recovery.

## CAPABILITIES OF LAPAROSCOPY IN THE PIG

### General Visualization and Complications

As in other species, most abdominal organs can be visualized in the pig using laparoscopy. Because of the amount of gut and sheer size of most major organs, the extent of visualization of a specific target site is directly related to the proper positioning of the animal. A slight alteration in the Trendelenburg angle can dramatically affect the observational field. The novice in large animal laparoscopy who is experiencing visual difficulty can alleviate much of the frustration by experimenting with variations in animal positioning. It should also be noted that the immobilized pig under the influence of the described anesthetic combinations tolerates various Trendelenburg angles quite satisfactorily without cardiac or respiratory distress.

Complications or technique problems are similar to those reported in previous chapters for other species. Infrequently, the operator may induce a bowel perforation upon insertion of a trocar-cannula. Although preferable, in the author's experience, it is not always necessary to subject the animal to immediate laparotomy to repair the puncture site, particularly if the smaller 6 mm in diameter trocar-cannula is being utilized. In all instances in which this has occurred, animals have recovered unevent-

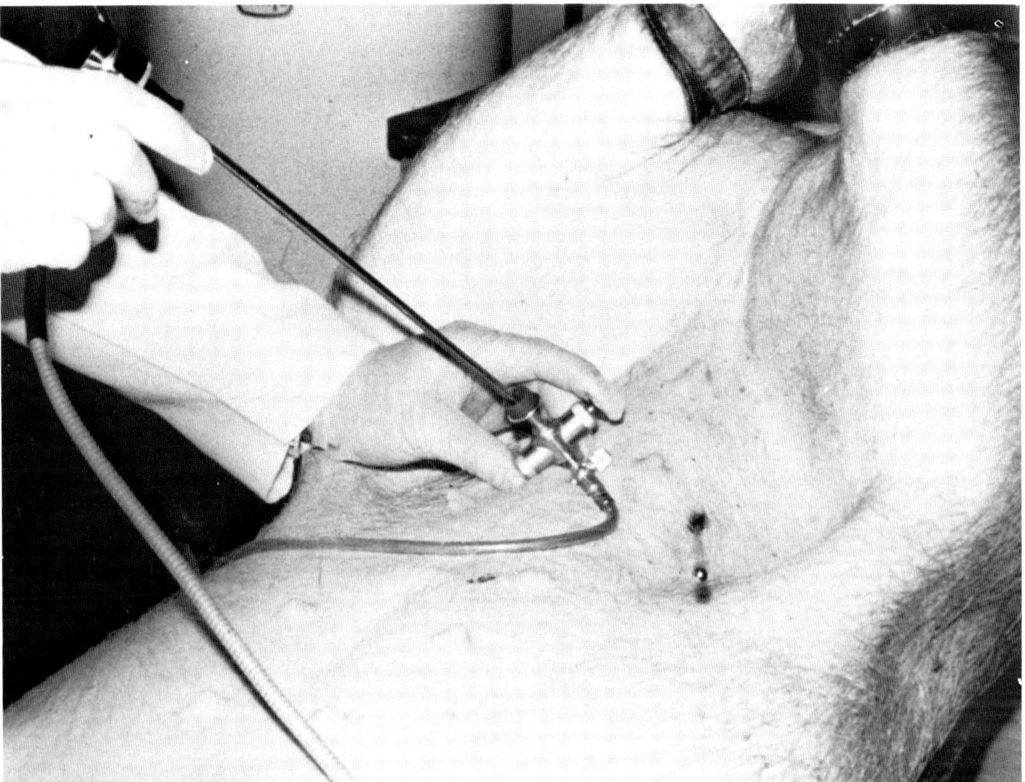

**Figure 7.6** Insertion of the laparoscope into the cannula. The gas hose is fixed directly to the sleeve of the cannula.

fully, even in several cases where small amounts of ingesta were noted to be leaking into the peritoneal cavity.

The pig can endure rather frequent laparoscopy. With respect to serial examination, response to anesthesia and not laparoscopy appears to be the limiting factor. Gilts have been subjected to laparoscopy as often as three times per week for two weeks using sodium pentobarbital as the single anesthetic agent.

## Clinical Aspects

Endoscopic techniques which have clinical application in other species such as the dog or cat (see Chapter 3) would likely, if needed, be adaptable to the pig. The author's experience in swine laparoscopy has been almost exclusively for reproductive organ evaluation. After identification of the gut, the elongated uterine horns are usually immediately observed. Minor manipulation of each horn with the accessory probe or forceps leads to the visualization of the ovary, which is usually located near the dorsolateral wall enclosed by the mesovarium or fimbria. Slight manipulation with the probe allows this mesentery to be removed for unobstructed observation of the ovary. The following types of reproductive studies have been successfully conducted using laparoscopy.

### DOCUMENTATION OF OVARIAN ACTIVITY

Ovarian structures, including preovulatory follicles, corpora hemorrhagica and/or corpora lutea (CL), are readily distinguishable using laparoscopy. The magnification

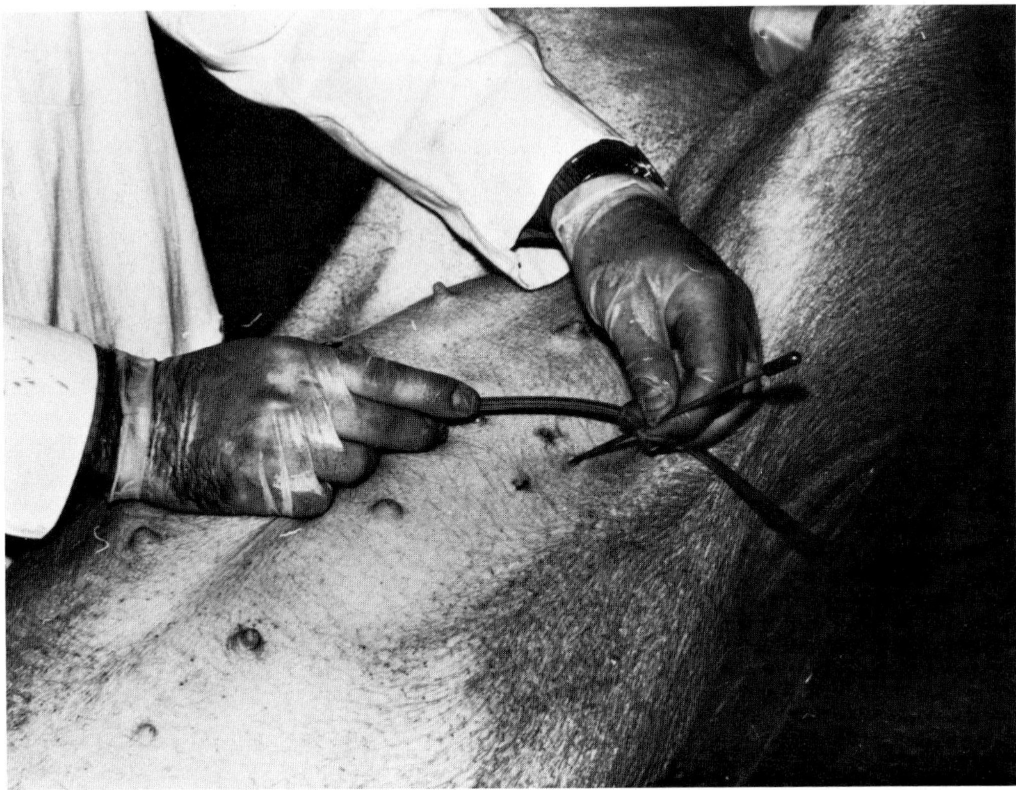

**Figure 7.7**   Insertion of the tactile probe directly through the abdominal wall without the use of an ancillary cannula.

characteristic of the rigid endoscope allows the study of subtle morphological alterations in follicular or luteal coloration and vasculature. Laparoscopy is a particularly efficient means of ascertaining ovulation rate. In one study, laparoscopy was used to count ovarian CL three to six days after expected ovulation. Five gilts were examined and then slaughtered one or two days after laparoscopy and the ovaries examined for the number of CL. There was no significant difference between the number of CL observed with laparoscopy and the number observed directly.

## PREGNANCY DIAGNOSIS

Pregnancy detection and the effects of pregnancy on reproductive tract morphology during gestation have been studied in pigs with laparoscopy (Wildt *et al.*, 1975). Twenty mature gilts, mated twice on the second day of estrus, underwent one laparoscopic examination at various stages of pregnancy. Confirmation of pregnancy was based on gross uterine appearance, including overall size, increase in uterine vascularization, and the detection of uterine conceptus sites. An additional nine pregnant gilts similarly mated served as controls. All gilts were killed between days 40 and 45 of gestation, the reproductive tracts recovered and the fetuses measured and weighed.

Pregnancy was easily detected in five gilts examined during the fourth and fifth week of gestation (days 28 to 33) because of the large size of the reproductive tract. Reproductive status was correctly predicted in 10 gilts examined between days 12 and 20 of gestation; six were pregnant. Correct predictions were made for only two of five gilts examined seven days after mating.

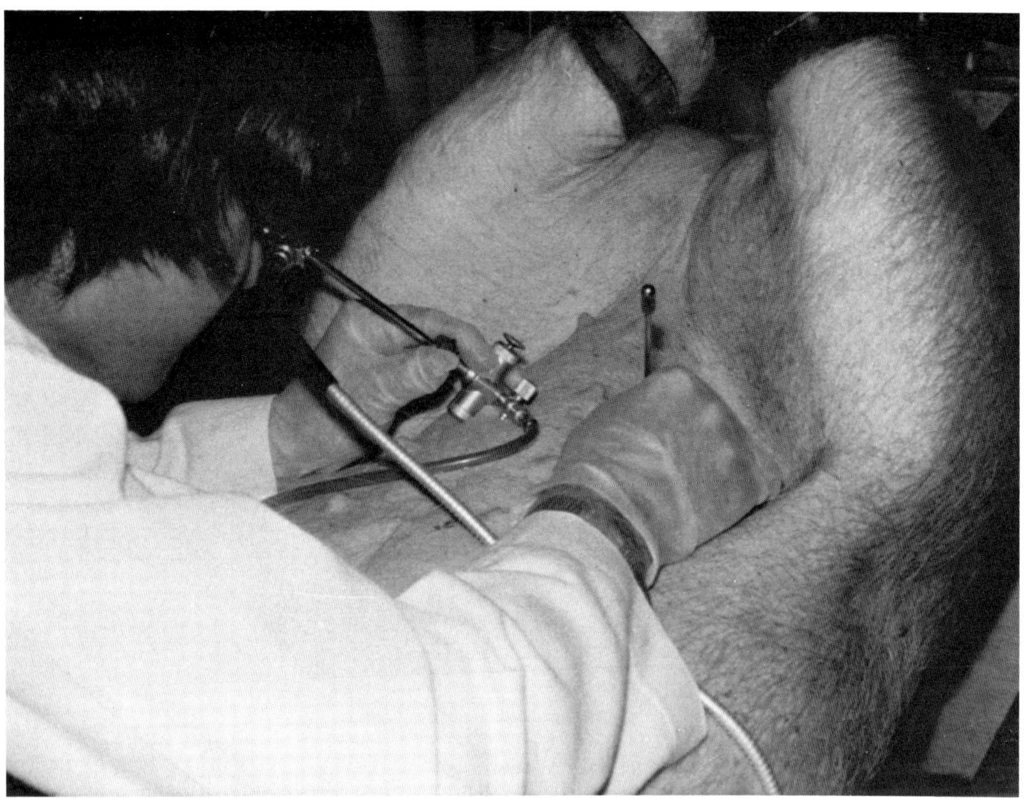

**Figure 7.8**  Combined laparoscopic observation-manipulation.

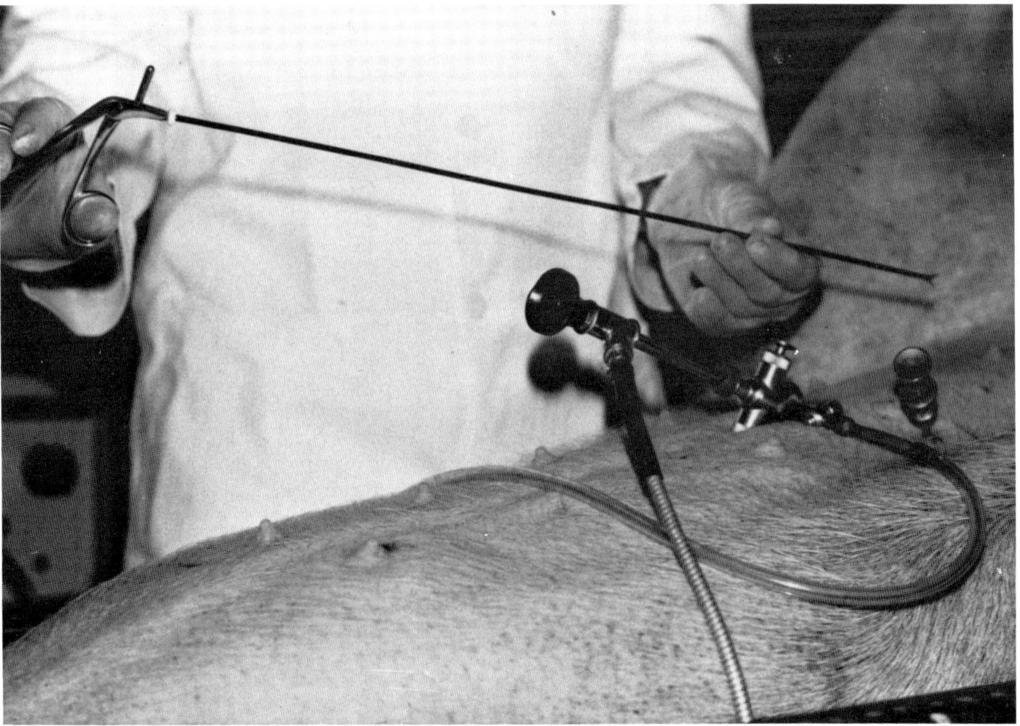

**Figure 7.9**  One type of ancillary forceps. The accessory trocar-cannula is *in situ* several cm lateral to the midline cannula.

The nine pregnant control gilts were compared with animals undergoing laparoscopy to determine the percent incidence of embryonic mortality. Fetal death was calculated from the numbers of normal fetuses and CL found at slaughter. The pigs undergoing laparoscopy had an 8% increase in fetal mortality, but this difference was not statistically significant. Mean fetal weights and crown-to-rump measurements were not different from those in the control group.

## ASPIRATION OF FOLLICULAR OOCYTES OR OVARIAN CYSTS

As in other species, transabdominal insertion of a sterile needle into the peritoneal cavity allows direct laparoscopic aspiration of ovarian follicles either for ova recovery or to alleviate a cystic condition. A 20 gauge needle, 4 to 8 cm in length is satisfactory to puncture the follicle. This technique requires that the ovary be supported at its hilus using an ancillary grasping forceps.

## UTERINE FLUID RECOVERY

Laparoscopy has been utilized as an alternative method for the collection of uterine secretions considered of importance to embryonic environment and viability. These techniques as performed in the pig are described in detail in Chapter 5.

# CONCLUSIONS

Laparoscopy in the pig allows repeated direct observation of the organs in the abdominal cavity with minimal surgical stress and trauma. Its application in this species appears more research than clinically oriented, although many of the clinical techniques applicable to other species could be adapted to the pig. To date, laparoscopy has served as a unique tool for swine reproductive research since it: (1) is a minor surgical procedure; (2) produces little or no adverse physical effects on either the cyclic or pregnant animal; (3) provides a practical method of diagnosing pregnancy, determining ovulation numbers and studying uterine morphology and activity; (4) provides the most practical method for collecting repeated uncontaminated samples of uterine fluids during any stage of the reproductive cycle.

**References**

Hulet, C. V., and Foote, W. C. (1968) A rapid technique for observing the reproductive tract of living ewes. *J. Anim. Sci.* 27:142–147.

Jarosz, S. J., Deans, R. J., and Dukelow, W. R. (1971) The reproductive cycle of the African Pygmy and Toggenburg goat. *J. Reprod. Fertil.* 24:119–123.

Jennings, S. (1971) General anesthesia of ruminants and swine. In: *Textbook of Veterinary Anesthesia.* L. R. Soma, ed., Williams & Wilkins, Baltimore, pp. 352–356.

Rossoff, I. S. (1974) *Handbook of Veterinary Drugs.* Springer Publishing Co., New York, p. 298.

Wildt, D. E., Fujimoto, S., Spencer, J. L., and Dukelow, W. R. (1973) Direct ovarian observation in the pig by means of laparoscopy. *J. Reprod. Fertil.* 35:541–543.

Wildt, D. E., Morcom, C. B., and Dukelow, W. R. (1975) Laparoscopic pregnancy diagnosis and uterine fluid recovery in swine. *J. Reprod. Fertil.* 44:301–304.

# CHAPTER 8

# Laparoscopy in Cattle*

## Duane P. Maxwell, M.S., and
## Duane C. Kraemer, D.V.M., Ph.D.

---

### INTRODUCTION

Laparoscopy has been used successfully in cattle to study and manipulate organs and tissues within the abdominal and pelvic cavities. Unlike other species previously described in this text, bovine laparoscopy is performed without general anesthesia and with the laparoscope inserted through either the right or left paralumbar fossa. In the fasted animal, laparoscopy can be accomplished rapidly and efficiently with minimal animal stress. However, considerable variation exists in an individual animal's response to the procedure and, in addition, entry into the abdominal cavity may vary slightly in each case. Proper equipment and a knowledge of the anatomy of the abdominal cavity greatly facilitate the laparoscopy procedure. However, the novice operator will discover that considerable practice is required to become a proficient bovine laparoscopist. Consequently, laparoscopy in cattle to some degree should be considered an art.

The primary objective of this chapter is to describe and illustrate procedures used for laparoscopic observation of the bovine abdominal cavity with particular emphasis on the reproductive tract.

### History of Bovine Laparoscopy

Laparoscopic technique in cattle has served many uses for observation of abdominal structures, with the main interest being for study of the reproductive organs. Liess (1936) described the use of the endoscope in the abdominal and thoracic cavities of cattle. This endoscope contained a small lamp in the terminal end and utilized a four volt battery power source. The optics were located immediately posterior to the lamp and gave a 70° field of vision at an angle of 135°. The abdominal cavity was observed from a paralumbar fossa approach and the thoracic cavity was entered through the fifth intercostal space.

Three different approaches were used in the cow by Megale *et al.* (1956) to enter the peritoneal cavity for laparoscopic examination of the reproductive organs; these in-

* The authors express appreciation to Joseph M. Massey for his assistance in development of the bovine laparoscopy techniques. This work was supported by project no. H-6143 from the Texas Agricultural Experiment Station, Texas A&M University, College Station, Texas.

cluded insertion through the vaginal fornix, paralumbar fossa, or through a chronically retained cannula in the paralumbar fossa. The vaginal fornix approach proved inadequate, mainly due to the rectum covering the laparoscope and obscuring the field of vision. The retained cannula was an effective means of serially passing the endoscope; however, the cannula occasionally became obstructed, necessitating reopening of the cannula with a blunt instrument. A right angle laparoscope, 9.9 mm in diameter, 60.9 cm in length and equipped with a miniature six volt incandescent lamp was used in this study.

A chronic cannula was also used in the experiments of Lamond and Holmes (1965) who developed an endoscope with increased diameter and multiple light bulbs. The latter modifications offered a greater field of vision and decreased reflection from peritoneal surfaces. These investigators also reported that vision was obscured by extensive fibrin formation which developed on the inner aperture of the cannula after a two day period.

Laparoscopic photography of the internal genitalia of the cow was first described by Megale (1967). A reflex camera was attached to a laparoscope similar to the telescope previously described by Megale *et al.* (1956). This photographic capability enabled the investigator to maintain a permanent record of the morphological changes of the bovine ovary during the reproductive cycle.

Until the development of fiber optic light transfer systems, these early endoscopes with miniature light bulbs were inherent with danger when used for extended periods. The major problem was heat generation which could dry out or traumatize surrounding tissue (Dziuk *et al.*, 1958). As in other species, the fiber optic systems revolutionized the safety and advantages of bovine laparoscopy and allowed prolonged abdominal observation with no concomitant heat production.

The laparoscopic technique similar to the one in current use in our laboratory was initially developed by Wishart and Snowball (1973). This study utilized a 180°, 50 cm in length, small diameter bronchoscope in association with a fiber optic light system. The ovary to be examined was usually observed from the contralateral lumbar fossa. To manipulate the reproductive tract, a probe was inserted through the flank on the side ipsilateral to the ovary.

Carbon dioxide was used to insufflate the peritoneal cavity in obese animals or in those individuals in which endoscope insertion was repeated several times over a short period. Gas insufflation can be used to avoid separation of the peritoneum from the abdominal wall during introduction of the cannula. Seeger (1977) recommended air as the preferable gas for insufflation. In the latter study, observation of the internal genitalia was made through a paralumbar fossa approach and the probe for organ manipulation was inserted in the ipsilateral fossa. A 10 mm in diameter laparoscope, 60 cm long, with a 130° angle was used.

To date, laparoscopy in cattle has been almost exclusively used in reproductive investigations for determining the timing and number of ovulations in single and multiple ovulating cattle (Wishart, 1972; Wishart and Snowball, 1973; Graves *et al.*, 1975; Roche, 1975; Rowe *et al.*, 1976; Schams *et al.*, 1976; Maxwell *et al.*, 1978).

## LAPAROSCOPIC PROCEDURE

### Laparoscopy Equipment

#### LAPAROSCOPES

Various types of endoscopes may be used in cattle. To facilitate adequate light transmission into such a large abdominal cavity, it is preferable that the laparoscope approximate 10 mm in diameter. A length of approximately 60 cm is desirable to permit the operator to effectively reach and view internal organs in the large animal from a paralumbar fossa insertion site. The 10 mm diameter gives the elongated laparoscope

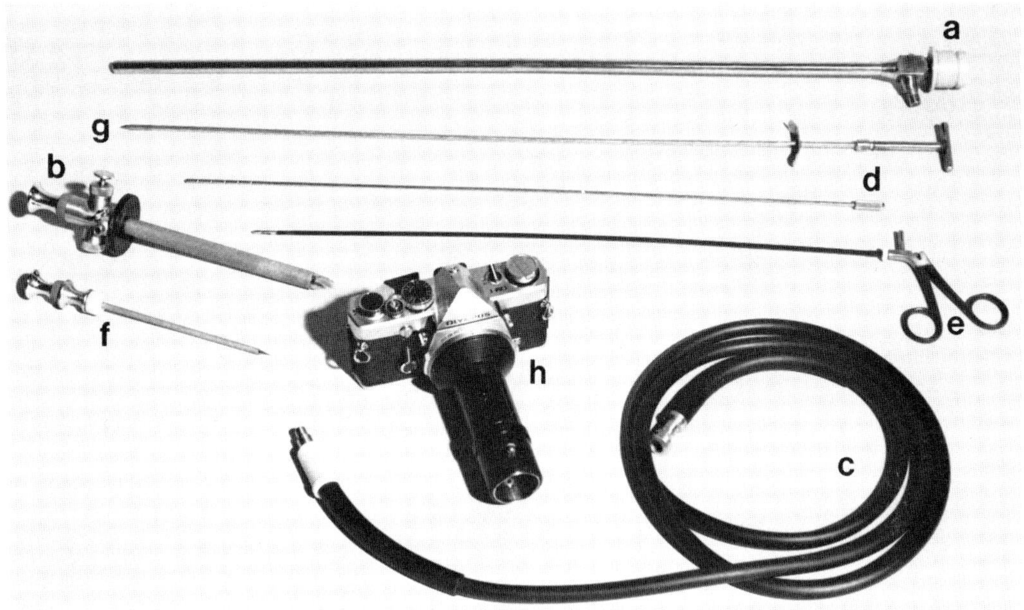

**Figure 8.1**  Laparoscopy equipment used in cattle: **(a)** 10 mm in diameter, 180° laparoscope, 67 cm in length; **(b)** laparoscopic trocar-cannula assembly; **(c)** fiber optic cable; **(d)** tactile probe; **(e)** grasping forceps, 45 cm in length; **(f)** accessory trocar-cannula assembly; **(g)** accessory trocar-cannula instrument for manipulation and aspiration; **(h)** Olympus OM-1 camera with specialized laparoscopic lens adapter.

sufficient strength to permit pushing the end of the telescope under heavy viscera, if necessary. Nevertheless, care must be exercised in using a laparoscope of this length, since it may be bent or damaged, especially in the event of extensive animal movement. A standard 10 mm in diameter laparoscope, although shorter than 60 cm, is usually adequate to view structures located in the vicinity of the ipsilateral paralumbar fossa. This eventually may result in some inconvenience. For example, in reproductive studies, the standard length laparoscope may be of insufficient length to visualize the contralateral ovary, necessitating reinsertion of the laparoscope in the opposite paralumbar fossa. Our laboratory uses a specially fabricated 67 cm long, 10 mm in diameter, direct forward viewing laparoscope (Eder Instrument Co., Inc.) for bovine laparoscopy (Fig. 8.1a). This particular field of vision has sufficed in our studies and gives a clear, wide field of vision needed when probing the large peritoneal cavity of the cow. A right or oblique angle laparoscope provides the capability of viewing the rear of an organ and has been used to such an advantage in the cow (Seeger, 1977).

For bovine laparoscopy, the standard length trocar-cannula assembly is sometimes too short to perforate all abdominal wall layers, including the peritoneum. Manufacturers of such equipment will generally fabricate a trocar-cannula unit of desired length. The specially made unit that corresponds to our 10 mm in diameter laparoscope is 23.5 cm long and consists of a pyramidal trocar and a fiberglass cannula with trumpet and insufflation sleeve (Fig. 8.1b). The trumpet valve of the cannula allows retention of insufflated gas in the absence of the trocar or laparoscope. If necessary, the insufflation sleeve allows for continual gas transfer into the abdominal cavity during the laparoscopy procedure.

## ILLUMINATION SOURCE

A light source (Fig. 8.2) and fiber optic cable (Fig. 8.1c) are used to transmit high intensity light to the laparoscope without heat transmission. Due to the large abdominal

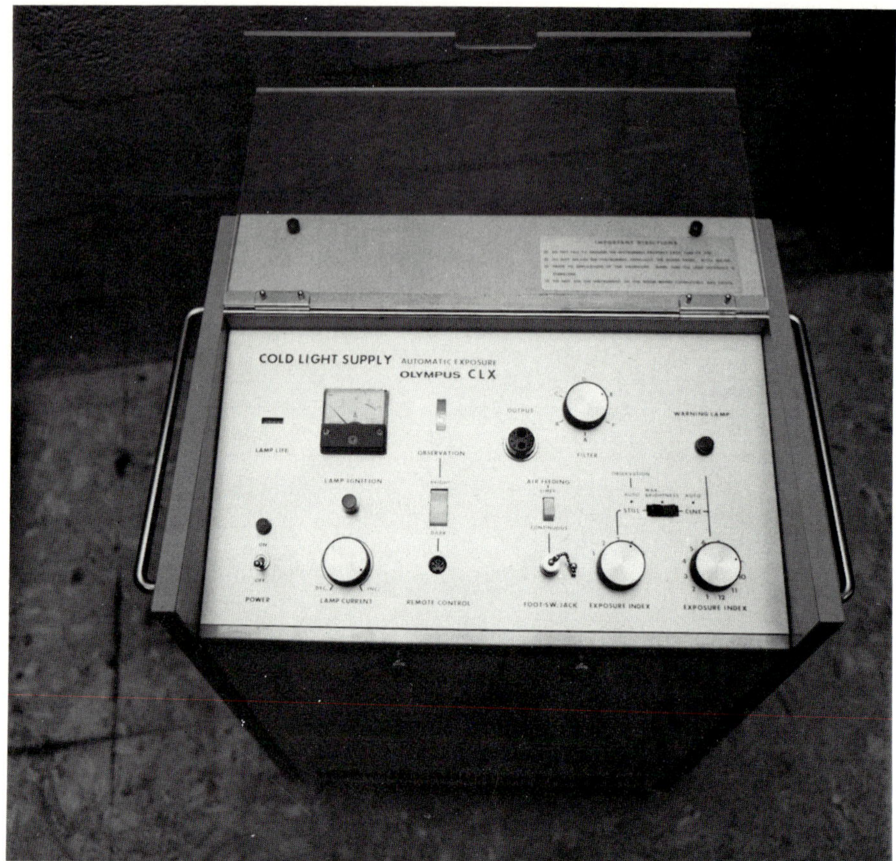

**Figure 8.2**   An Olympus CLX cold light supply with a 300 watt xenon lamp.

cavity, and consequently considerable light dispersion, an illumination source with at least 300 watts capacity is recommended for diagnostic observation of internal structures. More intense lamps or an electronic flash system are necessary for effective laparoscopic photography in cattle.

## ANCILLARY INSTRUMENTS

Abdominal and pelvic organs may be manipulated with a number of different types of instruments. The usual effective method of manipulation is with a straight probe (50 cm) (Fig. 8.1d) or grasping forceps (45 cm) (Fig. 8.1e) inserted through an accessory cannula (Fig. 8.1f). Our laboratory has developed an elongated trocar-cannula instrument (65 cm) (Fig. 8.1g). The hollow cannula with blunt tip is used as a probe and for aspiration of abdominal cavity fluids. Excessive manipulation with the laparoscope and ancillary probes over prolonged periods may result in fluid accumulation within the cavity which may obscure visualization. Use of this aspirating cannula can alleviate this problem. Like the laparoscope and trocar-cannula unit, many of these accessory instruments must be specially manufactured since the standard lengths used in human medicine are often too short for practical bovine laparoscopy. As more veterinarians and researchers become involved in laparoscopy of this species, manufacturers of endoscopy equipment will likely realize the need for the elongated instruments as standard equipment.

## Bovine Anatomy

Since proper placement and insertion of the trocar-cannula is one of the most critical factors in successful cattle laparoscopy, a brief review of the anatomy of this species is pertinent. The paralumbar approach into the abdominal cavity of the cow may be made from either the right or left side (Fig. 8.3). The paralumbar fossa is a potential depression in the upper part of the flank. Its boundaries are the last rib, an oblique ridge formed from the upper border of the internal abdominal oblique muscle, and the lateral border of the longissimus dorsi. After eating, the visceral mass of the animal is expanded and the depression of the paralumbar fossa is absent or only minimally observed. The fossa is distinct when the animal has been fasted.

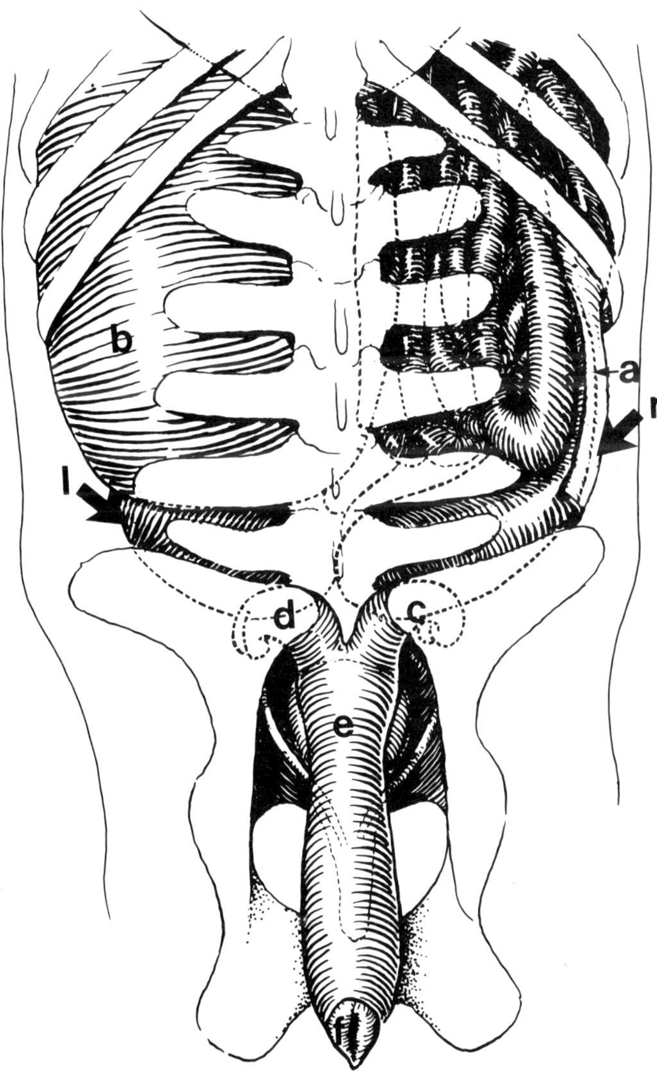



**Figure 8.3** A dorsal view of the caudal end of the bovine: **(a)** greater omentum; **(b)** dorsal sac of rumen; **(c)** right uterine horn; **(d)** left uterine horn; **(e)** uterine body; **(f)** vulvar opening. Arrows indicate the prescribed angle to direct the laparoscope to view the reproductive organs, either from the right (r) or left (l) approach.

The abdominal cavity is continuous with the pelvic cavity. The brim of the pelvis is the line of demarcation between these two internal spaces. To enter the abdominal cavity through the paralumbar fossa the laparoscope is passed through the external abdominal oblique muscle, the internal abdominal oblique muscle, the transverse abdominal muscle, the parietal peritoneum, and into the peritoneal cavity (Figs. 8.4 and 8.5). The peritoneum is a serous membrane lining the abdominal cavity (parietal peritoneum), all but the posterior part of the pelvic cavity, and covering most of the organs in these cavities (visceral peritoneum). The peritoneal cavity is a potential space between the parietal and visceral membranes. After feeding, when the visceral mass is extended, the peritoneal cavity is virtually absent. When the parietal peritoneum is penetrated by the trocar, care must be taken to avoid puncture of the greater omentum and entrance into the supraomental recess (Fig. 8.4).

The greater omentum (Fig. 8.4) is a double serous peritoneal membrane that extends from the rumen to attachments on the abdominal wall and adjacent organs. The greater omentum extends from the left longitudinal groove of the rumen as the superficial layer, and runs along the abdominal floor and attaches to the abomasum and the ventral border of the descending duodenum. The deep layer of the omentum attaches to the right longitudinal groove of the rumen and is continuous with the superficial layer of the caudal groove of the rumen, forming a free edge or fold which extends to the caudal flexure of the duodenum. A variable amount of small intestine and colon is located cranial to this free edge in the supraomental recess (Fig. 8.3).

There are several texts on anatomy of the bovine which may be helpful to the bovine laparoscopist (Dyce and Wensig, 1971; Getty, 1975; McLeod, 1965; Nickel et al., 1973; Papesko, 1978).

## Animal and Instrument Preparation

### RESTRICTING FEED INTAKE

Successful and rapid laparoscopy depends upon a large free peritoneal cavity. To decrease rumen volume and visceral mass, food and water are withheld a minimum of 24 hours. In dairy breeds and thin beef cows, 24 hours fasting is probably sufficient. In more obese or heavier muscled beef breeds, a more prolonged fasting period may be required. Roughage intake may be withdrawn for 72 hours and the diet limited to concentrated feed. If multiple laparoscopies are required, the animal should be maintained on a low roughage, high concentrate diet throughout the study period.

### RESTRAINT

In preparation for laparoscopy, the animal is restrained in a squeeze chute or stock, or secured to a stationary object. A docile cow which is accustomed to being handled may be secured by a simple head stanchion; however, it is recommended that all animals be placed in a squeeze chute (Fig. 8.6). This is for the protection of the laparoscopist and equipment, as well as the animal. Some animals become anxious or distraught during procedures which extend over 20 to 30 minutes.

Our laboratory routinely uses chemical restraint during laparoscopy, especially in beef cattle not accustomed to being handled. One of two types of agents is preferred: acepromazine (Ayerst Laboratories, 0.5 to 1.0 mg/kg) or xylazine (Rompun, Haver-Lockhart Laboratories, 0.02 mg/kg), both administered intramuscularly. The drug is injected immediately after placing the animal in the chute and generally results in an adequate tranquilizing effect within 15 minutes. Overdosing of either of these agents will cause the animal to lie down.

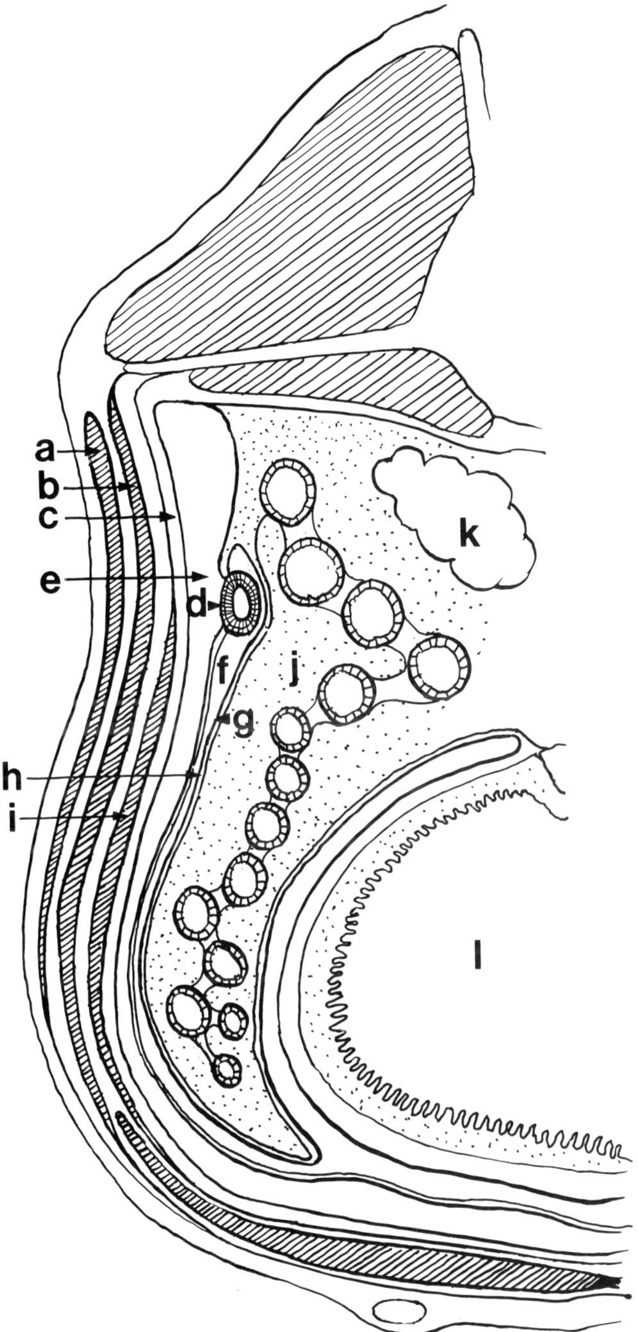

**Figure 8.4**  A craniocaudal cross-sectional view through the right paralumbar fossa in cattle: **(a)** external abdominal oblique muscle; **(b)** internal abdominal oblique muscle; **(c)** parietal peritoneum; **(d)** descending duodenum; **(e)** peritoneal cavity; **(f)** omental bursa; **(g)** superficial layer of greater omentum; **(h)** deep layer of greater omentum; **(i)** transverse abdominus muscle; **(j)** supraomental recess; **(k)** right kidney; **(l)** rumen.

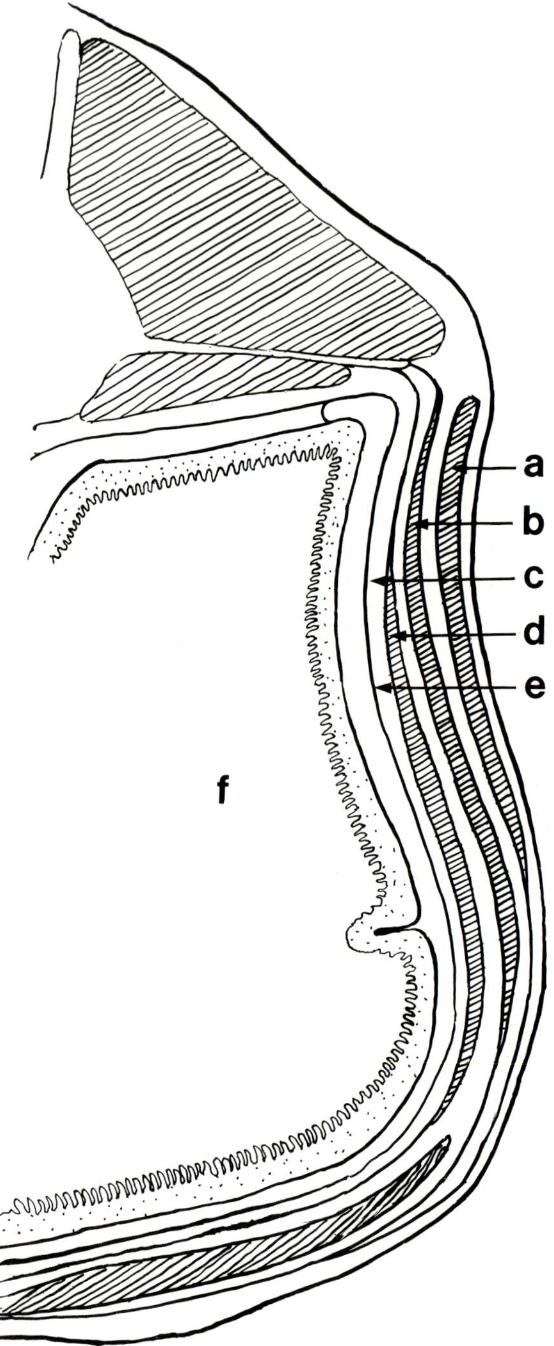


**Figure 8.5**   A craniocaudal cross-sectional view through the left paralumbar fossa in cattle: **(a)** external abdominal oblique muscle; **(b)** internal abdominal oblique muscle; **(c)** peritoneal cavity; **(d)** transverse abdominus; **(e)** parietal peritoneum; **(f)** rumen.

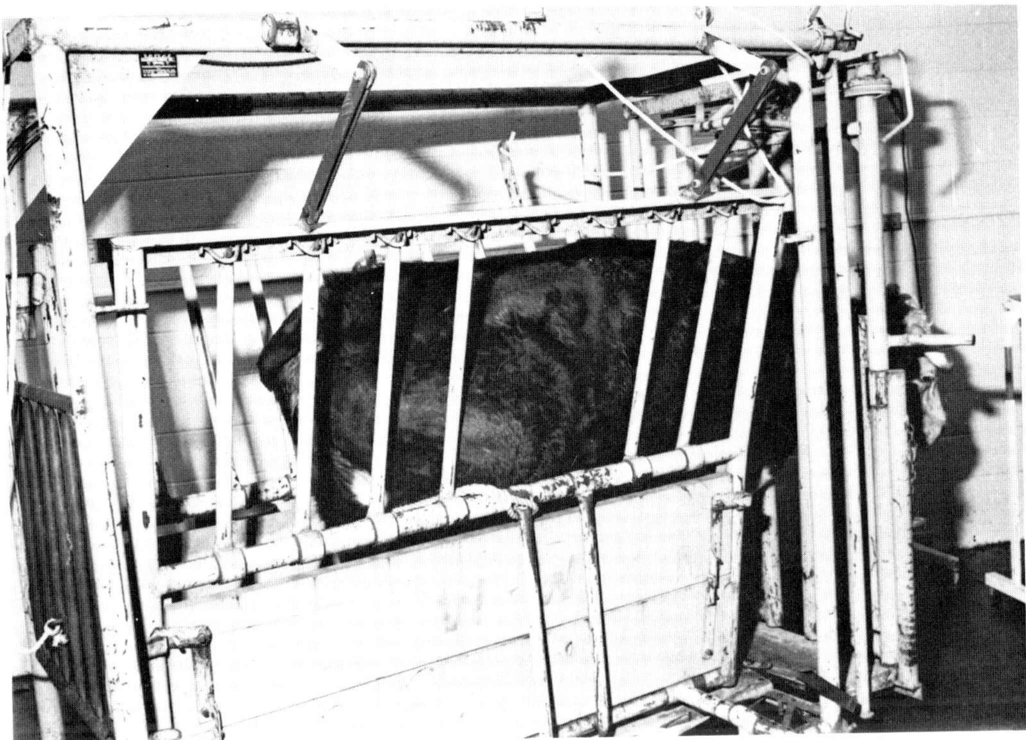

**Figure 8.6**  Cow restrained in squeeze chute with bars lowered to expose right paralumbar fossa.

After the animal is placed in the squeeze chute, the chute may be tilted at a slight angle (approximately 10°) to elevate the hindquarters (Megale *et al.*, 1956; Wishart and Snowball, 1973; Seeger, 1977). Tilting of the animal causes the visceral mass to slide slightly cranioventrally which enlarges the posterior portion of the peritoneal cavity. This procedure is especially beneficial in the obese, unfasted animal, but is probably unnecessary if the animal is of normal weight and feed has been withheld for 24 to 48 hours. It should be noted that some animals in the tilted position become restless, especially when held for extended periods of time.

Side bars on the squeeze chute must be adjustable to allow ample access to both the right and left paralumbar fossae. The operator should also have rope or a metal bar available to be placed between the chute walls and under the animal to prevent the animal from lying down (Seeger, 1977). To avoid contamination of the surgical field, the tail is tied away from the proposed site of laparoscope insertion.

## INSTRUMENT AND SURGICAL PREPARATION

Wet sterilization of laparoscopy equipment is recommended since autoclaving reduces the useful life of the endoscope as well as the rubber components of the cannulae. Because of the length of the procedure, gas sterilization is generally not practical when performing multiple laparoscopic examinations. In our laboratory, the surgical and laparoscopy instruments are presoaked in a solution of chlorhexidine (Nolvasan-S, Fort Dodge Laboratories) for a minimum of 20 minutes. Immediately prior to use, instruments are rinsed with sterile water or wiped dry with sterile gauze.

An area approximately 25 cm$^2$, including the paralumbar fossa (Fig. 8.7) is clipped free of hair using a no. 40 blade on a small animal clipper. The area is scrubbed three times using a providone-iodine scrub solution (Betadine scrub, Purdue Frederick, Co.) and rinsed with water. At this time, a local anesthetic is applied as described below. The area is then rescrubbed, rinsed, and providone-iodine solution (Betadine Solution, Purdue Frederick, Co.) is applied. Sterile drapes are not used.

## LOCAL ANESTHESIA

Two potential incision sites in the paralumbar fossa must be anesthetized with a local anesthetic drug. Our laboratory uses either 2% lidocaine (Xylocaine HCL, Astra Pharmaceutical Products, Inc.) with or without epinephrine or 2% procaine hydrochloride (Procaine HCL, Vitarine Co., Inc.). Although inherently more toxic, the onset of action of Xylocaine is usually more rapid and the duration of effect is more prolonged than with procaine. No undesirable side effects have been observed during laparoscopy using either drug.

The skin of the paralumbar fossa is innervated primarily by the dorsal and ventral rami of spinal nerves $T_{13}$, $L_1$, and $L_2$, and secondarily from $L_3$ and $L_4$. The underlying muscles and peritoneum are supplied by the ventral rami alone. One of three methods may be used to anesthetize the incision sites:

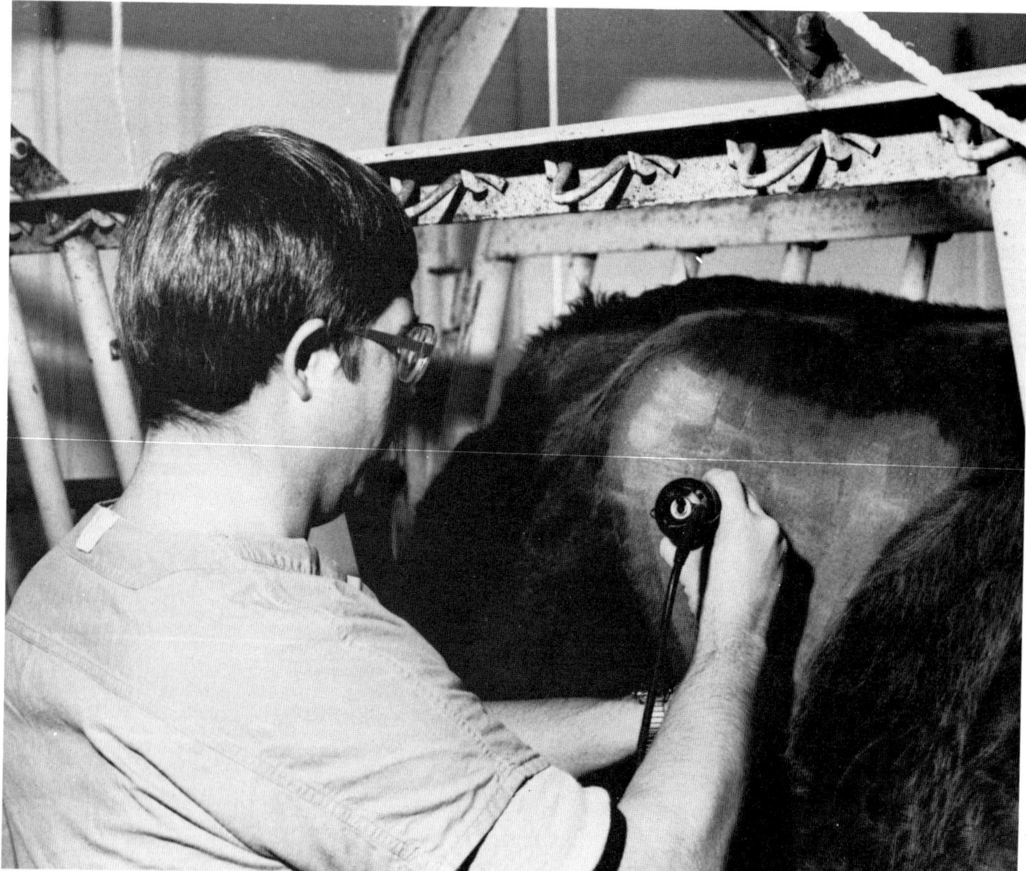

**Figure 8.7**  The right paralumbar fossa is clipped and then surgically prepared.

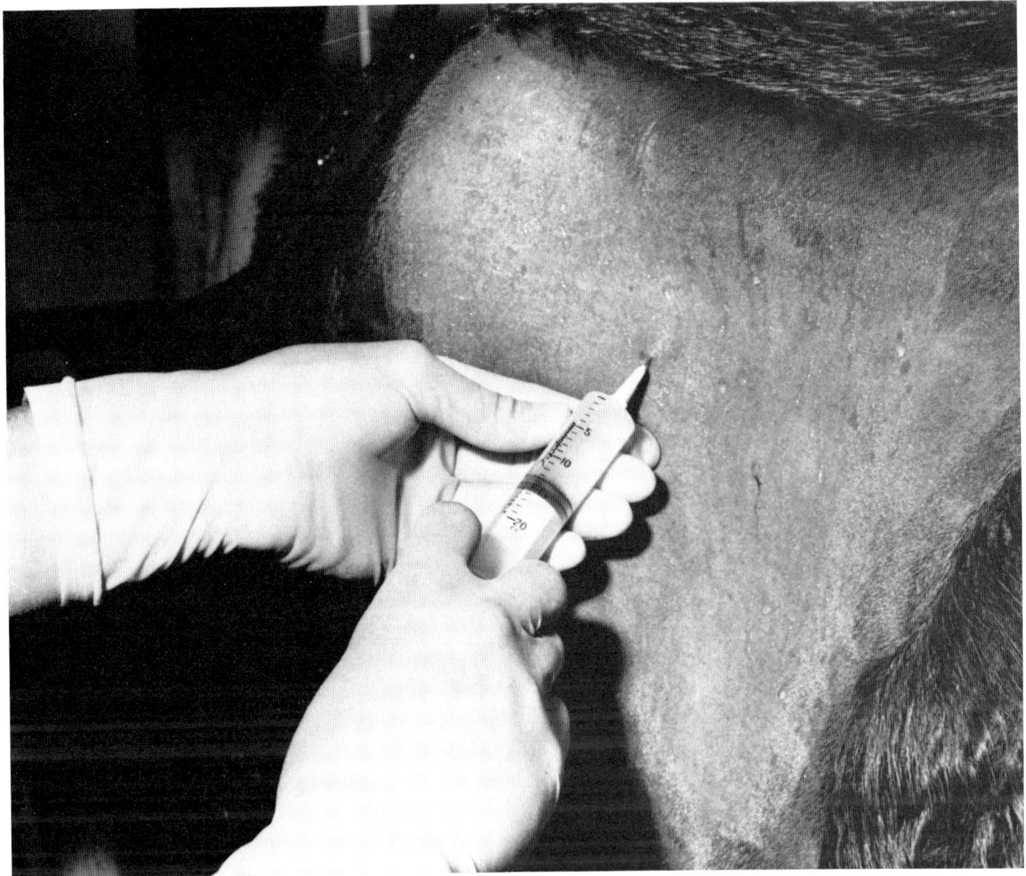

**Figure 8.8**   The proposed incision sites are infused with local anesthetic.

1. Approximately 15 ml of the anesthetic is infused through a 20 gauge, 1½ inch needle into each incision site to anesthetize the cutaneous, muscular, and peritoneal nerves. Care must be taken to infuse the deep muscles as well as the skin (Fig. 8.8).

2. Regional anesthesia of the paralumbar fossa may be accomplished by a paravertebral nerve blocking technique described by Frank (1955). The local anesthetic is injected close to the spinal column at the points of emergence of the nerve trunks from the intervertebral foramina (Figs. 8.9 and 8.10). Xylocaine is administered by inserting a 16 gauge needle through the skin and passing a 3 inch, 19 gauge needle through the larger needle into the area near the intervertebral foramina. The point on the skin for insertion of the needle to block the spinal nerve $T_{13}$ is located by tracing the posterior border of the last rib dorsally until the tubercle is encountered approximately 7.5 cm lateral to the median line. The points to insert the needles to block the first two lumbar nerves are located by following the depression between the first and second, and the second and third transverse lumbar processes until the respective points are reached approximately 4 cm from the median line.

As the Xylocaine is injected, the position of the point of the long needle is shifted approximately 1.5 cm in various directions in an effort to distribute the anesthetic over an area that includes the nerves. Ten ml of Xylocaine is injected in the area of spinal nerve $T_{13}$ and 5 ml at each of the spinal nerves $L_1$ and $L_2$.

3. A segmental lumbar epidural analgesia procedure has been reported recently for use in cattle (Skarda and Muir, 1979). This procedure has not been evaluated for use

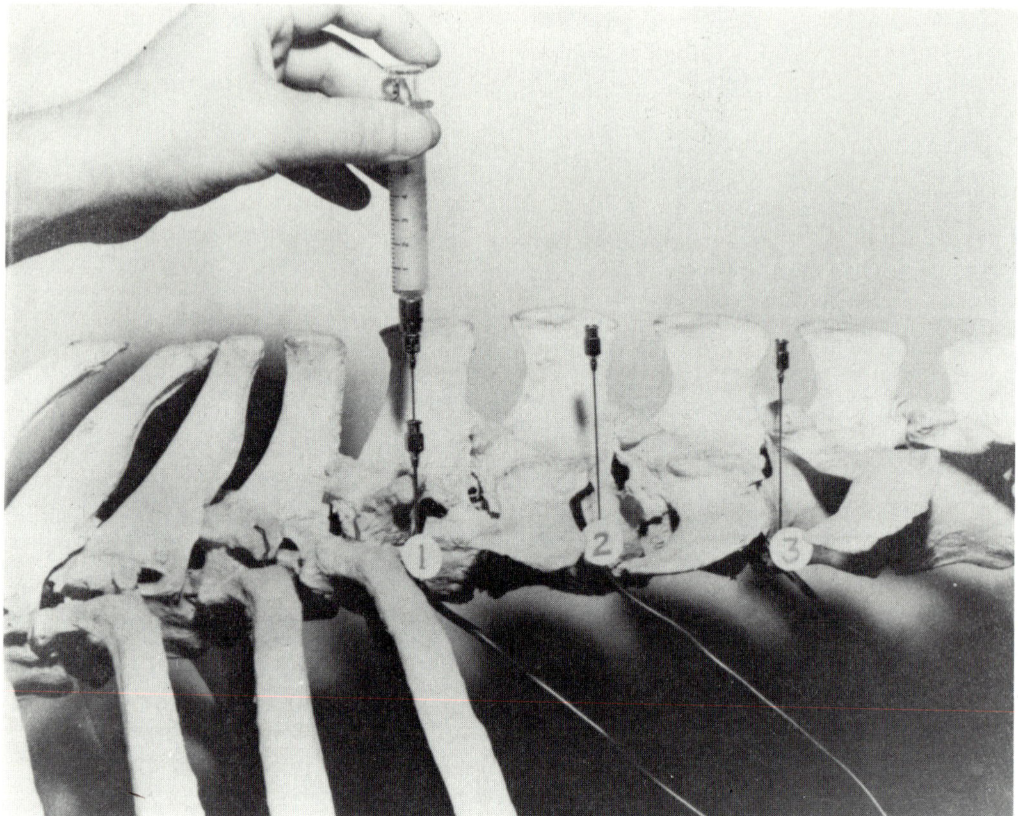

**Figure 8.9**   Lateral view of location for injection of local anesthetic for paravertebral block of the left paralumbar fossa.

with laparoscopy, but was recommended for standing surgical operations such as laparotomy, rumenotomy, and cesarean section. The dosage recommended was 5 to 12 ml of 5% procaine administered into the first lumbar interspace. Analgesia was achieved at dermatomes $T_{13}$ to $L_2$. There are several limitations to this procedure which must be considered. Ossification of the interarcuate ligament, which often accompanies advanced age, prohibits use of the procedure; migration of the anesthetic too far caudally will interfere with maintenance of the standing position; and migration of anesthetic too far cranially will interfere with respiration (this might be exaggerated if the posterior of the cow has been elevated for laparoscopy).

Combinations of the above methods of local or regional anesthetic block may also be used effectively.

## THE LAPAROSCOPIC EXAMINATION

### Paralumbar Fossa Approach

RIGHT APPROACH

To allow insertion of the trocar-cannula into the abdominal cavity through the right paralumbar fossa requires a 2.5 cm skin incision in the center of the fossa (Fig. 8.11a).

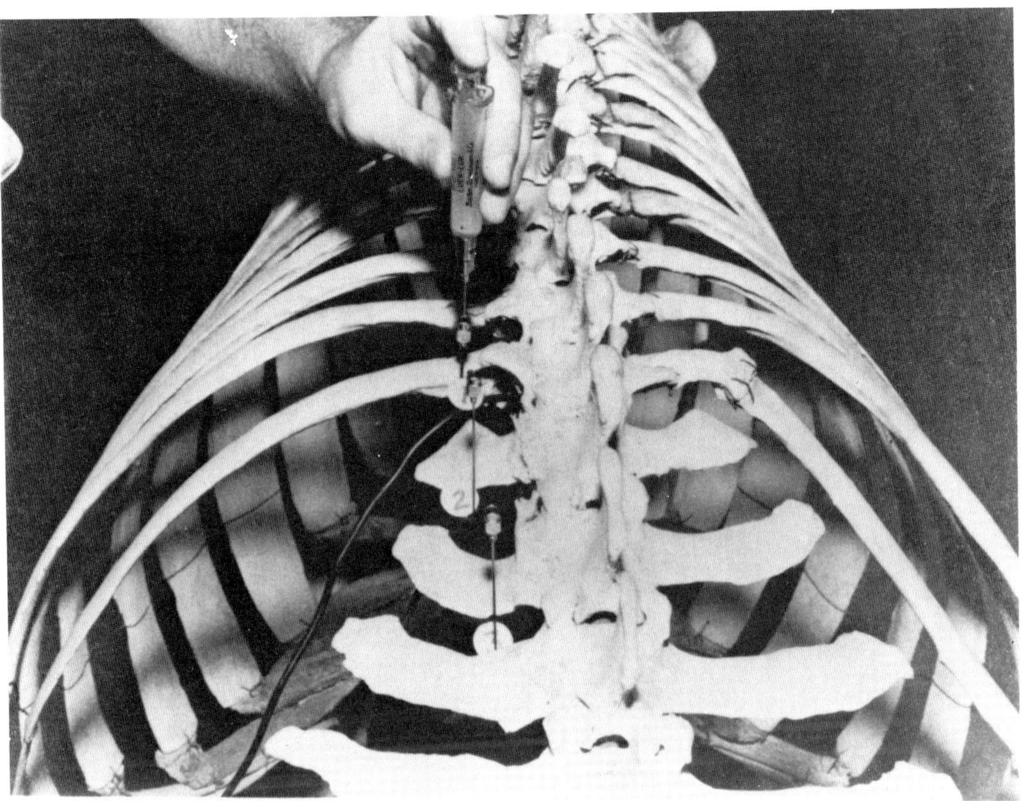

**Figure 8.10**  Dorsal view of location for injection of local anesthetic for paravertebral block of the left paralumbar fossa.

Approximately 8 cm caudodorsally from this site (Fig. 8.11b), a 1.5 cm skin incision is made for the accessory probe(s). The precise determination of the correct insertion sites is critical. If entry is made too far dorsal of the fossa center, there is an increased risk of trocar puncture of the descending colon and/or entry into the perirenal fat layer. Insertion of the trocar ventral to the center results in difficulty in observing the reproductive tract, predominately located in the pelvic cavity.

The laparoscopic trocar-cannula assembly is pointed at a slight caudal angle and then inserted through the center incision with a rapid, firm thrust (Fig. 8.12). The assembly is passed through the parietal peritoneum and into the peritoneal cavity. Care is taken to avoid puncture and insertion through the greater omentum, which could result in entry into the supraomental recess and possible intestinal damage. The trocar is removed from the cannula (Fig. 8.13), air is permitted to enter and expand the peritoneal cavity, and the laparoscope is inserted.

To facilitate exploratory movement of the laparoscope through the peritoneal cavity and to provide manipulatory capability, one or two accessory probes are inserted into the abdominal space. This can be accomplished by initially inserting the short accessory trocar-cannula assembly through the secondary 1.5 cm skin incision, removing the trocar and inserting the appropriate probe (Fig. 8.14). The elongated trocar-cannula probe device pictured in Figure 8.1g can also be inserted through this same incision without previous accessory trocar-cannula insertion. This cannula doubles as a probe and as a means of aspirating fluids that may collect during the examination. Other investigators have effectively manipulated the reproductive tract with a probe inserted

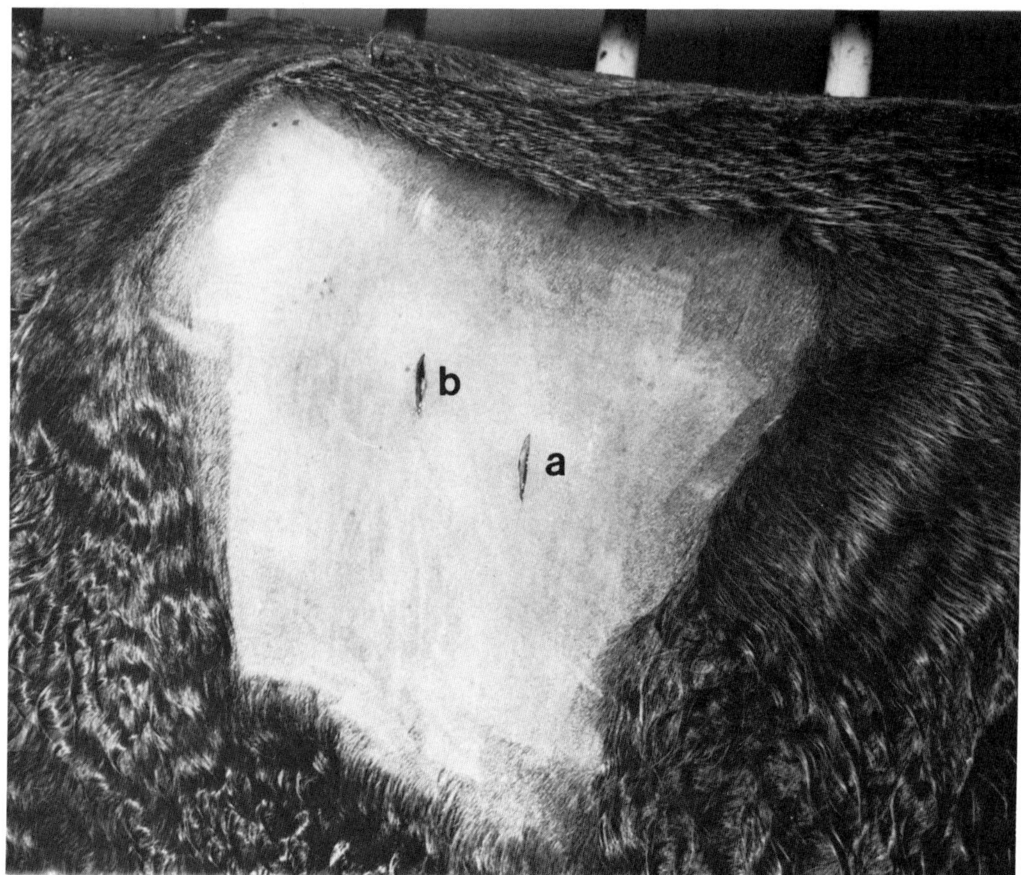

**Figure 8.11**  For the right approach two skin incisions are made in the paralumbar fossa: **(a)** the center of the fossa for insertion of the laparoscopic trocar-cannula; **(b)** 8 cm caudodorsal of the center incision, for insertion of the probes or accessory forceps.

through the contralateral paralumbar fossa and manipulated by an assistant or even the operator (Wishart and Snowball, 1973). The operator using this approach should laparoscopically observe probe penetration through the peritoneum to ensure that the greater omentum is avoided. This is especially important when using a long trocar-cannula probe device as depicted in Figure 8.1g. Unfortunately, it is difficult in the cow to detect or "feel" precisely the point at which the peritoneum is being punctured.

At this time in the examination, the inserted laparoscope is located between the parietal peritoneum (on the lateral side) and the greater omentum (on the medial side). To view the reproductive tract, the laparoscope is directed caudally (Fig. 8.14), around, and behind the free omental border (Fig. 8.3). Generally, the craniodorsal attachment of the broad ligament (Fig. 8.15) is initially observed. The laparoscope must pass to the medial side of the dorsal attachment, since the lateral side ends in a blind pocket consisting of the broad ligament medially and the parietal peritoneum (*Color Atlas*, Pl. 6, Fig. 2) laterally. This ligament (Pl. 6, Figs. 3, 4 and 5) is followed to eventually lead the viewer to the right uterine horn and adjacent ovary. The expanded portion of the peritoneal cavity may be observed in the direction of the pelvic cavity. In an obese or unfasted animal, this peritoneal space is absent, and instead is occupied by the enlarged small intestine and colon.

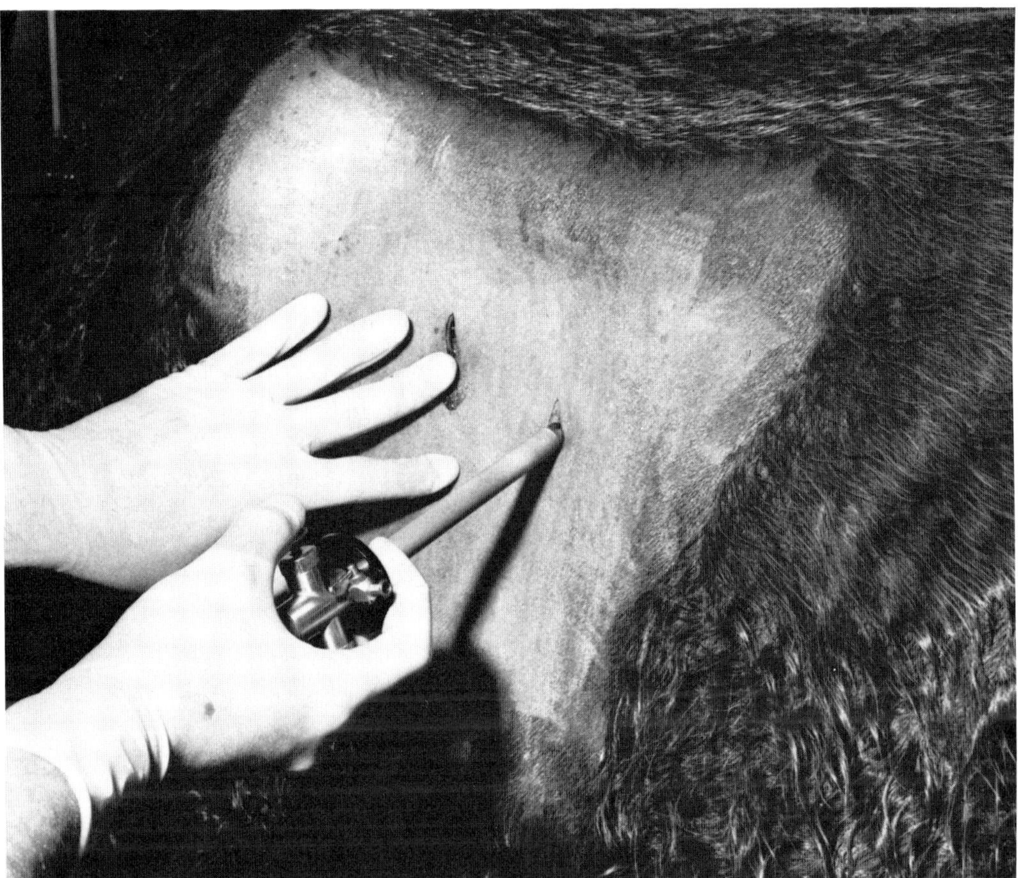

**Figure 8.12**  With the right approach, the trocar-cannula is inserted through the center incision, the point of the trocar directed slightly caudally.

The dorsal attachment of the broad ligament is the critical, visual landmark for guiding the operator to the ovary. Generally, at least one probe is necessary to manipulate the adjacent intestinal mass to observe each ovary fully. As could be expected considering its size, it is very tedious to locate the approximately 3 cm$^2$ ovary in the full visceral mass. This reemphasizes the need to remove feed from the animal for 12 to 48 hours prior to the laparoscopy procedure. Further details on specific endoscopic observation of the reproductive organs are provided later in this chapter.

Inadvertent insertion of the end of the laparoscope into the omentum does not produce serious visualization problems in most species. However, in cattle, such an occurrence is sometimes not easily resolved. The greater omentum is very thin and tears easily. Plate 6, Figure 6 illustrates the probe passing through a puncture in the greater omentum. Caution must be exercised to avoid ripping this tissue after it has been punctured. On subsequent entries into this area, the operator may be unable to determine precisely where the greater omental boundary lies, and therefore, the laparoscope may be repeatedly passed into the supraomental recess. An alternative problem is that the damaged omentum may adhere to the parietal peritoneum. When this occurs, the laparoscope cannot pass into the closed peritoneal cavity at this point, and so enters the supraomental recess.

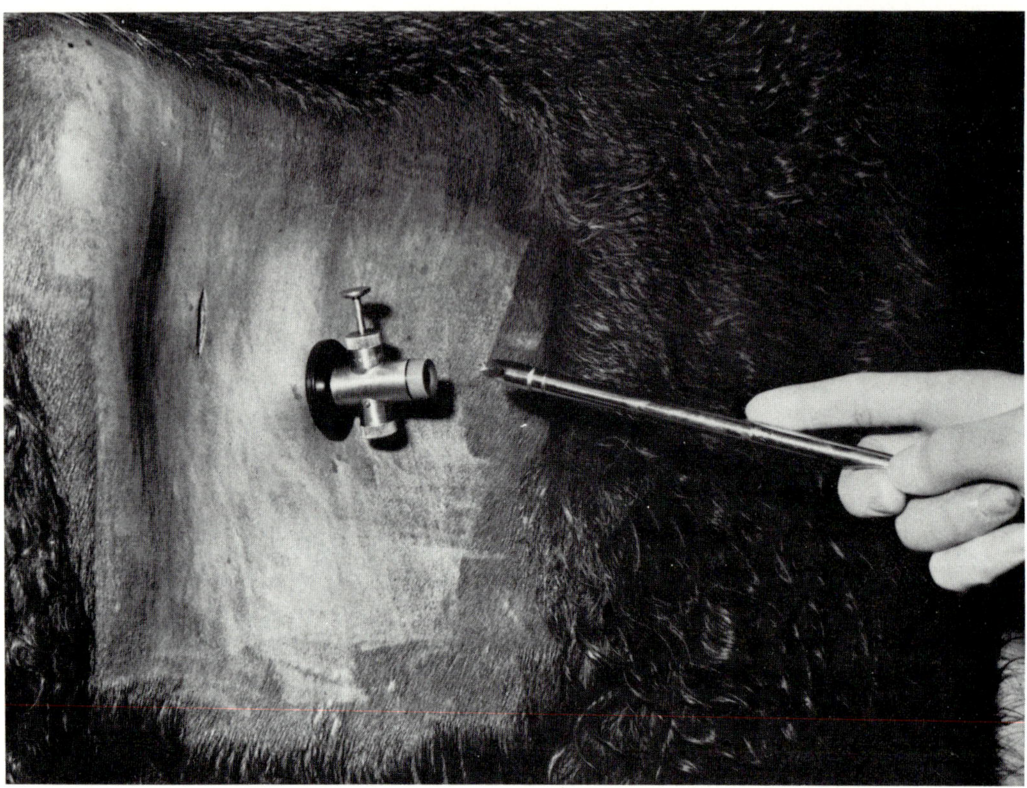

**Figure 8.13**    The trocar is removed leaving the cannula in place.

If the omentum is punctured and the laparoscope is inserted through the cannula into the supraomental recess, it is sometimes very difficult to pass the laparoscope back into the peritoneal cavity. The pocket encloses many fat containing mesenteries, small blood vessels and, in addition, the small intestine and colon. These structures and organs within this recess are easily damaged by trocar and laparoscope manipulation. Tearing of the mesenteries may produce minor hemorrhaging, which can obscure visualization if the tip of the laparoscope becomes coated with blood. Hemorrhage, as well as adipose tissue contamination may necessitate repeated withdrawal of the laparoscope to clean the lens tip.

There are two methods of directing the laparoscope back into the peritoneal cavity from within the omental pocket. The most efficient method is to slowly withdraw the laparoscope from the pocket until the greater omentum comes into view. The laparoscope is then reinserted caudally between the greater omentum and parietal peritoneum. A second method entails directing the laparoscope caudomedially through the supraomental recess. This technique may be aided by using an extremely long cannula which would pass through the supraomental recess and extend into the peritoneal cavity. The problem with this technique is that it is possible to puncture the colon when penetrating the unidentifiable mesenteries. However, inadvertent insertion of the trocar into the colon has not been reported to be dangerous unless the animal has diarrhea (Seeger, 1977).

Finally, it should be noted that, in some instances, the laparoscope may be inserted into the supraomental recess and despite all efforts, cannot be reintroduced into the free peritoneal space. In this circumstance, to salvage the examination, it is recommended that the laparoscope and cannula be withdrawn and reinserted via the left paralumbar approach (as described below).

## LEFT APPROACH

For general diagnostic observation of the peritoneal cavity, this laboratory prefers the right paralumbar fossa approach. Reasoning for such a preference is simple: the rumen generally occupies most of the left side of the animal. In certain circumstances, the operator may find it necessary to insert the endoscope via the opposite (or left) paralumbar fossa approach. Such an approach may be needed if the laparoscopist has poor visualization from the right fossa due to incorrect endoscope placement or a large visceral mass.

With the left paralumbar approach, it is especially critical that the animal be fasted for at least 24 to 48 hours to reduce rumen size. The left fossa is surgically prepared and the proposed incision sites are injected with local anesthetic. To avoid the rumen, the two incision sites are designated to the far dorsal caudal area of the paralumbar fossa (Fig. 8.16). After making the 2.5 cm incision, blunt dissection is performed with a pair of hemostats to spread the muscle layers and eventually puncture the parietal perito-neum. The use of blunt dissection decreases the chance of thrusting the trocar inad-vertently into the rumen. The laparoscopic trocar-cannula assembly is inserted through the opening in a dorsocaudal direction to aid in avoiding the rumen. The laparoscope is inserted into the cannula and the one or two accessory probes are inserted into the

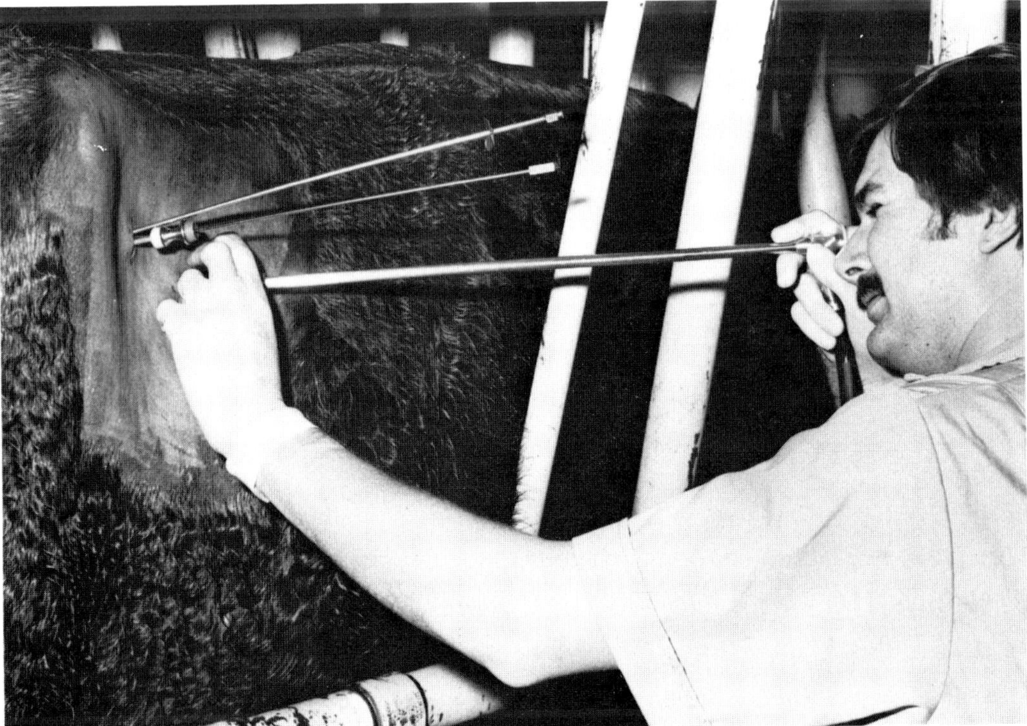

**Figure 8.14**　Laparoscopic observation through the right paralumbar fossa. Probes are inserted through the caudal incision site. To view the reproductive tract the laparoscope is directed caudally.

peritoneal cavity through the more caudal incision. To avoid ruminal puncture, the laparoscope should be used to monitor the entry of the probes.

An advantage to the left paralumbar approach is that the rumen supports the parietal peritoneum firmly against the left abdominal wall, facilitating puncture of this tissue layer. The parietal peritoneum on the animal's right side has a tendency to be flexible, shifting position because of visceral filling. This characteristic of flexibility sometimes results in the thrusted trocar tip pushing the peritoneum medially instead of perforating it. Another benefit of the left fossa approach is that the greater omentum does not affect visualization since it courses under the rumen and toward the right lateral side.

Once the laparoscope passes into the peritoneal cavity, the rumen may be observed ventrally and the parietal peritoneum covering the abdominal wall is observed dorsally. For examination of the reproductive organs, the laparoscope is guided over the caudal terminus of the rumen and directed toward the pelvic cavity. If the visceral mass of the animal is small, the reproductive tract is completely visible within the pelvic cavity. From the left fossa, the right ovary is more readily visible than the left ovary.

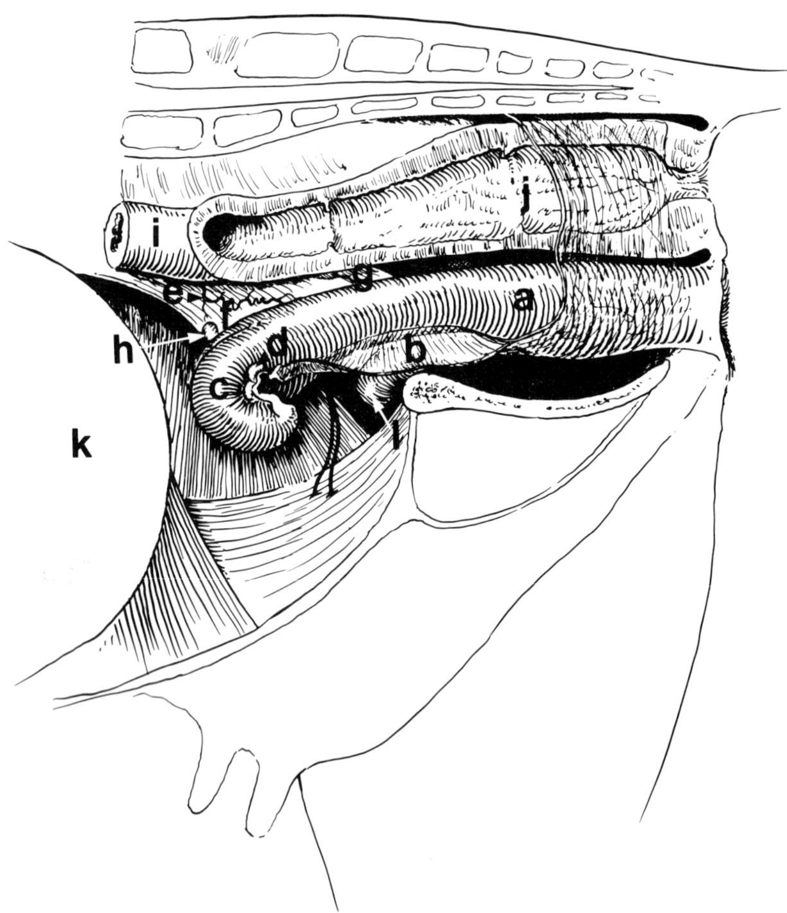


**Figure 8.15**   A lateral view depicting the bovine reproductive organs: **(a)** body of uterus; **(b)** left broad ligament of uterus; **(c)** left uterine horn; **(d)** left ovary; **(e)** right ovarian artery; **(f)** right broad ligament of the uterus; **(g)** right uterine artery; **(h)** right ovary; **(i)** descending colon; **(j)** rectum; **(k)** rumen; **(l)** urinary bladder.

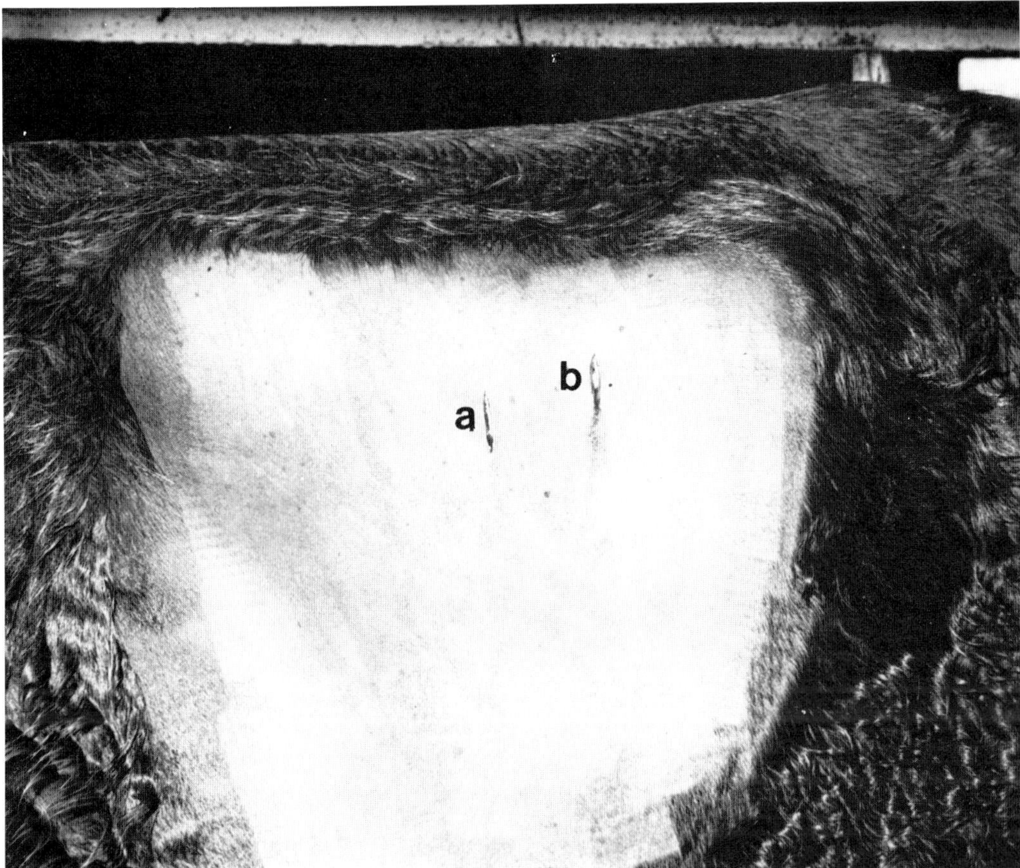


**Figure 8.16**  For the left approach, the incision sites are designated at a caudal location in the paralumbar fossa: **(a)** site for laparoscopic trocar-cannula insertion; **(b)** site for probe or forceps insertion.

## Gas Insufflation

Gas insufflation of the bovine peritoneal cavity is seldom used in our laboratory for laparoscopy. Our experience indicates little advantage in visualization from creating a pneumoperitoneum in such a large intraabdominal space. Gas insufflation, especially over prolonged examination periods, produces animal discomfort and restlessness, and may even result in animal collapse (Seeger, 1977). Therefore, the authors do not recommend insufflation for routine laparoscopy until methods are developed for preventing these undesirable side effects.

Insufflation has been reported as helpful to expand the peritoneal cavity of obese animals (Wishart and Snowball, 1973; Maxwell, 1977). In addition, this procedure may be beneficial if the peritoneum has separated from the abdominal wall, thus prohibiting the trocar tip from entering the abdominal space. Intraabdominal insufflation can force the peritoneum laterally, thus providing support for trocar penetration. For these reasons, the insufflation procedure, although not routinely recommended, is described.

In past studies, the bovine abdominal cavity has been insufflated with carbon dioxide ($CO_2$) (Wishart and Snowball, 1973; Seeger, 1977; Maxwell, 1977) or with air (Seeger, 1977). Both are obtained commercially as compressed gases. Seeger (1977) noted that compressed gas was irritating to the animal due to the cooling effect of decompression and, thus, recommended a noncompressed source of gas such as a hand operated pump. Gas has been passed into the abdominal cavity directly from the commercial tank or by means of a commercial insufflator. Our laboratory uses the Eder Insumat $CO_2$ Insufflator (Fig. 8.17). This unit allows a continued low volume of gas to be passed into the abdominal cavity. The pneumoperitoneum is produced by introducing the gas into the peritoneal space using one of three procedures: (1) the gas is transferred before trocar insertion using a Verres needle cannula (see Chapter 3 for the mechanics of this device). In this type of insufflation it is critically important that the needle be passed through the peritoneal layer or the gas can be unintentionally introduced between the abdominal wall and peritoneum, thus causing further separation of these two layers; (2) the gas is

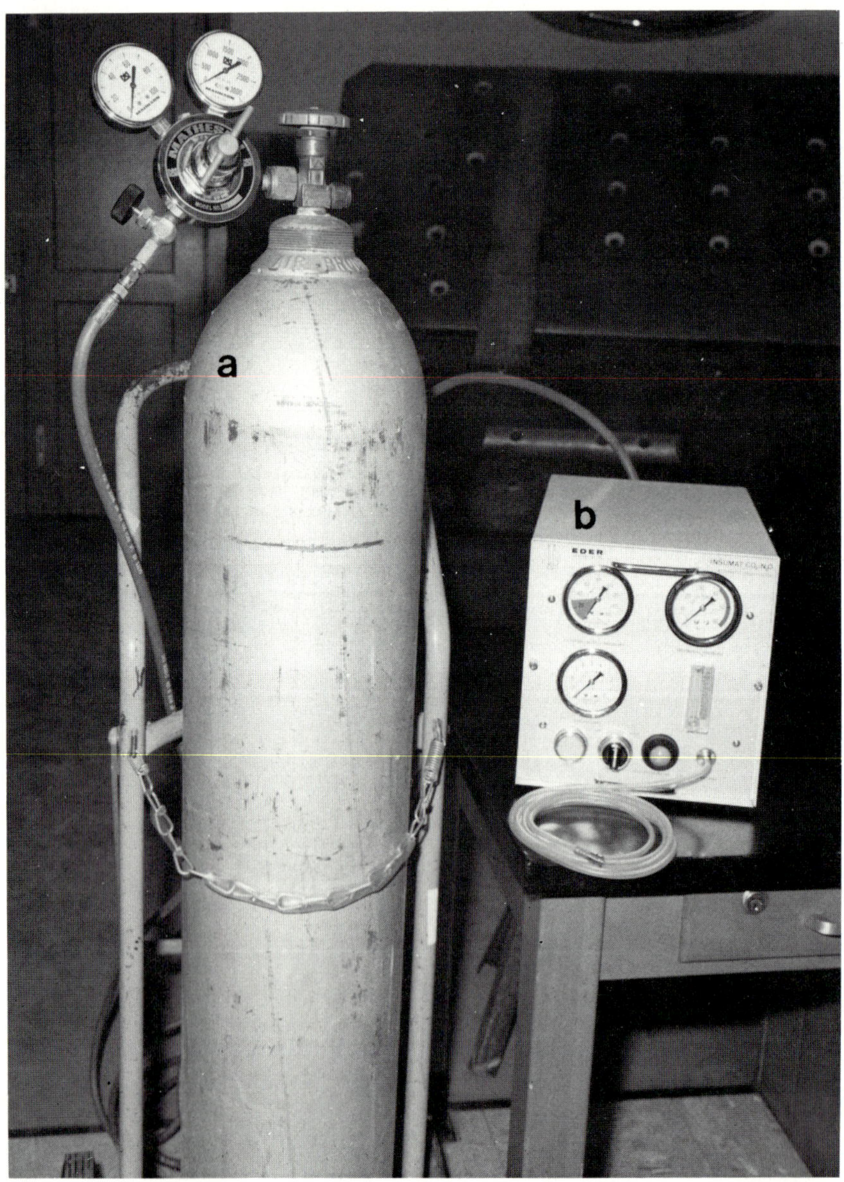

**Figure 8.17**   Compressed tank of $CO_2$ **(a)** and commercial insufflator **(b)**.

transferred through the cannula insufflatory sleeve after trocar insertion; (3) the gas is transferred using an elongated Verres needle or similar device inserted transvaginally into the pelvic cavity. In this technique the vagina is punctured dorsolateral to the cervix through the fornix. This method alleviates concern of false placement of the needle between the abdominal and peritoneal layers.

The volume of gas passed into the cavity varies widely and depends considerably on animal size, temperament, and gastrointestinal filling. When insufflation is employed in our laboratory, approximately 5 liters of gas are used.

## Photography

Intraabdominal photography by laparoscopy is more difficult in cattle than in smaller animals. Laparoscopy is performed in the standing animal which is sometimes tranquilized but never in a general anesthetized state. The animal is usually breathing deeply and moderately rapidly even when tranquilized. In addition, some animals are normally restless, especially those not conditioned to being handled and secured in a restraint chute. Further animal movement is sometimes induced by manipulation of internal structures, especially the broad uterine ligament. All of these animal movements can result in blurred or unclear photographs, especially when using slow shutter speeds.

Photographs are taken with a single lens reflex camera with a specialized, cylindrical lens adapter (Fig. 8.1h) which fits over the endoscope eyepiece (Fig. 8.1a). The light source used has a continuous illuminating 1000 watt photographic lamp. Shutter speeds used vary from $\frac{1}{30}$th to $\frac{1}{4}$th of a second. Shorter exposure times will often result in dark photographs. For color slides, ASA 200 film (Kodak Ektachrome 200 Daylight) has produced the most satisfactory results. For black and white prints, ASA 400 film (Kodak Tri-X Pan 135) is preferred. Use of the latter film allows the operator to use faster shutter speeds ($\frac{1}{125}$th to $\frac{1}{60}$th of a second).

The bovine laparoscopist should remain aware of the difficulty in illuminating such a large space as the cow's abdominal and pelvic cavity. With current fiber optic systems, it is not practical to obtain panoramic photographs of large areas of the cavity. The operator should confine the photographic field to closeups of individual organs or structures.

As in other species, electronic flash systems have produced high quality photographs in cattle. Seeger (1977) used a flash attachment for laparoscopic photography in bovine reproductive studies. The greater intensity of the flash permitted the operator to increase the camera shutter speed which helped overcome the problem of excessive animal movement.

## Details of Uterine and Ovarian Observation

### UTERUS

As indicated previously, at least one and sometimes two manipulatory probes are required for thorough examination of the reproductive tract. Often, the descending colon prevents visualization of these organs. For this reason, generally one probe is inserted to elevate the colon and a second probe utilized through the same incision site to maneuver the target organ into view.

The uterus lies almost entirely in the abdominal cavity. The body of the uterus (Pl. 6, Fig. 7) is approximately 3 to 4 cm long and each respective uterine horn is sheathed by a common peritoneal covering and by connective and muscular tissue, giving the false impression of being one body. The horns (Pl. 6, Fig. 7) gradually taper toward the uterine tube forming diverging spirals, first curving ventrally, then turning cranially, laterally, and dorsally. The ovaries (Pl. 6, Fig. 7) are usually located caudal to the ventral curve of the uterine horn.

## OVARIES

Average sized ovaries measure 3.5 to 4 cm in length and vary between 1 and 2.5 cm in width depending on the plane of measurement. Each of these organs is usually located near the lateral margin of the pelvic inlet, about 40 to 45 cm from the vulvular opening in an average sized cow. The ovary is suspended dorsally to the end of each respective uterine horn by the mesovarium and the ovarian ligaments which extend from the uterine ends of the ovaries to the mesometrium.

The ovary, when initially observed laparoscopically, is usually covered by a delicate appearing, translucent mesosalpinx (Pl. 6, Fig. 8). This vascular mesosalpinx, as well as the fimbriated (Pl. 6, Fig. 7) end of the oviduct, may be maneuvered to one side by manipulation with a probe. The uterine tube (oviduct) can then be observed transversing from the ovary through the medial portion of the mesosalpinx toward the uterus. The ovarian surface is generally uneven due to the presence of developing, mature, or regressing follicles and/or corpora lutea.

In our laboratory, laparoscopy has been used primarily to determine the time of ovulation and ovulation rate (number of corpora lutea per animal). In the cow which has been stimulated by exogenous gonadotropic hormone therapy, multiple follicles may be observed to develop, mature, and ovulate (Pl. 7, Fig. 1). The developing follicle morphologically appears as a small, pink colored swelling on the ovarian surface with its vesicular counterpart appearing as a clear protuberance (Pl. 7, Fig. 2) measuring as large as 2 cm in diameter (Pl. 7, Fig. 3). At ovulation, a small invagination appears on the follicular surface and the follicle forms a bright red, mushroom like eversion, the corpus hemorrhagicum (Pl. 7, Fig. 4). The latter eventually matures into a corpus luteum which appears as a bright red or orange papillum measuring as much as 3 cm in diameter (Pl. 7, Fig. 5). Approximately 15 days after ovulation, the corpus luteum pales to a yellow color and begins to slowly regress in dimension (Pl. 7, Fig. 6). The atretic corpus luteum regresses to a small yellow protuberance, the corpus albicans, and eventually is non-detectable by laparoscopy.

### Ova Recovery

Our laboratory has conducted preliminary investigations into the usefulness of laparoscopy for collecting unovulated bovine ova. The procedure is similar to the ovarian aspiration technique used in other species. The ovary is located and stabilized with an accessory forceps. We utilize a 3 mm in diameter aspiration cannula (Eder Instrument Co., Inc.) approximately 50 cm in length with a tapered 14 gauge tip. The cannula is inserted through the abdominal wall and the tip directed laparoscopically into the mature follicle. The hub of the cannula is attached to a continuous vacuum apparatus which allows aspiration of the follicular contents into the appropriate culture medium. Fig. 8.18 and Pl. 7, Fig. 7 show, respectively, an ovum collected by this technique and the collapsed follicular wall following aspiration.

### Frequency of Examination

The primary advantage of laparoscopy over other methods for observing and manipulating internal structures is the relatively reduced incidence of adhesion formation. Therefore, multiple observations can be made over a relatively short period of time without severe impairment of normal functions. Wishart and Young (1974) observed the ovaries of cows at four hour intervals from eight hours after the end of estrus until ovulation, which in some cases involved as many as four laparoscopy procedures within a 12 hour period. Our work has involved up to nine laparoscopies during a 48 hour period. The actual limits of the frequency and total number of laparoscopies which can be performed on an individual animal have not been established.

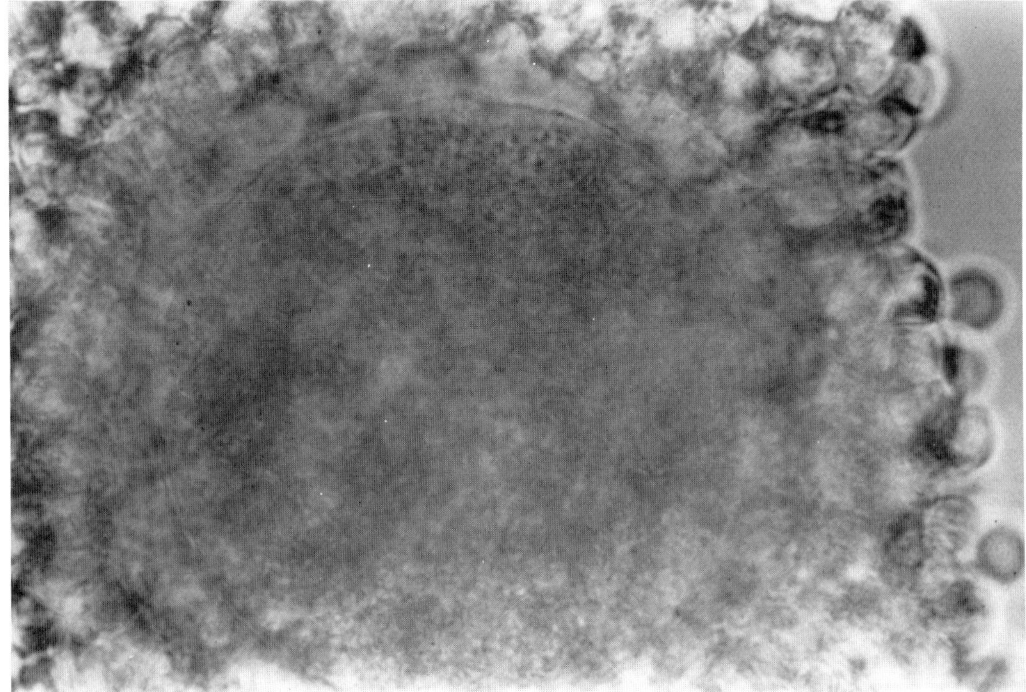

**Figure 8.18** Bovine oocyte collected from an ovarian follicle during laparoscopy.

## Termination of the Examination and Postoperative Care

When the laparoscopy procedure is completed, the laparoscope and probes are withdrawn and each incision site closed with a single mattress suture. In the event that nonsterile technique is used, systemic antibiotic (penicillin, fortified Longicil, Fort Dodge Laboratories, 1 ml/35 kg) is administered intramuscularly and a topical antiseptic (Topazone, Norwich-Eaton Pharmaceuticals) is applied to each incision site.

## CONCLUSIONS

Laparoscopy is an effective procedure for examination of abdominal organs for various diagnostic and research purposes in cattle. To date, this technique has had its most practical application in determining the timing and number of ovulations in cows. However, laparoscopy has also been used for diagnosis of reproductive tract abnormalities such as cystic ovaries and tubal obstruction. The feasibility of collecting follicular oocytes from cattle by laparoscopy has also been demonstrated. Certainly laparoscopy will also prove to be useful for biopsy of the liver, kidney, and other abdominal organs, for monitoring intestinal motility, and for diagnosing intestinal torsion. These and other additional applications will undoubtedly be developed as the use of laparoscopy becomes more extensive.

**References**

Dyce, K. M., and Wensig, C. J. G. (1971) *Essentials of Bovine Anatomy.* Lea and Febiger, Philadelphia.

Dziuk, P. J., Conker, J. D., Nichols, J. R., and Peterson, W. E. (1958) *In vivo* observation of the internal genital organs in the cow. *Tech. Bull. Univ. Minnesota Agr. Exp. Station* No. 222:65–67.

Frank, E. R. (1955) *Veterinary Surgery.* Burgess Publishing Co., Minneapolis, p. 5.

Getty, R. (1975) *The Anatomy of the Domestic Animals*. S. Sisson and J. D. Grossman, eds., W. B. Saunders, Philadelphia.

Graves, N. W., Dunn, T. G., Kaltenbach, C. C., Short, R. E., and Carr, J. B. (1975) Estrus and ovulation with $PGF_{2\alpha}$, SC21009, and GnRH. *J. Anim. Sci.* 41:354, abstract.

Lamond, D. R., and Holmes, J. H. G. (1965) Suitable endoscopy and laparotomy techniques for ovarian examination in the cow. *Aust. Vet. J.* 41:324–325.

Liess, J. (1936) Die endoskopic beim Rinde. Schaper, Hannover, Germany.

Maxwell, D. P. (1977) Determination of ovulation time in the superovulated and synchronized bovine. M. S. thesis, Texas A&M University, College Station, Tx.

Maxwell, D. P., Massey, J. M., and Kraemer, D. C. (1978) Timing of ovulations in the superovulated bovine. *Theriogenology* 9:97, abstract.

McLeod, W. N. (1965) *Bovine Anatomy, 2nd Edition*. Burgess Publishing Co., Minneapolis.

Megale, F. (1967) Endoscopic photography of ruminants. *Vet. Med. Small Anim. Clin.* 62:555–557.

Megale, F., Fincher, M. G., and McEntee, K. (1956) Peritoneoscopy in the cow: Visualization of the ovaries, oviducts, and uterine horns. *Cornell Vet.* 46:109–121.

Nickel, R., Schummer, A., Seiferle, E., and Sack, W. O. (1973) *The Viscera of the Domestic Animals*. Springer-Verlag, New York.

Papesko, P. (1978). *Atlas of Topographical Anatomy of the Domestic Animals*. Vol. 1., W. B. Saunders Co., Philadelphia.

Roche, J. F. (1975) Control of time of ovulation in heifers treated with progesterone and gonadotropin-releasing hormone. *J. Reprod. Fertil.* 43:471–477.

Rowe, R. F., Del Campo, M. R., Eilts, C. L., French, L. R., Winch, R. P., and Ginther, D. J. (1976) A single cannula technique for nonsurgical collection of ova from cattle. *Theriogenology* 6:471–483.

Schams, D., Toth, G., Schallenberger, E., Hoffman, A., and Karg, H. (1976) Relationship between hormonal parameters and ovarian morphology as observed by pelviscopy during the oestrous cycle in cattle. *Proc. VIII Int. Congr. Anim. Reprod. Artif. Insem.* 192–195.

Seeger, K. (1977) Laparoscopic investigation of the bovine ovary. *Vet. Med. Small Anim. Clin.* 72:1037–1044.

Skarda, R. T., and Muir, W. W. (1979) Segmental lumbar epidural analgesia in cattle. *Am. J. Vet. Res.* 40:52–57.

Wishart, D. F. (1972) Observations on the estrous cycle of the Friesian heifer. *Vet. Rec.* 90:595–597.

Wishart, D. F., and Snowball, J. B. (1973) Endoscopy in cattle: Observation of the ovary *in situ*. *Vet. Rec.* 92:139–143.

Wishart, D. F., and Young, I. M. (1974) Artificial insemination of progestin (SC21009)-treated cattle at predetermined times. *Vet. Rec.* 95:503–508.

# CHAPTER 9

# Laparoscopy in the Horse*

**Don M. Witherspoon, D.V.M., Ph.D.,
Duane C. Kraemer, D.V.M., Ph.D., and
Stephen W. J. Seager, M.R.C.V.S.**

## INTRODUCTION

Laparoscopy, while not used extensively, has been successfully adapted for use in the horse. The authors are aware of only four publications on the subject, two from Germany (Heinze *et al.*, 1972; Heinze and Klug, 1973) and two from the senior author's laboratory (Witherspoon and Talbot, 1970 a,b). More recently, Seager, Wildt, and Kraemer have experimented with the effectiveness of laparoscopy for detecting ovulation in the mare, but these results are yet unpublished.

As evident from the previous chapter, numerous studies have been reported on abdominal endoscopy in a similar sized species, the cow. One must consider why a scarcity of information exists concerning the efficacy of equine laparoscopy. The primary reason is that the clinician or researcher has generally been satisfied with relying on results from rectal palpation to determine the status of various abdominal organs. Although palpation is an indirect means of determining internal events, it requires no surgical intervention and is highly accurate when performed by the experienced person. This factor has limited experimentation or clinical use of laparoscopy in this species. Nevertheless, it is likely that inadequate published detail concerning the basic principles and potential of laparoscopy in the horse has contributed somewhat to its lack of application. Certainly, the use of laparoscopy for confirming questionable palpation results or performing organ biopsy under direct visualization justifies the further study and use of this technique in the equine.

This chapter presents a summary of the basic technique and instrumentation used in studies to date. As will be evident, a limited amount of detail is provided on clinical utilization, primarily because these frontiers are yet to be explored.

* D. M. W. wishes to express appreciation to Drs. Douglas Byars and Milton Adsit, University of Georgia, for their assistance. S. W. J. S. wishes to express appreciation to Drs. W. Zent, P. Thorpe, and E. Fallon, Lexington, Kentucky, for their interest and assistance. The authors thank Sylvia Charman Guthrie for photographing the laparoscopic procedures.

## EQUIPMENT AND PREPARATION FOR EXAMINATION

### Equipment

### LAPAROSCOPE

Laparoscopy can be performed using either a rigid or flexible endoscope. Studies have utilized the 9 mm in diameter peritoneoscope (Eder Instrument Co., Inc.) with either direct forward or forward oblique direction of view or the standard 10 mm in diameter, direct forward laparoscope (Richard Wolf Medical Instruments Corp.; Eder Instrument Co., Inc.). A standard length laparoscope, although only approximately 35 cm in length, is adequate to satisfactorily visualize the abdominal area ipsilateral to insertion. However, this length may preclude examination of organs near the contralateral abdominal wall, necessitating reinsertion of the laparoscope through the opposite paralumbar fossa. Smaller diameter rigid laparoscopes (i.e., 5 mm or less) should be avoided for horse laparoscopy. The limited visual field provided by this size instrument in such a large cavity often results in a prolonged and difficult examination. A flexible fiberscope can also be used in horse endoscopy (Fig. 9.1). The instrument of choice is the Olympus Colon 0 Fiberscope, Model CF, Type MB2 (Olympus Corp. of America) which is approximately 1.5 cm in diameter and 1 m in length. The observation range of this flexible apparatus exceeds that of the rigid laparoscope and, in addition, this device can be used to examine other anatomical regions, including the lumen of the rectum and uterus. The disadvantage of this instrument is that it requires a substantially longer incision for insertion than its rigid counterpart.

### TROCAR-CANNULAE, LIGHT SOURCE, AND ANCILLARY EQUIPMENT

Other equipment items are essentially similar to those described in other chapters. The standard length trocar-cannula assembly, originally developed for humans, may be

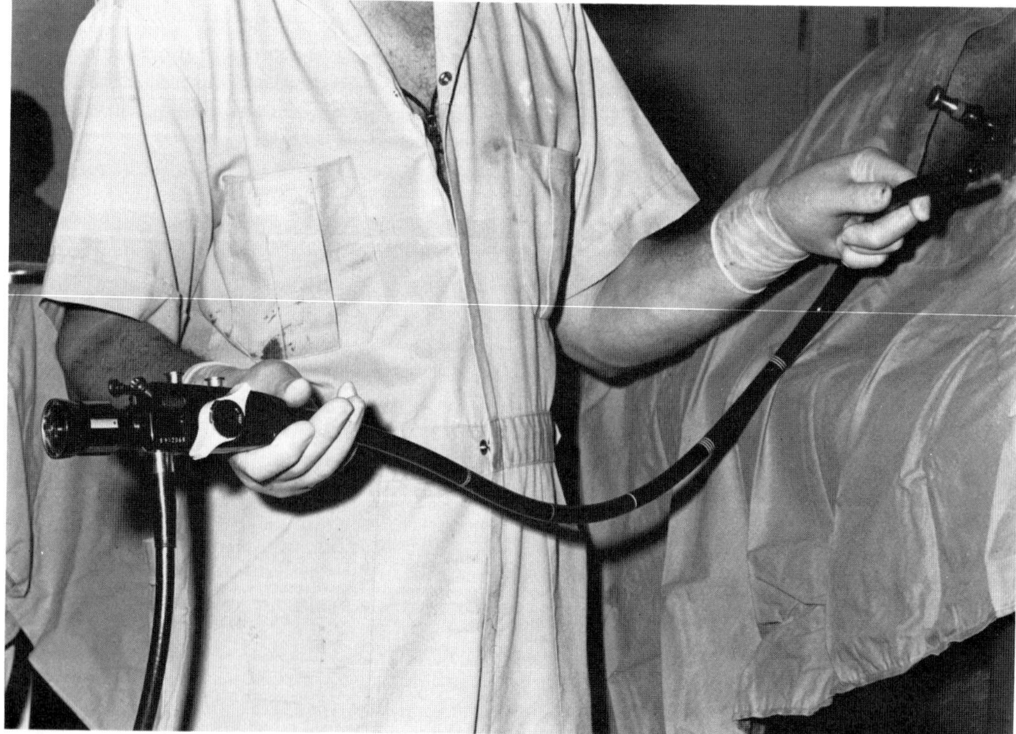

**Figure 9.1**  Flexible fiberscope. Instrument is adaptable for use with most standard light sources.

too short to allow perforation of all layers (skin, muscle, and peritoneum) in some horses, particularly obese or heavily muscled animals. This problem may be solved (as previously described for the cow) by requesting the manufacturer to elongate the standard trocar-cannula assembly. A total trocar length of approximately 24 cm is generally satisfactory.

It is recommended that the illumination source have both diagnostic and photographic lamp capabilities. Due to the large space requiring illumination in the horse and the larger diameter laparoscope used, the light supply fiber optic cable should have a diameter of 6 mm or greater. Laparoscopic photographs associated with this chapter have been obtained using an Olympus OM-1 camera, quick mount adapter and Kodak Ektachrome (ASA 200) color film.

Ancillary instruments inserted through an accessory cannula are useful in internal organ manipulation and tissue biopsy. Grasping forceps are manufactured for insertion through either 3 mm or 6 mm in diameter accessory cannulae. The operator should avoid using the former size instruments. Internal organs in the horse are obviously heavy and the smaller diameter 3 mm forceps are of insufficient rigidity to provide maneuvering or support capabilities. The larger, standard ancillary instruments that accommodate the 6 mm in diameter accessory cannula are of adequate size for performing internal manipulations.

Additional equipment required for preparation and examination includes hair clippers, instrument sterilization pan, scalpel, forceps, and suture.

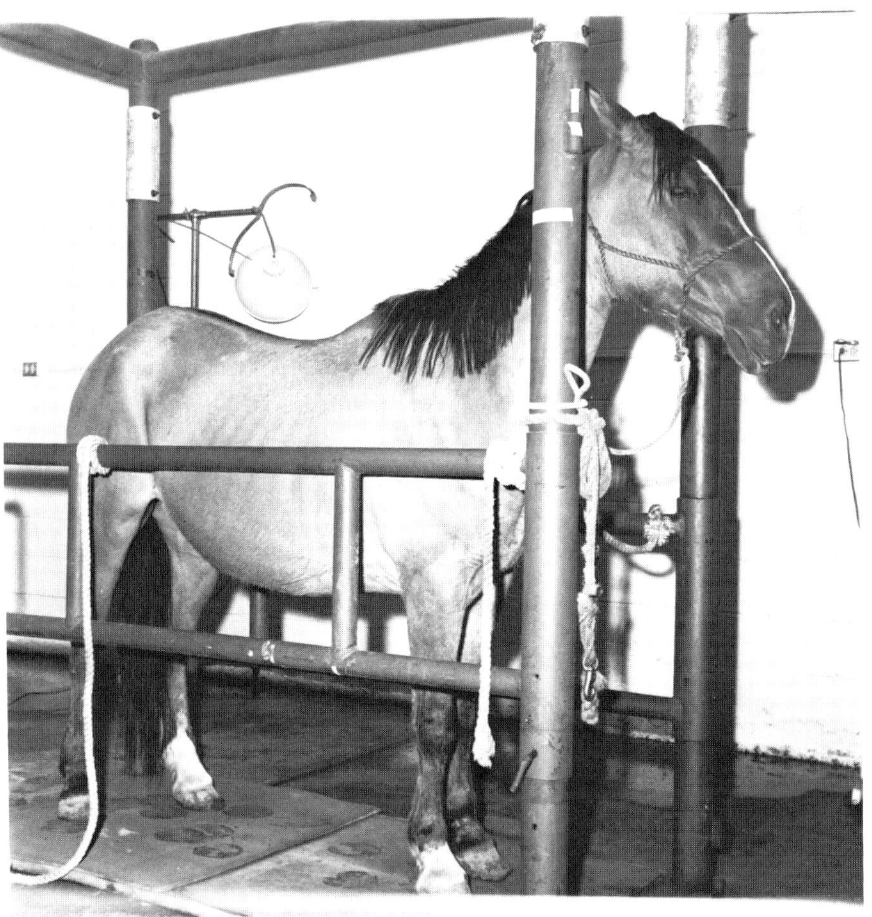

**Figure 9.2** Horse loosely restrained in stanchion.

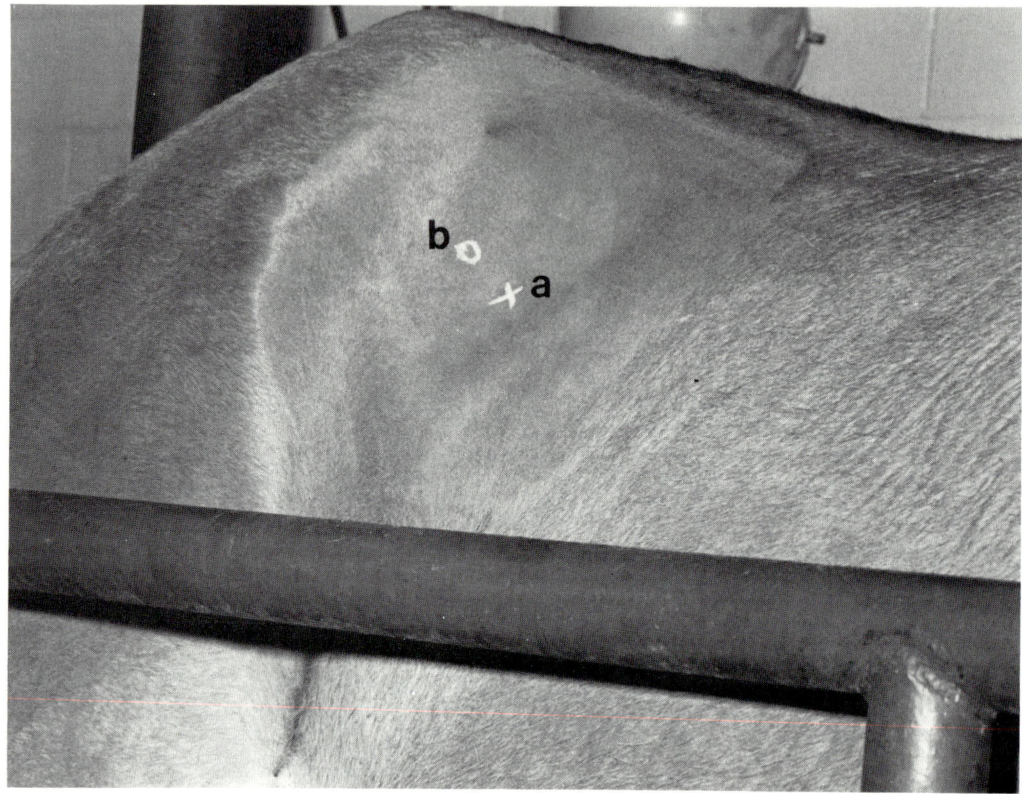


**Figure 9.3**  Paralumbar fossa area clipped. Marked areas are sites for laparoscope **(a)** and accessory instrument **(b)** insertion.

## Preexamination Procedures

The laparoscope and all ancillary instruments are chemically sterilized using the solutions and schedules recommended by the manufacturers. The authors' experience indicates that Cidex (Arbrook, Inc.), Amerase (Vestal Laboratories), or Nolvasan-S (Fort Dodge Laboratories, Inc.) are all suitable disinfecting agents. The rigid or flexible endoscopes discussed can be completely immersed in the chemical solution.

It is imperative that the horse be fasted for at least 24 hours prior to the laparoscoic examination. Water should also be withheld for a similar period, weather permitting. Failure to restrict food and water increases the possibility of traumatizing an abdominal organ upon insertion of the trocar-cannula and often complicates the viewing of an organ due to the need for displacement by a full cecum.

The horse is walked into a stanchion and loosely restrained to minimize movement (Fig. 9.2). A standard pipe stanchion is quite satisfactory (the classical "squeeze" chute or stanchion is usually not necessary). Neither horizontal nor vertical restraint bars of the stanchion should be located directly within or adjacent to the paralumbar fossa region. Such a design would make insertion of the instruments and comprehensive examination of the abdominal cavity difficult. In addition, unexpected quick movement by the horse against the restraint pipes during the examination might result in damage to the animal, the operator, or the delicate laparoscope.

Laparoscopy in this species is performed with the animal tranquilized and a local anesthetic administered at the laparoscope insertion site. For tranquilization, xylazine (Rompun, Haver-Lockhart Laboratories) or acepromazine (Acepromazine Maleate Injectable, Ayerst Laboratories) injected intravenously at the manufacturer's suggested dosage is recommended.

The tail of the horse is wrapped and tied on the side contralateral to the proposed incision site. Examination of the abdominal cavity by rectal palpation should precede each laparoscopy. This provides an initial indication of organ location and size and alerts the operator to any unusual masses or enlarged organs that may suggest a pathological condition. Special attention is given to the location of the spleen. In certain cases, the equine spleen extends caudally beyond the animal's left paralumbar fossa. Since this area is sometimes used for laparoscope entry, the operator must either select the contralateral fossa or insert the laparoscope dorsal to the splenic location.

## Surgical Preparation

The site for instrument insertion is approximately in the center of the paralumbar fossa. In horses weighing 300 to 450 kg, the proposed incision site is approximately 4 cm ventral to the point of the transverse processes of the lumbar vertebra and 3 to 5 cm caudal to the last rib (Fig. 9.3). Although laparoscopy can be performed safely in most species using nonsterile techniques, because of its susceptibility to infection the horse requires aseptic conditions for such an examination. The surgical site is prepared by clipping the hair 30 cm in each direction from the proposed incision site. The area is scrubbed with pre-op surgical scrub sponges (Pre-op-Iodophore Textured Surgical Scrub Sponge, Davis & Geck, American Cyanamid Co.) and rinsed with warm water six times. The scrub routine is then repeated three times, using sterile gloves and rinsing with sterile saline solution. An alcohol rinse is then followed by the application of 2% iodine

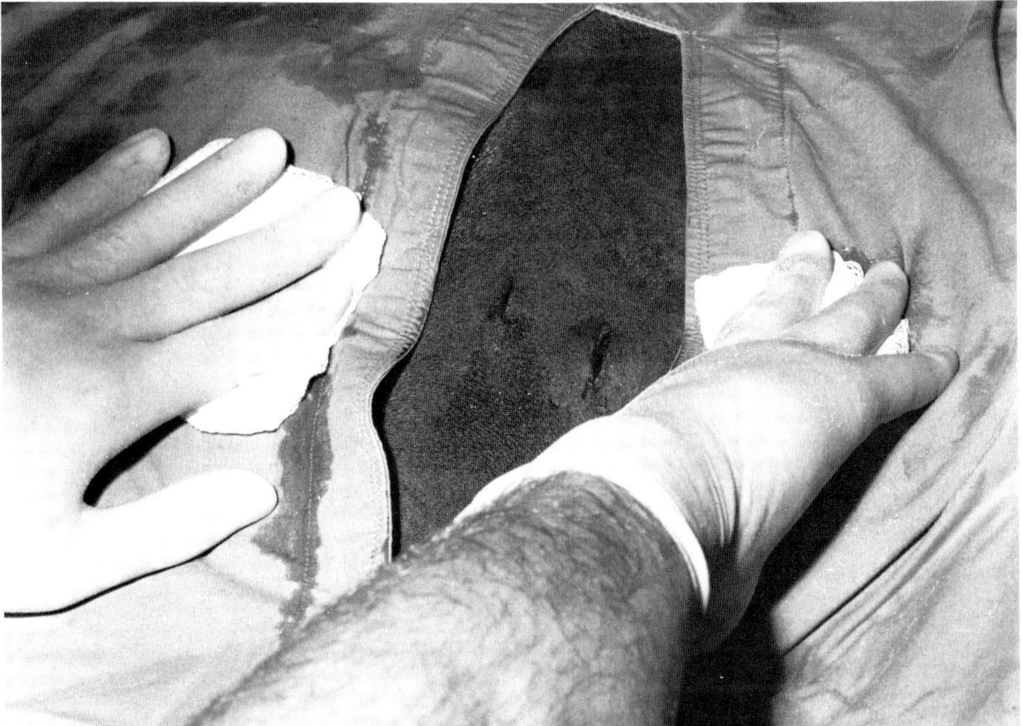

**Figure 9.4**  Paralumbar fossa area draped, infiltrated with local anesthetic, and incisions made.

solution over the area of the incision. The entire flank of the horse is draped with a sterile surgical drape.

There appears to be no advantage to producing a pneumoperitoneum in the horse, either prior to or during the laparoscopic examination. In fact, insufflation may be contraindicated as it may cause colic. Consequently, insufflatory equipment and associated procedures necessary in most other animals are excluded in equine laparoscopy.

The proposed incision site is anesthetized using 2.5% procaine hydrochloride (Haver-Lockhart Laboratories). Both the skin and muscle layers are sequentially infiltrated, with caution taken to not penetrate the peritoneum with the anesthetic. When the anesthetic effects are noted, a 3 to 4 cm incision (for insertion of the 10 mm in diameter rigid laparoscope) is made (Fig. 9.4). An incision 6 to 8 cm in length is required for the flexible endoscope. Muscle fibers are then separated by blunt dissection.

Two different methods may be used to penetrate the peritoneum and insert the endoscope. When using the rigid 10 mm in diameter laparoscope, it is preferable to penetrate the peritoneum with the corresponding trocar-cannula assembly. The trocar-cannula unit is inserted into the peritoneal cavity with the point directed slightly ventrally and at a 45° angle to the lateral body plane (Fig. 9.5). The trocar is removed and replaced with the laparoscope (Fig. 9.6). In the second method, an endoscopic cannula is not utilized and the incision is extended to approximately 8 cm in length. This procedure is favored when the flexible laparoscope is used. With this method the peritoneum is penetrated by blunt dissection. A rush of air is usually audible as the

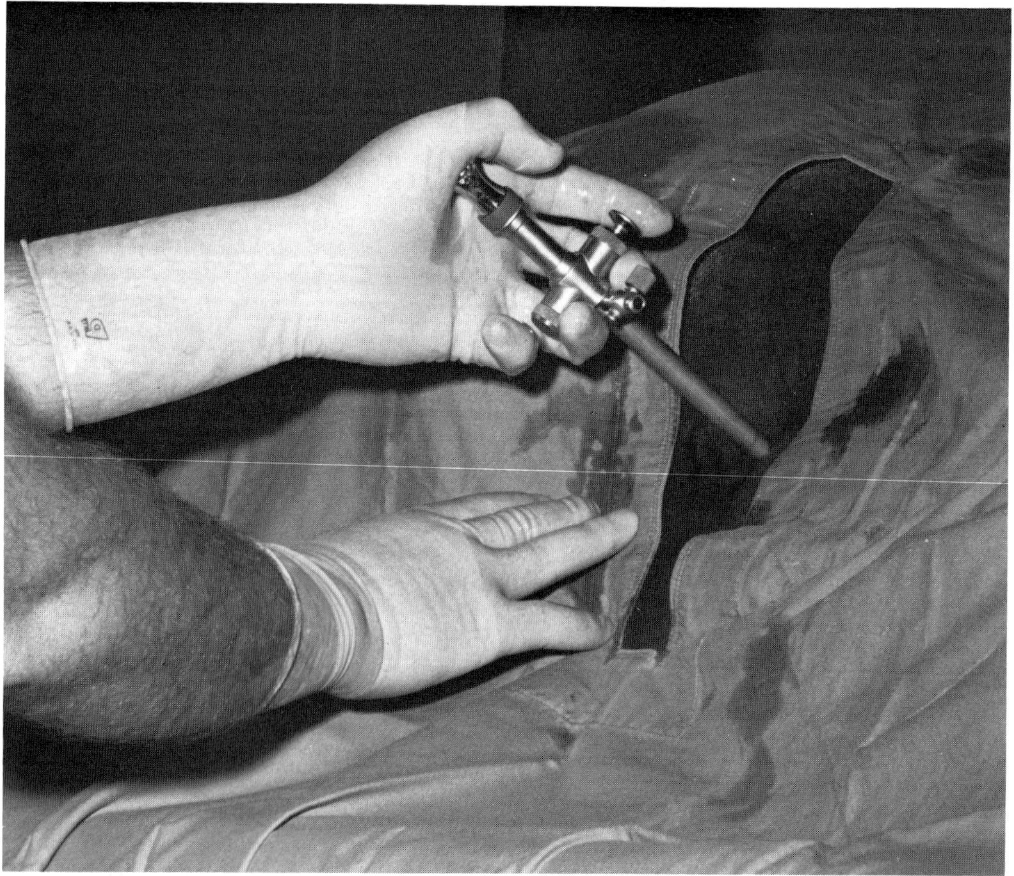

**Figure 9.5**   Insertion of the trocar-cannula through the cranial incision.

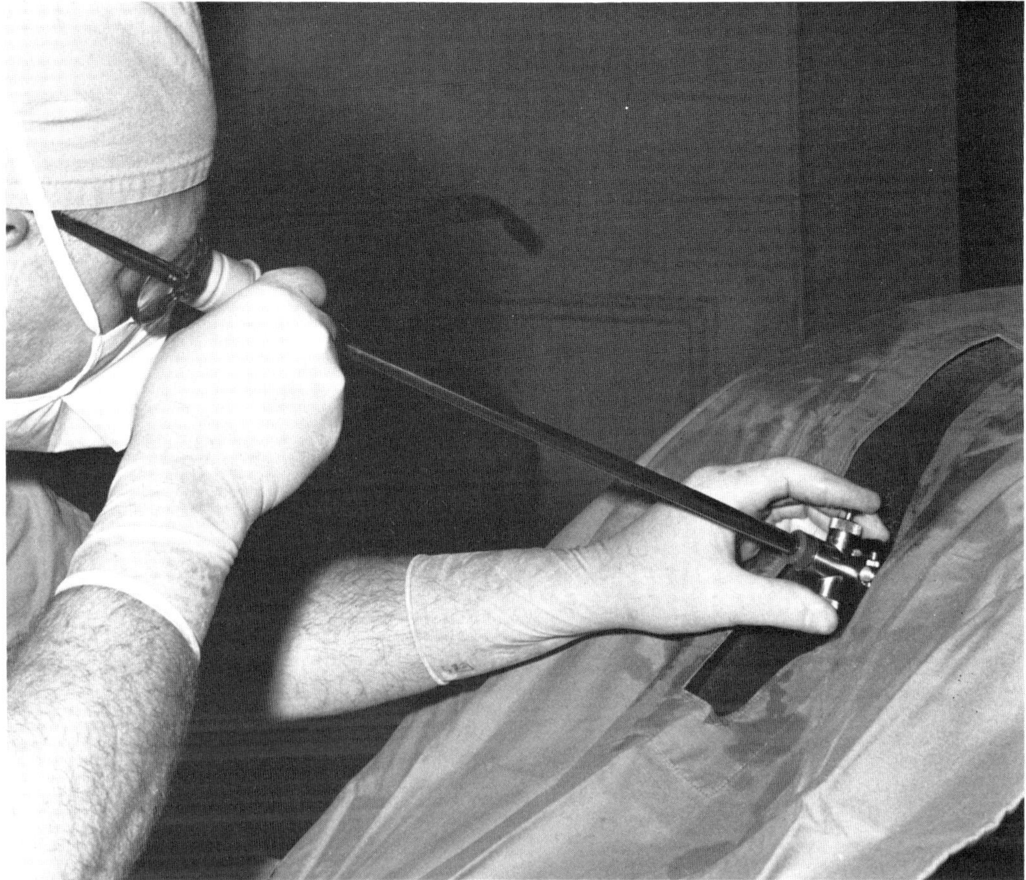

**Figure 9.6**   Observation through the rigid laparoscope.

peritoneum is perforated. The muscle and peritoneal layers are spread and the flexible laparoscope is inserted into the abdominal cavity (Fig. 9.7).

Use of the rigid laparoscope almost invariably requires adjacent accessory cannula and probe (Fig. 9.8) or forceps (Fig. 9.9) placement. Because of the relatively small operable area of the paralumbar fossa, the proposed site for insertion of the accessory cannula is rather limited and usually 4 to 6 cm to the left or right of the laparoscope. The distance between the laparoscopic cannula and the accessory cannula is important. The operator will discover that manipulation is extremely difficult if the two cannulae are located less than 4 cm apart.

An alternative approach to maneuvering the abdominal contents and assisting the operator's observation is rectal palpation. An assistant performs this with instructions from the laparoscopist and attempts to displace interfering organs or elevate the desired organ into the visual field.

## LAPAROSCOPIC PROCEDURE

### Clinical and Diagnostic Observations

A comprehensive understanding of the diagnostic and clinical capabilities of laparoscopy in the horse are yet to be determined. As previously indicated, the flexible

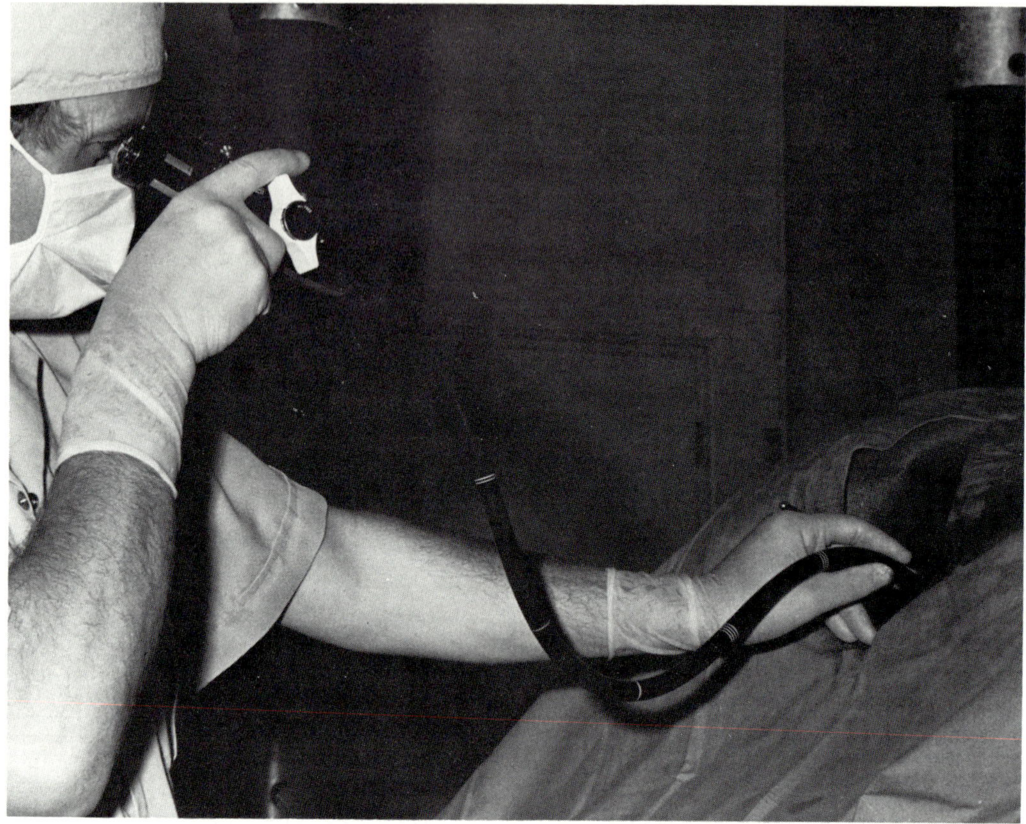

**Figure 9.7**    Observation through the flexible fiberscope.

endoscope provides an overall more inclusive observation range; however, both the flexible and rigid instruments are equally effective for examining certain organs, including the reproductive tract, bladder, spleen, lower small intestine, and colon.

A methodical approach is used in general diagnosis to assure that each organ is satisfactorily examined. Upon laparoscope insertion, the operator most likely will observe a natural airspace and then the convoluted small intestine (*Color Atlas*, Pl. 7, Fig. 8). Peristalsis, of course, causes this tissue to change position. By viewing first and again later, the laparoscopist can examine a greater portion of the gastrointestinal tract.

In the mare, the reproductive organs are easily observed, including the uterine body, horn, oviduct, fimbria, ovary, and ovulation fossa. Mares tend to vary in regard to the location of their ovaries. In most cases the ovary will be located caudal to the insertion site. In a few, however, it will be necessary to direct the laparoscope cranially to observe the ovary. Recently, Seager, Wildt, and Kraemer have used the rigid 10 mm in diameter laparoscope in preliminary studies for characterizing ovarian morphology. These investigators determined that this endoscope is effective for observing the ovary ipsilateral to the insertion site. Examination of the contralateral ovary has generally not been possible and has required the reinsertion of the laparoscope in the opposite side.

Ovarian activity in the mare is most visible in a specific anatomical locale, a groove, termed the ovulation fossa. Immediately adjacent, the very delicate appearing ovarian fimbria can be distinguished (Pl. 8, Fig. 1). The ovulation fossa of each ovary is most frequently positioned medially away from the direct view of the laparoscopist. The operator thus normally observes the inactive portion of the ovary (Pl. 8, Fig. 2). To

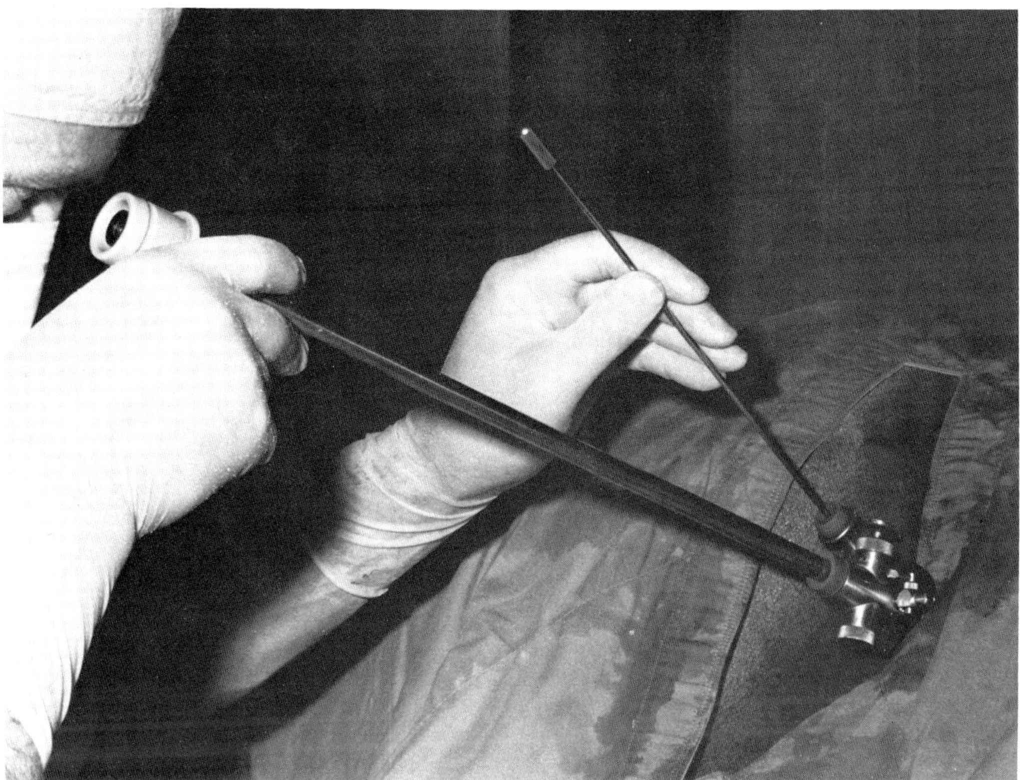

**Figure 9.8**   Manipulation with the accessory probe.

examine the ovulation fossa, the ovary must be rotated, using an accessory grasping forceps. Grasping the ovary itself appears to induce severe discomfort, even in mares heavily tranquilized. It is preferable that the fimbria be grasped and suitably maneuvered to bring the ovulatory fossa into view (Pl. 8, Fig. 3). The fimbria is less frail than it appears, and manipulating this tissue produces less animal stress. No apparent trauma has been induced. The ovulation fossa can be examined for follicular or luteal activity (Pl. 8, Figs. 4 and 5). The authors are unaware of any attempts to laparoscopically aspirate ovarian cysts in the mare; however, such a clinical procedure would appear feasible.

By directing the laparoscope caudally, the urinary bladder can be visualized. The flexible endoscope allows each ureter to be traced from the bladder to the respective kidney. The dorsal portion of the spleen is visible using either the rigid or flexible laparoscope. Splenic biopsy has been successfully performed in the horse, utilizing the rigid 10 mm in diameter laparoscope inserted through the left paralumbar fossa. An ancillary forceps (Palmer, Richard Wolf Medical Instruments Corp.) is inserted adjacent to the endoscope and used to obtain a tissue sample (Pl. 8, Fig. 6). Simultaneous electrocautery to prohibit postbiopsy hemorrhage has been unnecessary.

The flexible laparoscope has allowed additional examination of the gastrointestinal tract, beyond simple viewing of the small intestine. The dorsal surfaces of the left and right large colon are visible as well as the lower colon. The angulation of these structures prevents detailed observation. A limited portion of the cecum can also be observed in the right quadrant of the abdominal cavity.

Some technique problems exist, which are similar to those experienced in other species. Fogging may occur at the distal end of the laparoscope unless the instrument is

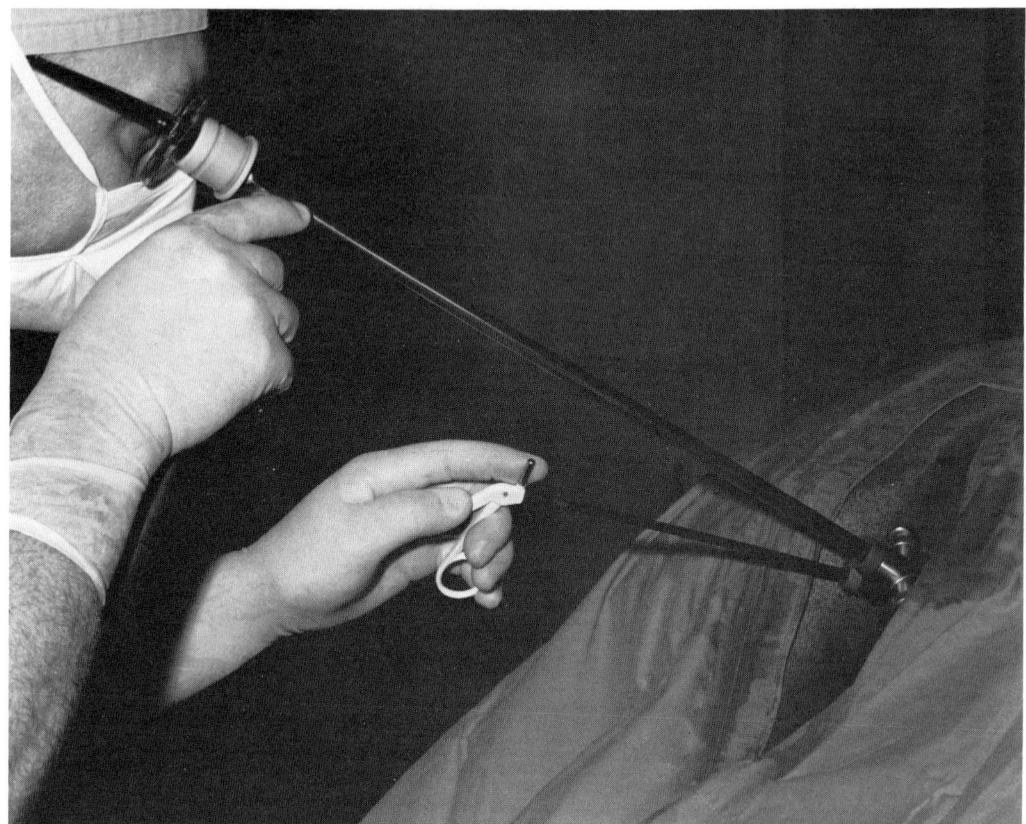

**Figure 9.9**  Manipulation with the accessory forceps.

near body temperature when initially inserted. Rinsing the endoscope in warm, sterile saline may alleviate this problem. Obesity in horses, as with other species, severely limits viewing potential. Vast abdominal deposits of fat dramatically reduce the number and extent of organs that can be visualized.

## Termination of the Examination and Postoperative Care

After completing the examination, all instruments are withdrawn from the peritoneal cavity. If entry through the peritoneum is made in the dorsal third of the paralumbar fossa, it is unnecessary to close the peritoneum with sutures. If the incision is more ventral or much longer than the laparoscope diameter, then one or two sutures are used to repair the peritoneum. The muscle layers are then sutured. These internal closures are performed using absorbable suture (1-0 chromic on an atraumatic ¾ circle needle). The skin is repaired using a nonabsorbable suture such as 1-0 braided silk. The horse should receive tetanus toxoid at the time of laparoscopy and a broad spectrum antibiotic injection daily for 72 hours as a prophylactic measure against peritonitis. Food and water can be given when the animal has sufficiently recovered from the effects of tranquilization. After the examination the horse should be walked to promote passage of gas par rectum and observed for some hours for signs of developing colic. If such symptoms occur they should be treated by routine procedures.

### Use of Endoscopes Outside the Abdominal Cavity

Both flexible and rigid fiber optic systems are becoming popular as diagnostic tools for examining areas outside of the abdominal cavity. The flexible endoscope has had other applications in equine medicine, particularly for examination of various portions of the gastrointestinal and respiratory tracts. The rigid endoscopes are also being utilized more outside the equine abdominal cavity for direct observation within the uterus (hysteroscopy), urinary tract (cystoscopy), and within joints (arthroscopy). A paper on the latter subject has been recently published (Hall and Keeran, 1975).

## CONCLUSIONS

The field of equine laparoscopy is currently not as advanced as in other smaller, domestic or laboratory animals. The pioneering efforts, nevertheless, have indicated the feasibility of this technique for reproductive study and as a diagnostic aid to confirm speculations made by rectal palpation. The effectiveness of laparoscopy for diagnosing and solving various pathological and oncological states in the horse remains to be tested. It is most likely that continued efforts by both equine research and clinical investigators will soon provide the specific information required to perform many of the sophisticated laparoscopic procedures currently routine in other species.

**References**

Hall, M. E. and Keeran, R. J. (1975) Use of the arthroscope in the horse. *Vet. Med. Small Anim. Clin.* 70: 705–706.

Heinze, V. H., and Klug, E. (1973) Endoskopische Beobachtungen an der inneren Genitalorganen (Pelviskopie) bei pferd und Esel. *Die Blauen Hefte fur den Tierarzt.* 50:550–560.

Heinze, V. H., Klug, E., and von Lepel, J. D. (1972) Optische Darstellung der inneren Geschlechtsorgane bein Equiden zur Diagnostik und Therapie. *D.T.W.* 79:49–51.

Witherspoon, D. M., and Talbot, R. B. (1970a) Ovulation site in the mare. *J. Am. Vet. Med. Assoc.* 157: 1452–1459.

Witherspoon, D. M., and Talbot, R. B. (1970b) Nocturnal ovulation in the equine animal. *Vet. Rec.* 87: 302–304.

# CHAPTER 10

# Laparoscopy in Zoo Mammals*

**Mitchell Bush, D.V.M.,**
**Stephen W. J. Seager, M.R.C.V.S., and**
**David E. Wildt, Ph.D.**

## INTRODUCTION

The laparoscope is a valuable diagnostic aid and research tool in zoological medicine (Bush *et al.*, 1978; Wildt *et al.*, 1978). The clinical diagnosis of illness in a zoological patient is a continual challenge. Many nondomesticated species characteristically mask overt signs of clinical disease, an adaptation from the wild to prevent attraction of predators. This presents problems in detecting the initial stages of illness and illustrates the need for continually testing new and improved modes of making clinical diagnoses. Stress factors, disposition, and potential danger of handling many zoological patients require immobilization of the animal even for such routine manipulatory procedures as physical or radiographic examination, and the collection of blood. Laparoscopy, if indicated, can be safely performed concurrently as an additional diagnostic aid to visualize and biopsy selected abdominal organs.

As with domestic species, application of laparoscopy to zoological research is continually expanding. Its initial use has been oriented to reproductive research, particularly the documentation of ovarian function. Much of the information obtained by laparoscopy serves as baseline data to facilitate both natural and artificial insemination breeding programs. More recently, other physiological-anatomical areas have received attention, particularly sequential observation and biopsy of various organs, including liver, kidney, and spleen. In this manner, laparoscopy offers a "new" means of studying the effects of nutrition and aging as well as a technique for characterizing pathological changes associated with chronic diseased states. Not only can laparoscopy provide early confirmation of a suspected diseased condition, but it also allows the operator to more fully study and understand the intermediate progressive changes in an illness instead of simply observing the terminal result at necropsy.

* The authors wish to thank the staff of the Houston Zoological Gardens, Houston, Texas; St. Louis Zoological Park, St. Louis, Missouri; and Gladys Porter Zoo, Brownsville, Texas, for their cooperation. The authors appreciate the assistance of Dr. S. Kennedy, College of Veterinary Medicine, University of Tennessee, Knoxville, Tennessee; and P. Schmidt, S. Charman Guthrie, G. Kinney, and C. Platz, Baylor College of Medicine, Houston, Texas.

The authors' respective laboratories have conducted collaborative investigations for four years concerning the effectiveness of laparoscopy in zoo mammals. The basic laparoscopy procedure, although utilized in a wide variety of mammalian species, is remarkably similar, illustrating the versatility, practicality, and simplicity of the procedure. The following chapter does not emphasize laparoscopy for any one species but discusses the applicability of this technique for zoo mammals in general.

## ANIMAL PREPARATION AND EQUIPMENT

### Animals, Anesthesia, and Restraint

As with any surgical procedure, it is advantageous to evaluate the animal prior to anesthesia. Often in zoo mammals, because of the risk and stress in handling, precise animal evaluation can only be made after inducing anesthesia. Our laboratories generally utilize this method and perform a limited physical examination. This serves as a base from which the animal can be examined further. Clinical evaluation of zoo patients prior to a laparoscopic procedure generally requires more care and effort than similar examinations of common domestic animals. Thus, once the decision is made to immobilize the animal, the clinical personnel should be organized to obtain maximal information from the procedure. Two immobilizations may be required—the first to evaluate general patient status and the second to perform the laparoscopic examination. If the initial examination indicates that the health of the animal will not be compromised by laparoscopy, then the latter examination may be conducted immediately.

In all zoo mammals examined to date, laparoscopy has been performed on animals under general anesthesia. The choice of anesthetic drug is dependent on the species examined. A comprehensive discussion of anesthesia is beyond the scope of the chapter and only a brief description is given here. The most common preparations used in a wide variety of mammals are dissociative anesthetics including ketamine hydrochloride (Ketaset, Bristol Laboratories), phencyclidine hydrochloride (Sernylan, BioCeutic Laboratories), or tiletamine-zolazepam combination (Telazol, Parke, Davis and Co.) alone or in combination with other drugs, including tranquilizers and/or xylazine (Rompun, Haver-Lockhart Laboratories). In hoofstock and some large bears, etorphine (M99, D-M Pharmaceuticals, Inc.) may be the drug of choice. After induction, anesthesia can be maintained by inhalation anesthetics, including halothane (Fluothane, Ayerst Laboratories) or methoxyflurane (Metofane, Pitman-Moore, Inc.). For further details on anesthetic drugs and methods and routes of administration in exotic species, the reader should refer to several recent textbooks (Young, 1975; Harthoorn, 1976; Fowler, 1978a,b).

### Equipment

The instrumentation used in the laboratories of the authors is the same as that previously described in Chapter 3. In brief, this consists of three rigid laparoscopes, 10, 5, and 2.7 mm in diameter, corresponding trocar-cannula assemblies, and an ancillary biopsy, manipulatory, and cautery forceps (Richard Wolf Medical Instruments Corp.). An automatic insufflator is employed to produce and maintain a pneumoperitoneum and heavy duty light projector provides illumination for visualization. Still photographs are obtained with an Olympus OM-1 SLR camera and 100 mm lens. The laboratory of the senior author uses 3/4 inch color videotapes for documentation using a portable color television camera (Sony Trinicon Color Camera DXC 1600, Atsugi, Japan) and a color video-cassette recorder (Sony Umatic VO 2800, Atsugi, Japan). More details on laparoscopic videotaping of intraabdominal anatomy and activity are provided later in the chapter.

The endoscopic instruments described are of standard type and length originally fabricated for use in humans. Although these devices are readily adapted to most species, examinations in certain animals can be greatly facilitated by special modifications provided by the manufacturer. The primary problem is in large mammals, particularly large felidae, the great apes, and hoofstock. Standard trocar-cannula units may be of insufficient length to successfully perforate all layers of the abdominal wall. In addition, an elongated Verres needle (150 mm in length) may be required to ensure proper placement of insufflated gas into the peritoneal cavity proper. Operators who suspect such a potential problem should consult with the equipment manufacturer.

In many instances, financial limitations will necessitate that the zoo clinic purchase a single endoscope. Authors of previous chapters have urged the potential laparoscopist to carefully consider specific needs and this is particularly sound advice for the zoological clinician likely faced with examination of very diverse sizes of animals. Although the large diameter laparoscopes (i.e., 8 to 10 mm) offer an exceptional viewing field and greater photographic potential, a smaller diameter instrument (i.e., 4 to 7 mm) will likely provide more versatility and practicality to a general zoological practice or research program. Our laboratories generally restrict use of the 10 mm in diameter endoscope to species weighing greater than 15 kg. The operator should carefully examine all pertinent equipment from several manufacturers before purchase.

## Surgical Preparation of Patient and Equipment

Because of the ecological and economical value and often rarity of many zoo mammals, laparoscopy is considered analogous to major surgery necessitating the same preparations and precautions. All clinical evaluations are performed using sterile technique. Instruments are immersed in a germicidal solution of chlorhexidine (Nolvasan-S, Fort Dodge Laboratories) as described in Chapter 3.

Anesthesia in zoological mammals produces certain inherent risks due to the animal temperament, anatomical and physiological differences, drugs used, method of administration, and the general lack of knowledge of the science of anesthesiology in such animals. Physiological status, including pulse, respiration rate and depth, tissue perfusion, and body temperature are intensely monitored during anesthesia and the laparoscopy examination. Proper evaluation of these findings will alert the anesthetist to the status of the animal and allow early detection and treatment of potential problems. The patient's position (head down) during laparoscopy and the production of a pneumoperitoneum causes increased pressure on the diaphragm which can compromise respiration and potentiate gastric reflux inducing secondary inhalation pneumonia. These problems can be minimized by intubating the patient with a cuffed endotracheal tube so that respiration can be assisted when indicated. If gastric reflux should occur, the tube will help prevent aspiration of stomach content. As in cattle and sheep, in captive wild hoofstock the rumen presents a special problem. These animals are fasted at least three days. After anesthesia, these species are also intubated to assist respiration and prevent inhalation pneumonia.

Laparoscopy in zoo mammals is best performed in a well equipped surgical suite. This facilitates sterility and ensures access to appropriate equipment to respond to unexpected complications and emergencies. Following induction of anesthesia, the animal immediately undergoes the described evaluation procedures. The urinary bladder is palpated and, if distended, expressed or catheterized. With the exception of hoofstock, (discussed later) other zoo mammals must at least initially be restrained in the supine head down position (Fig. 10.1). Although most species can be accommodated on a standard surgical table, some ingenuity may be required to accurately position extremely large species. Size of some animals may even preclude transfer to the clinic area. For example, the authors have laparoscopically examined several adult bears (300 to 400 kg), lions, and gorillas in the cage quarters with the anesthetized animal restrained on a sloping sheet of plywood.

The ventral abdomen is clipped and/or shaved and the skin prepared for sterile

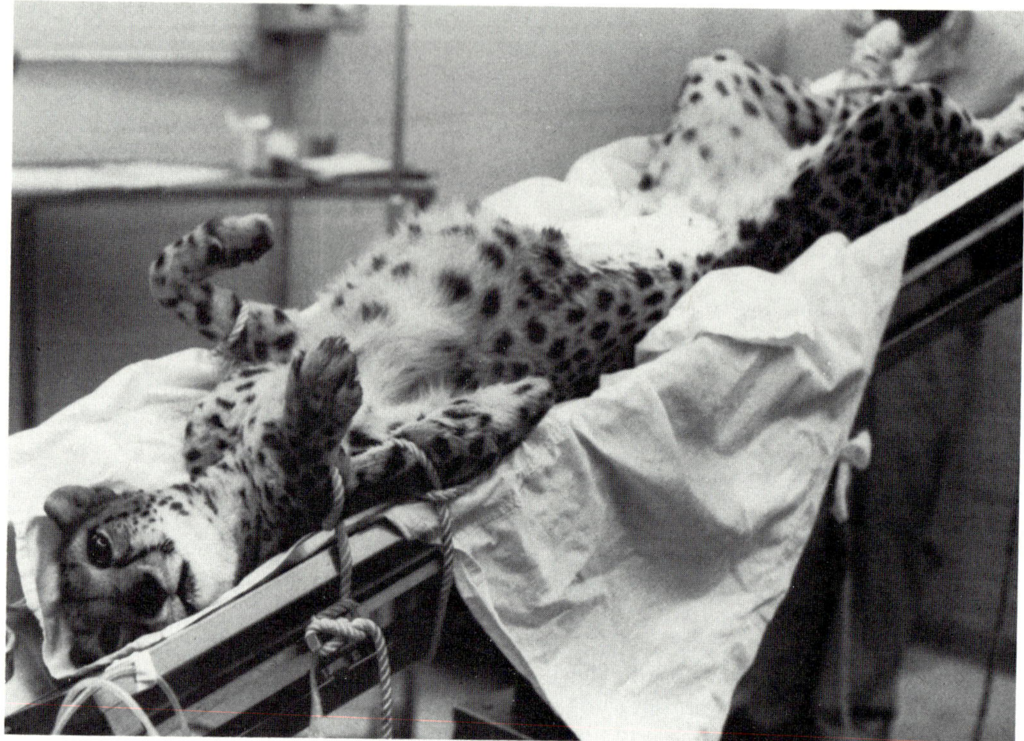

**Figure 10.1**   Cheetah restrained in a head-down supine position at an angle of approximately 45°.

surgery using germicidal soap (Betadine Surgical Scrub, Purdue Frederick Co.), tincture of Zephiran (Winthrop Laboratories), and tamed iodine (Pharmadine, Sherwood Pharmaceutical Co.). The animal is then covered with a sterile drape. The clear plastic drape is preferable to the cloth type since the former facilitates monitoring animal respiration, position, and degree of insufflation.

## CAPTIVE WILD HOOFSTOCK

Laparoscopy in domestic cattle and horses is challenging and, as expected, similar zoo hoofstock can present additional technique problems. As previously described in this text, the domestic cow and horse are subjected to laparoscopy in a standing position, sometimes with the rear quarters elevated. Laparoscopy in large, nondomesticated hoofstock is complicated because the patient will not tolerate such a manipulatory procedure in a restrained standing position. Therefore, patients must be anesthetized and placed in either the lateral recumbent or supine head down position. In the former, ruminants are positioned on the left side and the right paralumbar fossa region designated as the site for laparoscope insertion. The operator should be aware that, because of displacement of abdominal contents, a comprehensive examination of internal organs is not possible, even with considerable insufflation. Generally, from the paralumbar approach, one ovary and a portion of the uterus and gut may be viewed. In nonruminants, it may be necessary to reposition the animal on its right side and reinsert the laparoscope in the left fossa to allow observation of the contralateral portion of the cavity. The operator may experiment with various positions to ultimately achieve visualization of the target organ. For example, the senior author has attempted paralumbar laparoscopy with the anesthetized animal in a sternal position. Unfortunately, the resulting pressure on the abdominal wall compresses the cavity contents dorsally, restricting the viewing area. Even with these problems, a limited examination can provide useful information.

Some ruminants, especially those weighing less than 35 kg in body weight (i.e., gazelles), can be restrained in the conventional supine Trendelenburg position. This allows pelvic organs to be viewed in a relatively normal manner. The experienced operator can also place larger size species in this position. Figure 10.2 illustrates laparoscopy in a blesbok weighing approximately 100 kg. The reader should refer to Chapter 6 for descriptions of specific procedural techniques for ultimately visualizing various abdominal organs in ruminants in the Trendelenburg position. Using such a procedure, the operator should be concerned with two major factors: (1) avoiding rumen content reflux by fasting the animal and the insertion of an endotracheal tube; (2) insertion of the endoscopic trocar-cannula at a far caudal site adjacent to the mammary gland to avoid perforation of the rumen.

Other techniques should be considered to aid laparoscopy of hoofstock. Animals are fasted for 72 hours and water withheld for 18 to 24 hours prior to examination to reduce rumen size. Insertion of a stomach tube may be beneficial to relieve gaseous distension within the rumen. The urinary bladder is catheterized and internal air space increased by insufflation. The examination may be facilitated by the utilization of a specialized cannula assembly and one or more manipulative forceps or probes. Lastly, when

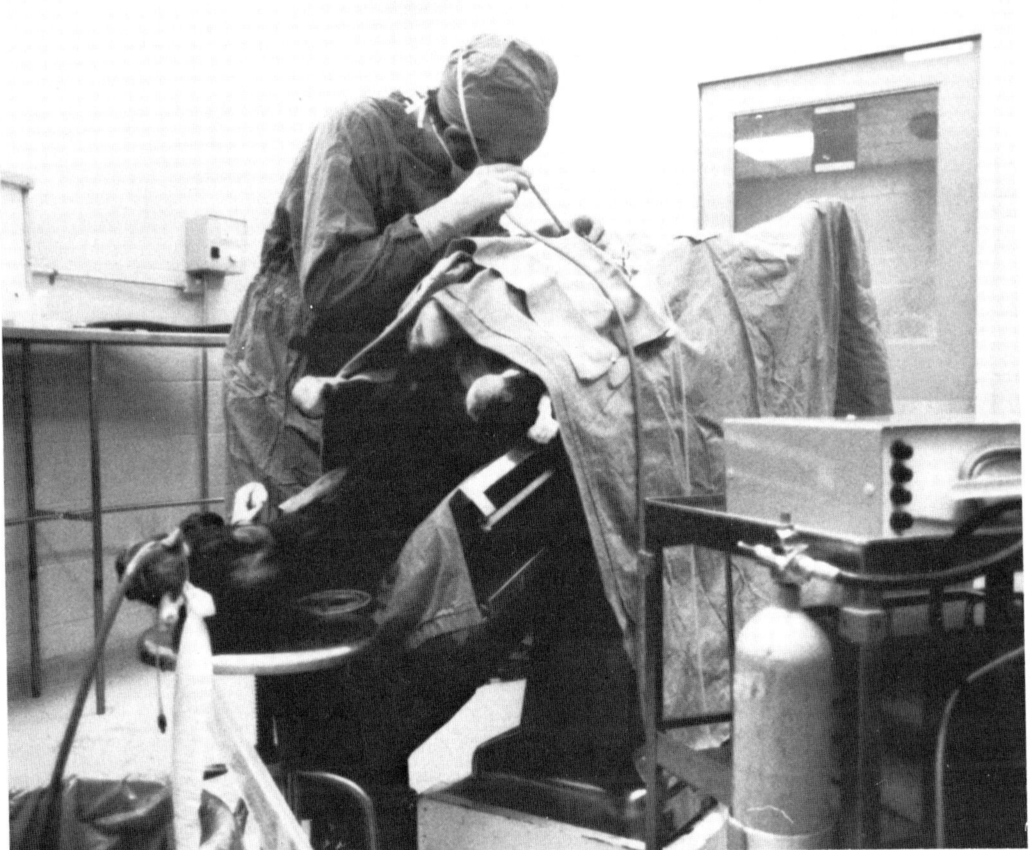

**Figure 10.2**  Midventral laparoscope approach in a blesbok.

performing laparoscopy with the animal in the lateral recumbent or sternal position, anatomical location and organ displacement can be provided by an assistant performing a simultaneous rectal examination. Such a procedure is particularly beneficial for reflecting the expansive colon laterally or dorsally, increasing the viewing space.

## LAPAROSCOPIC TECHNIQUE

### Operative Procedure

A basic understanding of the patient's abdominal anatomy is necessary before any laparoscopy examination. With a wide variety of species available in zoological practice or research, the operator must make a concerted effort to learn the comparative anatomy necessary for performing a safe examination.

A pneumoperitoneum is produced in all zoo mammals; however, insufflation techniques may vary due to animal size or anatomy. For most species, the standard Verres needle technique in conjunction with an automatic insufflator is the most efficient. The commercial insufflator designed for use in humans provides a relatively slow transfer of gas. In large animals, for example the adult bear, the time required for establishing a pneumoperitoneum may be prolonged, thus infringing on the critical anesthesia interval. The experienced operator can resolve this problem by insufflating directly from a tank of compressed gas. Additional precautions are required using this high pressure procedure (see Chapter 3).

Either 100% carbon dioxide ($CO_2$) or 5 to 10% $CO_2$ in air is used to establish and maintain the pneumoperitoneum. Gas is infused until the abdomen is distended, making the skin slightly tense to touch, but not compromising respiration. The intraabdominal pressure gauge of the insufflator should never record greater than 30 mm of mercury.

The site of laparoscopic trocar-cannula insertion is dictated by species size, abdominal anatomy, the area to be viewed, and the length of the laparoscope. For small and medium sized animals (for example, the size of the cheetah, jaguar, or less) insertion is at or near the umbilicus. This positioning allows the operator visual access to the pelvic organs as well as the cranial abdominal cavity contents. In larger animals (i.e., the lion, tiger, or bear) the puncture site is altered in the direction of the organs to be examined. A skin incision (1 to 2 cm) is usually made at the midline. In some obese patients, some difficulty may be experienced with this approach when passing the laparoscope through or by the falciform ligament. In such cases, a paramedian insertion method may avoid such a problem.

The trocar-cannula is inserted through the skin incision and the underlying abdominal layers at a 30° angle to the body plane with the assembly directed caudally. Elevating the skin with thumb forceps and using a slight rotating motion of the trocar aids the insertion procedure. The trocar is then removed and replaced with the laparoscope.

As in domesticated species, ancillary manipulation can greatly facilitate the examination. In small to medium sized animals, the 120 or 150 mm Verres needle can be used to maneuver internal organs. An accessory trocar-cannula can also be inserted lateral to the ventral midline to allow subsequent insertion of a grasping, cautery, or biopsy forceps.

### Termination of the Procedure

At the end of the laparoscopic examination, the pneumoperitoneum is relieved by removing the laparoscope and evacuating the gas slowly through the open cannula. If the gas is relieved too rapidly, there is the potential for vascular collapse, with sudden redistribution of abdominal pressure and blood flow. In addition, there is a greater tendency for fat or omentum to herniate through the incision site. The cannula and Verres needle are withdrawn and the cannula puncture site closed by a routine two layer (peritoneum, skin) suture method. Topical wound care is usually unwarranted and, in fact, may draw the animal's attention to the surgery site. Postoperative antibiotics are not indicated unless sterile technique was not maintained. Because of the recovered patient's temperament and potentially dangerous nature, further postoperative care in zoo mammals is minimal.

## CAPABILITIES OF LAPAROSCOPY

A total of 162 examinations have been performed in 32 different zoological species. Few complications and no deaths have been recorded. Serial laparoscopy has been performed in several species, including 16 examinations in a single jaguar and 14 examinations in a cheetah.

### Diagnostic Capabilities

The diagnostic capabilities of laparoscopy have been discussed in detail throughout this text. Most zoo mammals are not unique; laparoscopy offers excellent visualization of the reproductive organs (*Color Atlas*, Pl. 8, Fig. 7), bladder, kidney, spleen (Pl. 8, Fig. 8), liver, gallbladder, and various portions of the stomach and intestinal tract. The major diagnostic uses by the authors have been concerned with reproductive study or ascertaining gross organ status in diseased or apparently unaffected states. Each of these categories is discussed and illustrations provided.

### EVALUATION OF REPRODUCTIVE ORGANS

Little information exists on basic reproductive parameters in most exotic species. In the past, data from domestic animals have been used to extrapolate assumptions concerning zoo mammals. With the continued endangerment of many rare species, such assumptions are no longer valid. Unfortunately, more speculation will not help solve breeding problems or alleviate pathological conditions.

**1. Determining Reproductive Anatomy and Function.** Laparoscopy is an effective tool for analyzing cyclic alterations normally occurring in the reproductive organs of little studied zoo mammals. Even though these species are more susceptible to imposed stress compared to domesticated animals, they have been successfully subjected to serial laparoscopic examinations. These studies are designed to relate changes in ovarian morphology to estrous behavior, serum levels of reproductive hormones, and vaginal cytology. Our laboratories have employed laparoscopy for conducting such investigations in the jaguar (Pl. 9, Fig. 1), lion (Pl. 9, Fig. 2), cheetah, and tiger.

To illustrate the lack of basic knowledge in zoo mammals, the literature contains no specific information on the type of ovulatory response experienced by most wild felidae. It is *assumed* that the wild cat is similar to the domestic cat and that ovulation occurs only following a mating stimulus (induced ovulatory response). Laparoscopy has allowed the collection of preliminary data indicating that the jaguar and lion are indeed induced ovulators. However, laparoscopy of some isolated unmated cheetahs and tigers soon after exhibiting behavioral estrus has shown surprising results. Ovaries contain unmistakable ovulation sites (corpora lutea) indicating, at least in these cases, that ovulation was spontaneous in the absence of a copulation.

As another example, a curator wished to initiate a reproductive control program in a pair of Kodiak bears which were "overproducing" offspring. Progesterone administration to the female was prescribed, and it was determined that the effect of such treatment on the ovary would be monitored by laparoscopy. Subsequent examination revealed that each of the bear's ovaries was completely encapsulated in an ovarian bursa or pouch and not visible to the operator (Pl. 9, Fig. 3). Subsequent laparoscopy in the spectacled and polar bear confirmed this unique reproductive anatomical arrangement to exist in at least three members of the Ursidae family. Such results demonstrate the paucity of baseline knowledge currently known in the rather common zoo species and illustrate the potential of laparoscopy in helping to establish such data.

**2. Assisting Natural or Artificial Perpetuation of Species.** A major directive for zoos is to propagate species within the collection. Such a program strives for a self sustaining population so that it is unnecessary to replenish the collection with animals from the wild. Consequently, a greater responsibility is incurred in maintaining endangered species by captive breeding. Success in this endeavor requires not only satisfying the animal's social, nutritional, and health requirements, but understanding basic reproductive control mechanisms to sustain optimum reproductive potential. Species selected for breeding may initially undergo diagnostic laparoscopy to ensure a sound and anatomically intact reproductive tract. More important, this technique serves as an adjunct tool for the development of exogenous hormonal therapy necessary to induce ovarian activity and estrous behavior. For example, hormone treatments for inducing estrus in the anestrous domestic cat have been modified and used successfully in the jaguar and cheetah (Pl. 9, Fig. 4). Laparoscopy offers the most effective means to repeatedly evaluate the extent of ovarian follicle development during and after hormone treatment. As breeding programs expand and further federal restrictions are placed on legal animal transport between zoos, researchers will rely heavily on the procedures for collecting and freezing spermatozoa and performing artificial insemination. Detection of time of ovulation laparoscopically allows more precise timing for sperm deposition via artificial insemination, thus improving considerably the chances of obtaining optimum conception rates.

**3. Discovery of Abnormal Reproductive States.** It is currently impossible to estimate the incidence or effect of abnormal or pathological conditions on fertility in zoo mammals. The authors have encountered, and in some cases resolved, abnormal states using laparoscopic technique. With direct visualization of the ovary, oviduct, and uterus, gross abnormalities can be easily detected, including cystic follicles, polycystic ovaries, pyometra, and pelvic adhesions possibly contributing to infertility. Cystic follicles have been diagnosed in the white Bengal tiger (Pl. 9, Fig. 5) and African lion. In the latter case, the female was anorectic and demonstrating chronic behavioral estrus. Laparoscopy allowed confirmation of the abnormal state and, based on this diagnosis, prescription of effectual treatment. After hormonal therapy, reexamination by laparoscopy gave an accurate evaluation of the effectiveness of treatment.

Reproductive problems have also been examined in female gorillas which have failed to reproduce for five or more years. In one animal, laparoscopic visualization was impaired by extensive pelvic adhesions which were speculated to contribute to poor reproductive performance. Minor adhesion development was also noted in the second individual; however, reproductive anatomy appeared sound and luteal tissue remnants on both ovaries indicated that this female's ovaries were cycling normally.

## EVALUATION OF OTHER ABDOMINAL ORGANS

A major advantage of laparoscopy is that only minor surgical intervention is required to determine the gross appearance of most abdominal organs and tissue. As in the human, animal laparoscopy allows the operator to easily evaluate organ status and determine the degree of a diseased condition prior to performing major surgery. Such a technique has wide application in zoo medicine and research. As an example, the cheetah is often afflicted with chronic, progressive liver disease (Lombard et al., 1968). Laparoscopy has been used to diagnose and monitor the gross and microscopic (via biopsy) changes associated with this disease. In a like manner, laparoscopy is useful in oncology to detect or confirm tumor development and progression. Plate 9, Figure 6 illustrates a seminoma which infiltrated the abdominal cavity of a clouded leopard.

## Biopsy and Surgical Capabilities

In addition to viewing an organ directly, laparoscopy allows simultaneous biopsy of selected sites. This advantage stimulates considerable opportunities in the areas of histopathology, electronmicroscopy, histochemistry, and bacterial, fungal and/or viral cultures. The laparoscopic biopsy is less traumatic in that it requires less surgery than the open biopsy, requires less surgical time, and produces fewer postoperative adhesions and complications. In addition, the potential for repeated or serial biopsy of the same organ exists, providing the opportunity for the gathering of sequential data.

### BIOPSY OF THE LIVER, SPLEEN, AND OVARY

Biopsy equipment and insertion techniques have been previously described in this text for the domestic dog and cat (see Chapter 3). These procedures and corresponding comments are equally applicable to zoo mammals. For hepatic, splenic, and ovarian biopsy a grasping type biopsy instrument is preferred. This type of device provides adequate tissue for histopathological examination and, if necessary, can be used to obtain multiple samples from the same organ. A biopsy forceps is usually serrated on the cutting edge, minimizing postbiopsy hemorrhage. Bleeding is not a common problem and, if it occurs, the biopsy forceps can be attached to an electrosurgical unit to allow coagulation of the bleeding site. A second method involves covering the hemorrhaging area with absorbable gelatin (Gelfoam, Upjohn Co.). This gelatin is placed in the jaws of a forceps, transferred down the accessory cannula, and applied directly to the bleeding site.

Tissue samples have been obtained from a variety of species using the grasping forceps technique. Of particular interest has been the sequential collection of liver samples in cheetahs with degenerative liver disease (Pl. 9, Fig. 7). Biopsies are taken at selected intervals and the histopathological course of this disease is monitored in an attempt to determine the etiology and progressive changes of this anomaly.

### BIOPSY OF THE KIDNEY

For sampling renal tissue, a biopsy needle works most satisfactorily. A brief discussion of this procedure is presented in Chapter 3. Again, laparoscopy allows direct examination of the desired site, guidance of the biopsy unit, and post-biopsy observation of the target organ for complications such as excessive bleeding. The technique employs a 13 gauge, 8 cm in length trocar-cannula needle (Special Needle, Becton, Dickinson and Co.) and has been used to successfully and repeatedly obtain kidney tissue samples in the cheetah (Pl. 9, Fig. 8), tiger, lion, and binturong. It has been particularly useful as an aid in documenting renal disease and correlating tissue findings to urinalysis and serum chemical values.

The animal is subjected to routine laparoscopy. After the operator is assured of adequate pneumoperitoneum, instrument insertion, and visualization, the surgical table is leveled and the animal rotated so that the target kidney is elevated slightly dorsally. Access to the right kidney is easier since the spleen may have to be manipulated to approach the left kidney. Depending on the species, the kidney proper is either directly observed or, in the case of felidae, its contour is visible under the perirenal fat layer. The latter case may be confirmed by palpation of the suspected renal outline using a Verres needle or manipulatory forceps. With the animal repositioned, the biopsy needle can be inserted through a surgically prepared and draped area in the paralumbar fossa and then laparoscopically directed to the kidney (Pl. 9, Fig. 8). The trocar-cannula needle is pushed into the kidney parenchyma, the trocar removed, and a 20 ml syringe (containing 7 to 10 ml of heparinized saline) attached to the needle hub. The needle is then advanced into the kidney while negative pressure is produced and maintained with the syringe. This is usually sufficient to aspirate a uniform core of renal tissue. The needle is then partially withdrawn from the kidney. Generally, before complete removal from the kidney the needle is redirected at a slightly different angle to collect a second sample. Some hemorrhage will occur, but usually ceases within several minutes. The operator should laparoscopically observe the biopsied site to ensure that hemorrhage does not progress.

The plunger is removed from the syringe and the core of tissue retrieved. The operator should be aware that the tissue sample does not always pass completely into the syringe barrel. The needle should be flushed with saline to detect any tissue adhered to the internal wall of the cannula.

## SURGICAL PROCEDURES

In our laboratories, laparoscopic surgery in zoo mammals has primarly been limited to alterations in reproductive function. Although infertility problems are all too prevalent in many zoo species, some specimens are overly prolific. A surplus of animals results and compatible adult pairs of opposite sexes must be maintained separately for fear of unwanted pregnancy. Castration or ovariohysterectomy is undesirable since such procedures eliminate endogenous hormone secretion responsible for maintaining secondary sex characteristics desirable for exhibit animals.

One remedy for this overpopulation problem has been vasectomy of the male. Laparoscopy has been used to perform internal vas deferens occlusion (internal vasectomy) and has been shown to be a positive alternative to the external inguinal approach. Basically, laparoscopic vas occlusion and ligation offers the advantage of being a rapid procedure and eliminating the postsurgical complications associated with an incision in the inguinal region. The male animal is subjected to routine laparoscopy and the laparoscope directed to the far caudal and lateral corner of each side of the abdominal cavity. Each vas deferens is easily identified, grasped with an electrocoagulation forceps, and 2 to 3 cm cauterized. The forceps are replaced with ancillary scissors and a section of the cauterized vas severed (Pl. 10, Fig. 1) and then removed from the cavity (Pl. 10, Fig. 2). Such a procedure has been conducted successfully in crabeating foxes and African lions. The latter animals were electroejaculated to obtain semen samples before and after laparoscopic sterilization. Preoperative ejaculates contained normal concentrations of spermatozoa; postoperative ejaculates were void of any live or dead sperm. Both male foxes and lions have been paired with adult females and no offspring have resulted.

Similar sterilization procedures require investigation in selected females. It may be necessary that a male be housed with numerous females, some of which for genetic reasons or pathological conditions are undersirable for perpetuating the species. This was the case in a troop of macaque monkeys housed together, in which one adult female consistently became pregnant and required repeated infant delivery via caesarian section. The animal was subjected to laparoscopy and the oviduct coagulated using a cautery forceps. This procedure was considered safe and effective since this was essentially the same procedure utilized extensively in women for over a decade. However, similar laparoscopic sterilization procedures in species other than primates deserve considerably more investigation prior to widespread utilization.

## Use of the Laparoscope Outside the Abdominal Cavity

Although beyond the scope of this text, the individual considering the purchase of laparoscopy equipment should also be aware of its potential uses outside the abdominal cavity. Small diameter laparoscopes designed for arthroscopy or internal joint observation in humans are feasible for use in larger zoo mammals. The endoscope can also be used for examination of various body openings, including the oral cavity, respiratory system, and vagina. When observing the vaginal vault, the urethral orifice, vaginal mucosa, and cervical os are visible. Direct visual control with the endoscope aids in the insertion of culture, insemination, or irrigation instruments into the cervix and/or uterine body. The laparoscope may also be employed to view the posterior pharynx, larynx, and trachea. In examining these areas, it is imperative that the patient be adequately anesthetized and a mouth gag be in place to protect the telescope. Only short examinations should be conducted within the trachea since the tidal volume of the lung will be reduced as a result of the occluding laparoscope.

## Laparoscopic Photography

Combined laparoscopy-photography is an excellent means of documenting findings and providing teaching material. A photography record is particularly valuable in zoological medicine and research because of the wide variation in patients, many of which are rare. The novice will soon discover the importance of photographed observations as an important reference for self use or illustration to colleagues and students.

Laparoscopy is adaptable to various types of photography, including 35 mm still photographs, television videotape, and both 8 and 16 mm film. Most of the authors' experience has been concerned with the former two procedures. Basic technique for 35 mm laparoscopic photography used in our laboratories has been discussed previously (see Chapter 3). Several additional points of information may be noted. The SLR camera can undergo three rather inexpensive modifications to either assist the operator in obtaining greater quality photographs or to provide a method of identifying the resulting pictures. Internally, the standard viewing screen of the camera can be removed and replaced with a clearer or brighter screen plate. Most standard screens are excessively dark, making precise identification of the target organ through the camera-laparoscope unit difficult. The clear screen, although not directly improving picture quality, allows a brighter field of view. This type of viewing screen is inexpensive and can be installed easily by the operator. A second useful camera modification is a standard release cable. This flexible cable, 15 to 20 cm in length, screws into the camera shutter release and allows an assistant to expose the film (Fig. 10.3). The operator can then concentrate on steadying the camera and maintaining the proper visual field. When the time is correct, the operator instructs the assistant to release the camera shutter by means of the cable. This procedure reduces camera motion, allows the utilization of longer exposure times, and definitely can improve photograph quality.

Difficulty often arises in the accurate identification of resulting photographs. This problem can be alleviated by an identification device which attaches to the back of the camera body (Richard Wolf Medical Instruments Corp.). This device identifies each exposure permanently with a letter and/or number. The operator instructs an assistant keeping a written record on the letter-number sequence being used and also indicates a description of the target site being photographed. Upon receiving the processed photographs, the letter-number sequences in the written record are merely referred to for individual picture identification.

Impressive documentation of observations can be achieved using videotape recording. The laparoscopist affiliated with an academic institution with television camera and recording facilities may be surprised at the rather limited modifications required to perform laparoscopic video-recording. Either a black and white or color camera unit may be utilized. The former provides sharper contrast of internal organs; however, the color provided by the latter unit obviously provides a more natural indication of the character of the abdominal cavity content.

Our experience has generally involved a portable minicamera with standard 100 mm zoom lens. This unit is very lightweight (3.5 kg) and can easily be held in one hand. The camera is attached to the eyepiece of the laparoscope using the same mounting adapter employed for attaching the SLR camera 100 mm lens to the endoscope (Fig. 10.4).

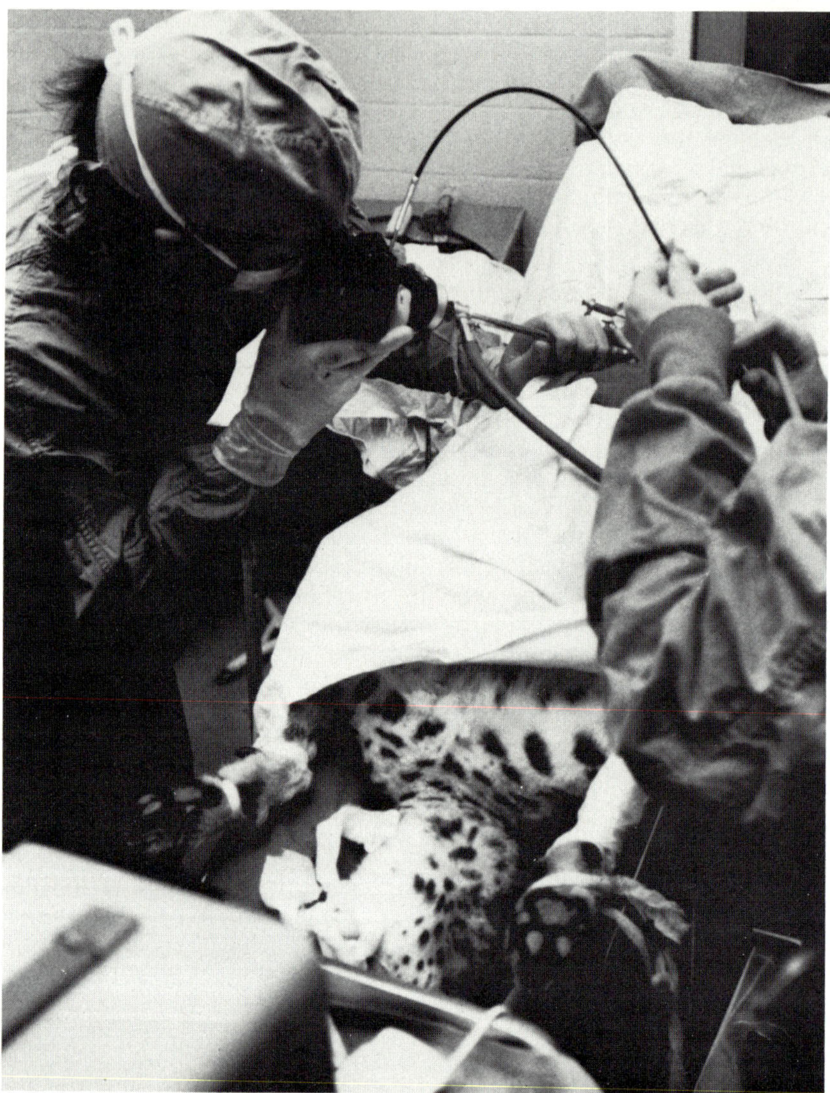

**Figure 10.3**   Laparoscopic still photography in the cheetah. An assistant operates the shutter release cable.

In laparoscopic examinations in which photographs are desired, we first switch the light source to the photographic intensity. Still photographs are usually taken initially, using the SLR camera attached to the laparoscope. This camera is detached and the mounting adapter removed and attached to the television camera. The latter unit is associated with both a videotape player/recorder and a television monitor. The operator supports the laparoscope-cannula unit as an assistant attaches and then holds the television camera (Fig. 10.4). The videotape recorder is started and the operator, by viewing the television monitor, maneuvers the laparoscope to the target site to be photographed. After brief practice, the operator can become quite adept at performing internal manipulation and even surgical and biopsy procedures by direction provided by observation of the television monitor.

It should be noted that the quality of the resulting videotape is directly affected by the quantity of internal illumination. Hence, improved quality is provided by a larger

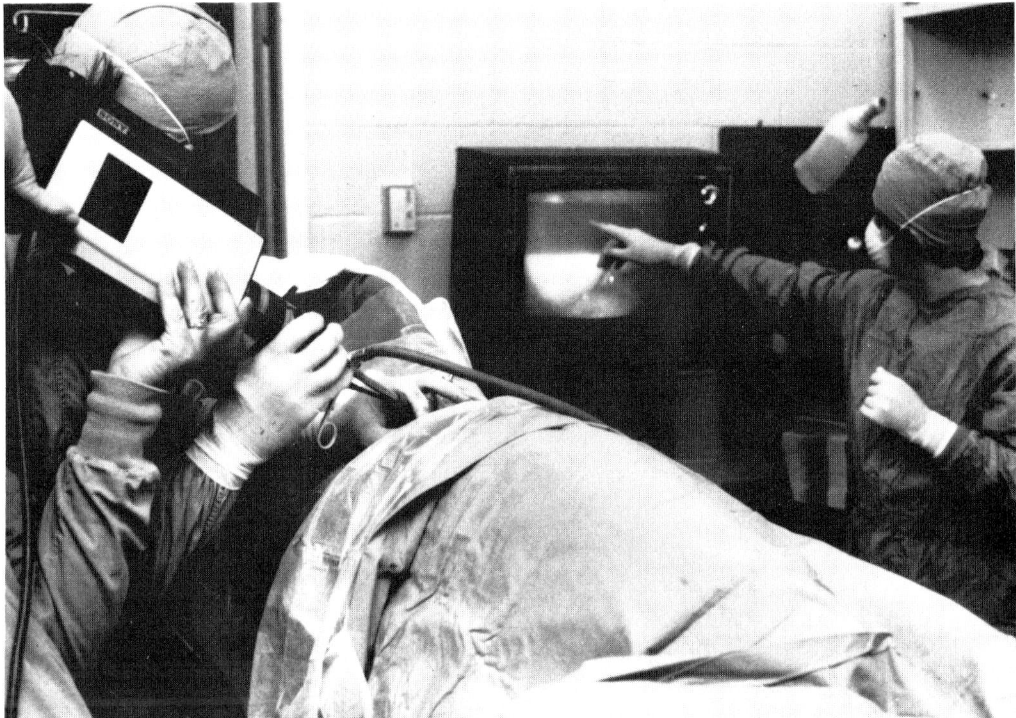

**Figure 10.4** Videotape recording through the laparoscope. The operator steadies the laparoscope while an assistant attaches and supports the camera. Internal manipulations are made by viewing the monitor seen in the background.

diameter laparoscope. Adequate recordings have resulted from using the smaller, 5 mm in diameter endoscope. Video-recording units are also available with microphone and voice recorders which allow documentation of important comments made during the examination. Following laparoscopy, these audible recordings can be referenced and information converted into written data records. The videotape can subsequently be edited, reproduced, or narrated, all of which allow this type of photography to be an extremely valuable documentary technique for medical, research, or teaching purposes.

It should be realized that still and television camera equipment is not sterile; therefore, minimum exposure to the surgical field should be allowed. If the operator has handled a camera during the photographic session, he should change to sterile gloves prior to continuing the examination or closing the incision sites.

### Laparoscopic Records

Because of numerous variations in zoo mammal anatomy, physiology, and reaction to anesthetics, it is vitally important that information be properly documented. This data should include detail on method and success of anesthesia, insufflation volume, site of trocar insertion, organs observed, anatomical considerations, photographs obtained, and complications. These records will not only aid the laparoscopist in succeeding examinations but will be of use to other colleagues performing similar studies.

## CONCLUSIONS

The art and sciences of laparoscopy in zoological medicine and research are coming of age. This technique is readily adaptable to a variety of species. Since anesthesia induction is routinely required for most manipulative procedures in zoo animals, and since laparoscopy adds little additional risk, the use of this technique provides an additional diagnostic aid when indicated. Additional advantages are achieved by the effectiveness of this procedure in assisting the collection of basic physiological data, particularly that associated with reproductive function. Such information on the use of laparoscopy will be directly valuable in establishing either natural or artificial breeding programs. In short, the value of laparoscopy in a zoo program is significant. Hopefully, this chapter has aided others who will be ultimately responsible for determining the full potential of laparoscopy in zoological medicine and research.

### References

Bush, M., Wildt, D. E., Kennedy, S., and Seager, S. W. J. (1978) Laparoscopy in zoological medicine. *J. Am. Vet. Med. Assoc.* 173:1081–1087.

Fowler, M. E. (1978a) *Restraint and Handling of Wild and Domestic Animals.* Iowa State University Press, Ames, Ia.

Fowler, M. E. (1978b) *Zoo and Wild Animal Medicine.* W. B. Saunders Co., Philadelphia.

Harthoorn, A. M. (1976) *The Chemical Capture of Animals.* Baillière Tindall, London.

Lombard, L. S., Fortna, H. M., Garner, F. M., and Brynjolfsson, O. (1968) Myelolipomas of the liver in captive wild felidae. *Pathol. Vet.* 5:127–134.

Wildt, D. E., Bush, M., Whitlock, B. S., and Seager, S. W. J. (1978) Laparoscopy: A method for direct examination of internal organs in zoo veterinary medicine and research. *Int. Zoo Yearb.* 18:194–197.

Young, E. (1975) *The Capture and Care of Wild Animals.* A Ralph Curtis Book, Hollywood, Fla.

# CHAPTER 11

# Laparoscopy in Birds and Reptiles

## Mitchell Bush, D.V.M.

### INTRODUCTION

Laparoscopy in birds has developed as a technique for sex determination in species without consistent visible sexual dimorphism (Bush *et al.*, 1978a; Bush *et al.*, 1978b; Harrison, 1978). The proper pairing of birds by sex in a zoological collection is an obvious prerequisite for a successful captive propagation program. This is especially true for the Gruiformes, Falconiformes and Psittaciformes in which visual differences are not present in many species, making definite sex identification practically impossible even for an experienced aviculturist. Prior to the use of laparoscopy, various surgical techniques, including laparotomy, were used (Berthold, 1969; Ingram, 1977). Such methods are more traumatic since a larger surgical area of exposure is required for adequate viewing. Use of the laparoscope allows the operator to displace less tissue and also adds a magnification capability to enhance viewing. Laparotomy techniques also tend to be limited to larger birds, whereas laparoscopy can be performed on large as well as small species. More recently, avian laparoscopy has evolved from a management tool for sex determination to a diagnostic aid in evaluating medical problems.

Reptilian laparoscopy is an even more recent science; our laboratory has utilized the laparoscope in various species of snakes and turtles for both diagnostic and research purposes. There are indications for this procedure in resolving certain medical problems in circumstances in which physical examination, radiology, and hematology fail to establish a definitive clinical diagnosis. As in birds, sex of certain reptiles is difficult to establish based on external, physical characteristics. Potentially, laparoscopy may be used to determine sex based on direct gonadal inspection, thus facilitating the accurate management of breeding pairs.

This chapter focuses on basic laparoscopy techniques utilized successfully in our laboratory in both birds and reptiles. Little information is presented on ancillary procedures since such methodology is yet to be developed in these animal groups.

### AVIAN LAPAROSCOPY

#### Animals, Anesthesia, and Restraint

Any surgical procedure requiring anesthesia, such as laparoscopy, is accompanied by certain risks. These can be reduced by careful evaluation of the patient prior to laparoscopy. A comprehensive medical examination minimizes complications by identifying birds that are debilitated or have concurrent disease. If available, a history of previous medical problems is examined. During the physical examination the bird is placed in a quiet environment and observed for alertness and stance. The bird is handled and its nutritional status evaluated by palpation of the pectoral muscle. The appearance of the skin and feathers is noted and abdominal palpation and oral examination are also performed. Further evaluations may be indicated, such as radiology, examination of the feces, and clinical hematology, including determinations of packed cell volume, total protein, and white blood cell count.

If a bird with obvious or potential problems is identified, laparoscopy may be postponed until the problem is corrected and the patient is considered a better surgical risk. If the laparoscopic examination is designed to evaluate a sick bird, the physical examination may provide a more comprehensive understanding of underlying problems, thereby improving the operator's basic knowledge and choices regarding the most effective course of anesthesia and surgery.

Preoperative fasting varies with the size of the bird. Usually, smaller patients (50 to 500 gms) are not fasted because of concern of inducing hypoglycemia. Larger birds, especially those with a large crop or stomach, are fasted to allow emptying of the crop and upper digestive tract. This prevents regurgitation during anesthesia and inadvertent trocar puncture of an enlarged stomach. Raptors, in particular, should not be examined for two days after consuming a large meal.

The decision on whether to use anesthesia during avian laparoscopy is left to the discretion of the laparoscopist. A method using manual restraint for laparoscopic sexing of birds has been reported (Harrison, 1978). This may be adequate for a rapid sexing procedure in which the operator is very familiar with the particular species' anatomy and the laparoscope is inserted only momentarily to identify the gonad. The author feels that it is safer to perform laparoscopy in an anesthetized patient. This is especially true when the technique is being learned, performed on a wide variety of birds with differing anatomy, or when examining a small sized bird. Anesthesia is considered mandatory if diagnostic laparoscopy is being conducted alone or in conjunction with the sexing procedure. Obviously, anesthesia helps alleviate patient stress and eliminates patient struggling. If the distraught, manually restrained bird is exhibiting excessive movement, it is difficult to maintain proper anatomical positioning to allow clear internal visualization. In addition, the struggling patient can increase the incidence of instrument induced contusions and lacerations of the abdominal contents.

Classically, avian anesthesia has presented more risks and problems than are encountered in mammals. This trend is being reversed now due to the development of newer and safer drugs and techniques for anesthesia, in conjunction with close physiological monitoring and supportive care. The choice of anesthesia varies with the preferences and previous experience of the laparoscopist. The author recommends low dosages of ketamine hydrochloride (Ketaset, Bristol Laboratories) ranging from 20 to 35 mg/kg (0.02 to 0.035 mg/gm) of body weight. This regimen generally produces anesthesia adequate to facilitate laparoscopy. After injecting the drug intramuscularly into the pectoral muscle, the bird is placed in a dark, quiet environment until the maximal anesthetic effect is observed—usually 8 to 12 minutes. Minor motor activity of the limbs may be observed, but this is controlled simply by an assistant restraining the patient during laparoscopy. Occasionally, supplemental anesthesia may be required either by a second dose of ketamine hydrochloride or by placing the bird on inhalation anesthesia. For the latter procedure, either a halothane (Fluothane, Ayerst Laboratories)-nitrous oxide mixture or methoxyflurane (Metofane, Pitman-Moore, Inc.) administered using an endotracheal tube is satisfactory. Induction and maintenance of anesthesia using halothane has been used with success; however, during induction an occasional bird may suffer fatal cardiac arrest. Unfortunately, external cardiac massage is not possible in birds due to the rigid anatomical configuration of the chest. For this reason, the author no longer performs halothane induction and restricts the use of this anesthetic for supplemental or maintenance anesthesia. In birds, ketamine hydrochloride produces a surgical plane of anesthesia for 15 to 40 minutes which is adequate for most laparoscopic examinations. It is important to minimize heat loss during anesthesia, especially in smaller sized birds. Such a loss produces additional patient stress and prolongs the recovery interval. Hypothermia is avoided by placing the bird on a heated water blanket on the surgery table and by using a minimal amount of water and alcohol during presurgical preparation.

## Equipment

The basic equipment required for avian laparoscopy includes a light source, fiber optic cable, and a small diameter laparoscope with corresponding size cannula and trocar. The use of secondary puncture equipment or a large diameter operating laparoscope (see Chapter 3) is not routinely applicable, but if necessary, could be used in larger birds over 2 kg.

The laparoscope of choice is an instrument ranging from 2.0 to 2.7 mm in diameter. Such an endoscope is more commonly referred to as an arthroscope (Richard Wolf Medical Instruments Corp., Karl Storz Endoscopy-America, Inc.) or Needlescope® (Dyonics, Inc.). A larger diameter laparoscope such as the 5 mm in diameter instrument can be used in large birds such as cranes. This size endoscope is also used when photography is desirable, since photographic documentation through the arthroscope or needlescope is often difficult. The greater diameter instrument simply transfers more light to the target organ, thus facilitating photography.

Our laboratory utilizes a 2.7 mm in diameter arthroscope (Fig. 11.1) in most birds and a 5 mm in diameter laparoscope when photography is planned. The arthroscope and corresponding trocar-cannula assembly is designed for internal observation of joints in

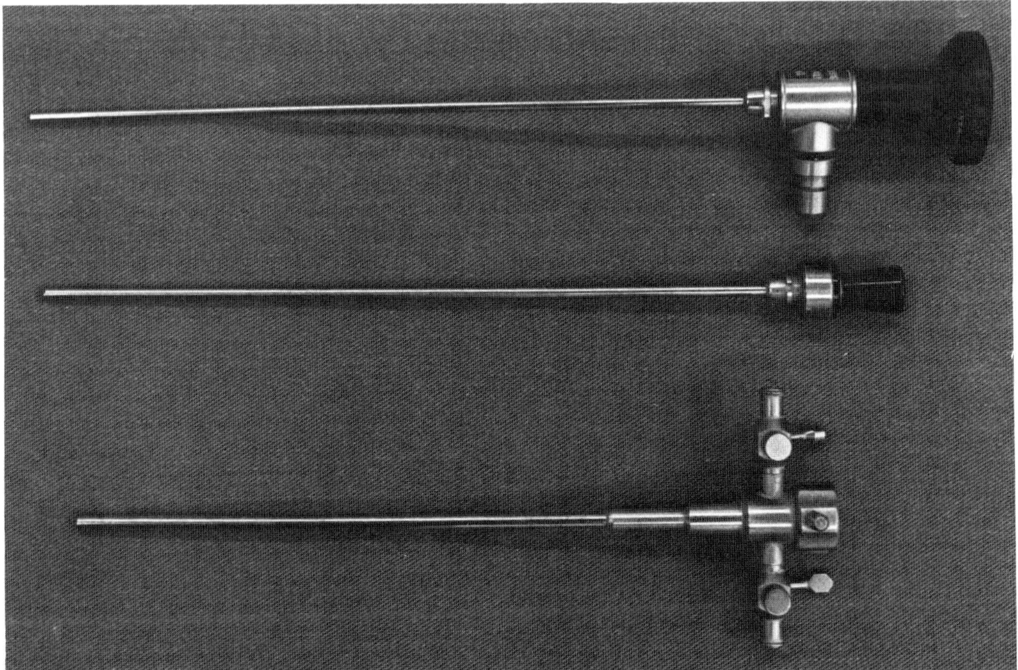

**Figure 11.1** Laparoscope (arthroscope) 2.7 mm in diameter and corresponding trocar and cannula.

humans, but works well in birds. As will be described later, the endoscope may be singularly inserted into the abdominal cavity or passed into this area by means of the conventional trocar-cannula device. The arthroscopic trocar-cannula unit differs slightly in appearance from that used with most laparoscopes (Fig. 11.1). This unit's pyramidal trocar aids in insertion through the abdominal muscles and lessens the severity of an organ puncture or laceration if it should occur. The cannula has no trumpet valve but does contain attachment sleeves designed to allow flushing and draining of fluid and/ or insufflation of air. These sleeves are not used during routine examination in birds.

A standard endoscopic light source and fiber optic cable can be used to generate illumination. Because of an interest in photographic documentation, our laboratory utilizes a light source with both diagnostic and photographic (1000 watt) lamp capabilities. The internal photographs associated with this chapter were taken with an Olympus OM-1 camera and 100 mm lens attached to the 5 mm in diameter laparoscope. Film type used is the same as described for zoo mammals (see Chapter 10). Further details on still and videotape photography in avian species will be provided later in the chapter.

## Equipment and Surgical Preparation

Avian laparoscopy is performed using sterile instruments and technique. The laparoscopic instruments are either sterilized by gas sterilization (ethylene oxide) or cold sterilization (chlorhexidine, Nolvasan-S, Fort Dodge Laboratories). When several birds are scheduled for laparoscopy, cold sterilization of instruments between patients is the only practical method of maintaining asepsis. If this procedure is used, it is best to warm the sterilization solution which will help prevent fogging of the laparoscope's distal lens when the endoscope is inserted into the bird's warm abdominal cavity. Before entering the abdominal cavity, the instruments are rinsed of the disinfectant solution using sterile water or saline.

Following induction of a surgical plane of anesthesia, the bird is placed on the warm surgical table on its right side with the wings reflected dorsally (Fig. 11.2). The left leg is displaced either cranially or caudally to expose the area behind the last rib. The bird can be taped in this position, although it is more advantageous if this support is provided

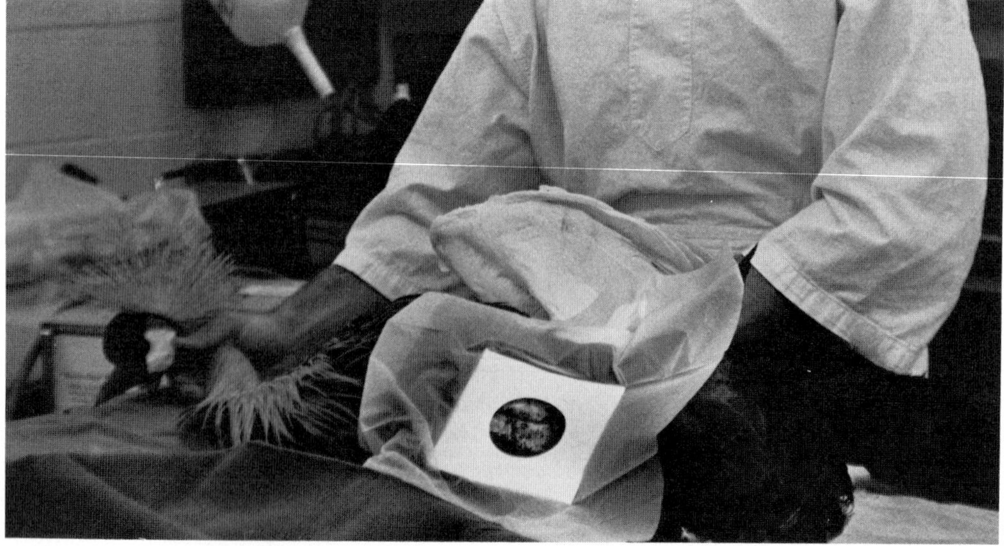

**Figure 11.2**  Anesthetized bird lying on its right side with the left wing reflected dorsally.

by an assistant. This same position is used for the laparoscopic sexing procedure or for general diagnostic exploration. The left side approach developed as a result of early endoscopic attempts to identify avian sex. Female birds have only a functional left ovary and a rudimentary right gonad. Hence, the left approach is often used so that the operator may clearly visualize the morphology of the closely located left ovary. If indicated in a general diagnostic effort, the bird can be placed on its left side and the laparoscope inserted using the right side approach.

Due to variations in anatomy, displacement of the leg varies markedly with different species. The objective of leg displacement is to expose the site for insertion of the laparoscope. This critical area is designated the sternal notch (Fig. 11.3), which is a "V" formed where the last sternal rib joins the sternum or slightly dorsal to this site caudal to the last rib. When palpated, this area forms an indented fossa. From this site, the inserted laparoscope can be easily manipulated to view the various internal organs (Fig. 11.4). The feathers are carefully plucked from the sternal notch area and the site is surgically prepared using aqueous benzalkonium chloride solution (Zephiran, Winthrop Laboratories) and tamed iodine (Pharmadine, Sherwood Pharmaceutical Co.). The area is covered with a small opening sterile plastic drape which allows monitoring of the bird's respiration and antomical position throughout the procedure (Fig. 11.2).

### Laparoscopic Techniques

## OPERATIVE PROCEDURES

Positioning is very important, especially in small birds, to assure a consistent anatomical relationship that is easily recognized by the operator. The author prefers a true lateral position with the bird restrained as described above. A small skin incision (5 to 10 mm in length) facilitates the insertion of the trocar-cannula. If skin bleeding occurs, it is important that this be controlled prior to insertion of the laparoscope. Even a drop of blood can obscure the field of view directly, or when exposed to air flow from the air sacs can produce a foam which may necessitate premature termination of the exami-

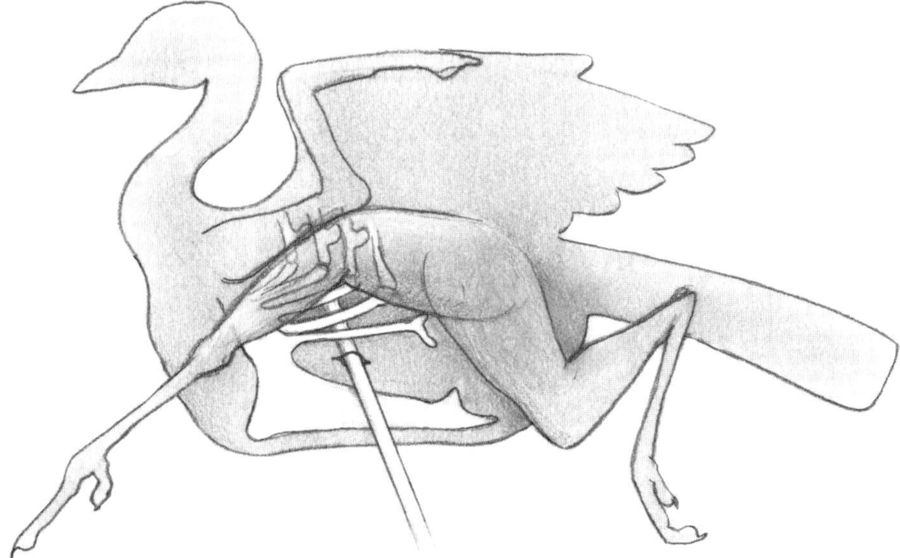

**Figure 11.3** Drawing indicating either anterior or posterior leg positioning to expose the sternal notch, the site for laparoscope insertion.

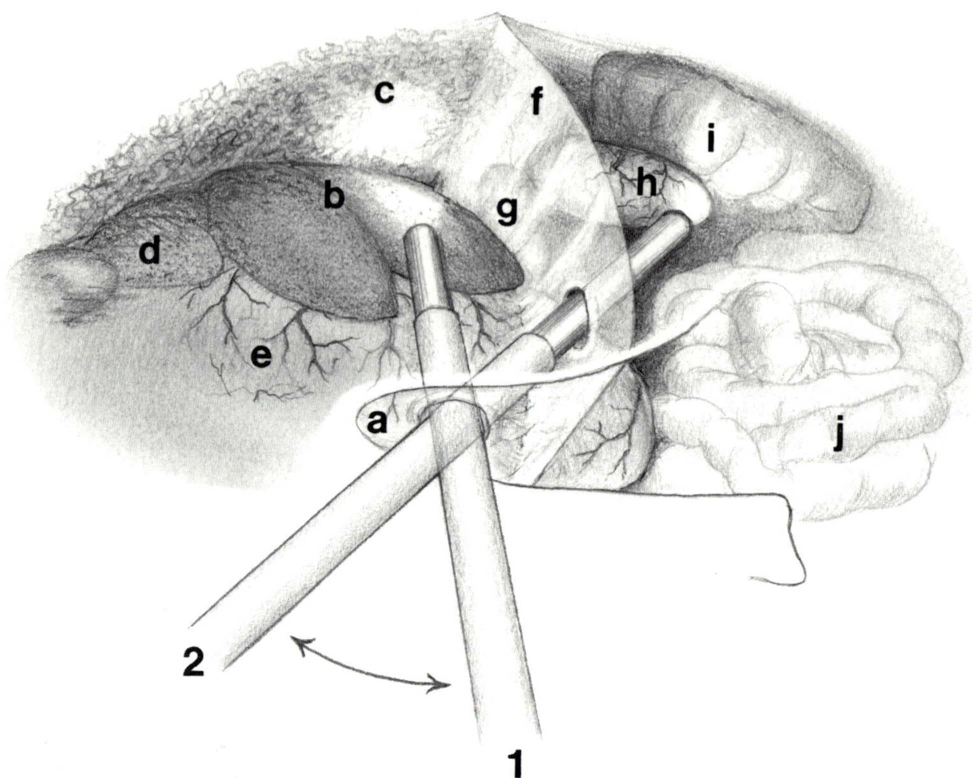


**Figure 11.4**   Positioning of the laparoscope through the sternal notch **(a)** to view various organs. In position 1 the laparoscope is inserted into the anterior thoracic air sac to view the liver **(b)**, lungs **(c)**, heart **(d)**, and stomach **(e)**. In position 2 the laparoscope is inserted through the air sac membrane **(f)** entering the left abdominal air sac to view the adrenal **(g)**, gonad **(h)**, kidney **(i)**, and intestines **(j)**.

nation. The trocar-cannula assembly is inserted through the skin incision using controlled pressure until the abdominal cavity is entered. During insertion, the plane of the trocar-cannula is parallel to the thoracic-lumbosacral vertebrae with the point of the trocar directed cranially (Fig. 11.5). Often, a "pop" is felt as the trocar perforates the abdominal wall. Following penetration, the trocar is withdrawn and the cannula supported until the laparoscope is inserted (Fig. 11.6) and its position verified visually.

Birds are ideal patients for laparoscopy because the presence of air sacs eliminates the need for insufflation and the lack of a diaphragm allows viewing many more organs than in mammals. However, to adequately visualize the abdominal contents, the operator must invariably penetrate the air sac membrane. This is done routinely in avian laparoscopy and produces no complications. During initial insertion, the trocar-cannula unit may not perforate the air sac, which may necessitate replacing the trocar and advancing it further to enter the appropriate air space.

During the examination, more control of the laparoscope can be achieved with the operator sitting and positioning both elbows on the table. This provides stability, aids in visualization, and minimizes inadvertent trauma, which could result from accidental instrument movement. Internal viewing may be enhanced by slightly withdrawing the laparoscope within the cannula. This prevents tissue from contacting the terminal lens of the laparoscope and also provides a slightly enlarged visual area, both of which aid viewing in a confined space. In addition, with the endoscope retracted, the end of the

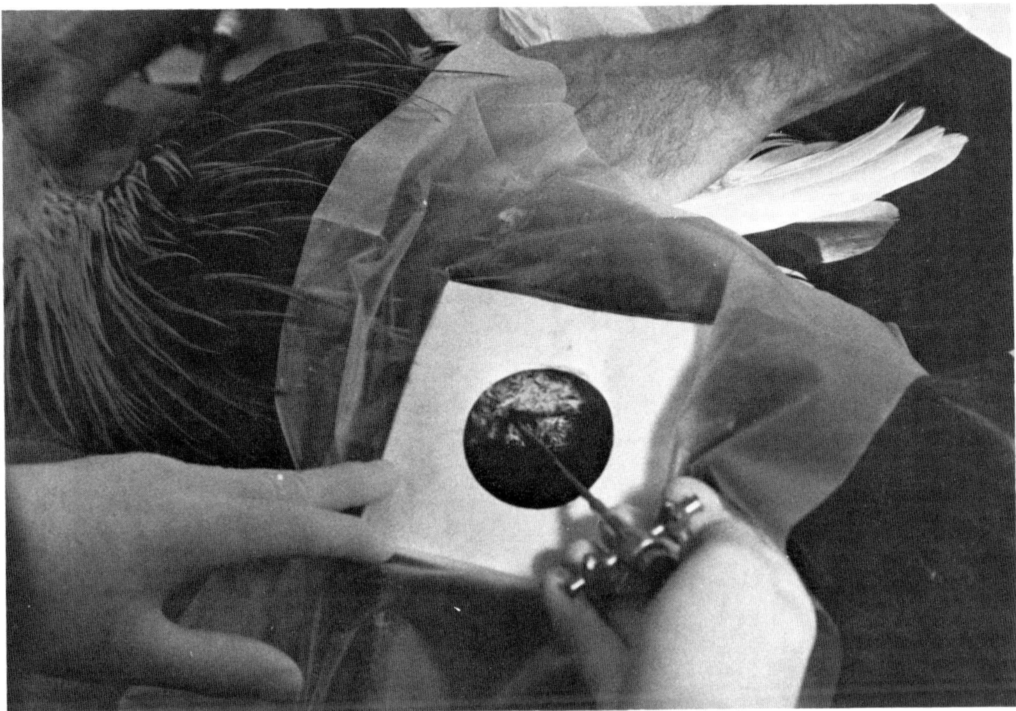

**Figure 11.5**   Insertion of the trocar-cannula assembly through the sternal notch.

cannula can be used to manipulate and displace tissue without obscuring the distal viewing lens.

The trocar-cannula approach is used in birds weighing more than 500 grams. In smaller birds or under circumstances in which hepatomegaly is suspected, the laparoscope alone is inserted through the abdominal wall. In this procedure, delicate ophthalmic instruments are used to perform careful blunt dissection of the abdominal wall at the sternal notch. By separating the muscles along the fibers, an opening (approximately 5 mm) is made through which the laparoscope is inserted. Birds weighing as little as 50 grams have been examined by this technique. Again, care must be exercised to control hemorrhage during this procedure to avoid curtailing the examination due to lack of visibility. Additional caution must be used when the small diameter laparoscope alone is inserted in this fashion. The cannula normally provides considerable stability and support for the endoscope. When the latter is used alone, the operator must avoid bending this delicate instrument, since this can dislodge an internal lens or, more drastically, result in laparoscope breakage.

Using either of the above insertion approaches, the laparoscope usually enters the anterior thoracic air sac (*Color Atlas*, Pl. 10, Fig. 3) in which the liver (Pl. 10, Fig. 4), heart (Pl. 10, Fig. 5), lungs (Pl. 10, Fig. 6), and bronchi are seen. To visualize the posterior wall of the anterior thoracic air sac, the laparoscope is directed caudodorsally from the site of insertion. The kidney and gonads may be visualized through the transparent sac. However, the operator will sometimes discover that the air sac is opaque due to fat infiltration or air sacculitis. In this case, the laparoscope is used to penetrate the posterior wall of the sac, avoiding surface vessels and underlying organs. This is accomplished by pressing the terminus of the instrument against the sac membrane and then retracting until a small slit is observed through which the laparoscope is advanced into the left abdominal air sac. Inside this space, the gonads (Pl. 10, Figs. 7

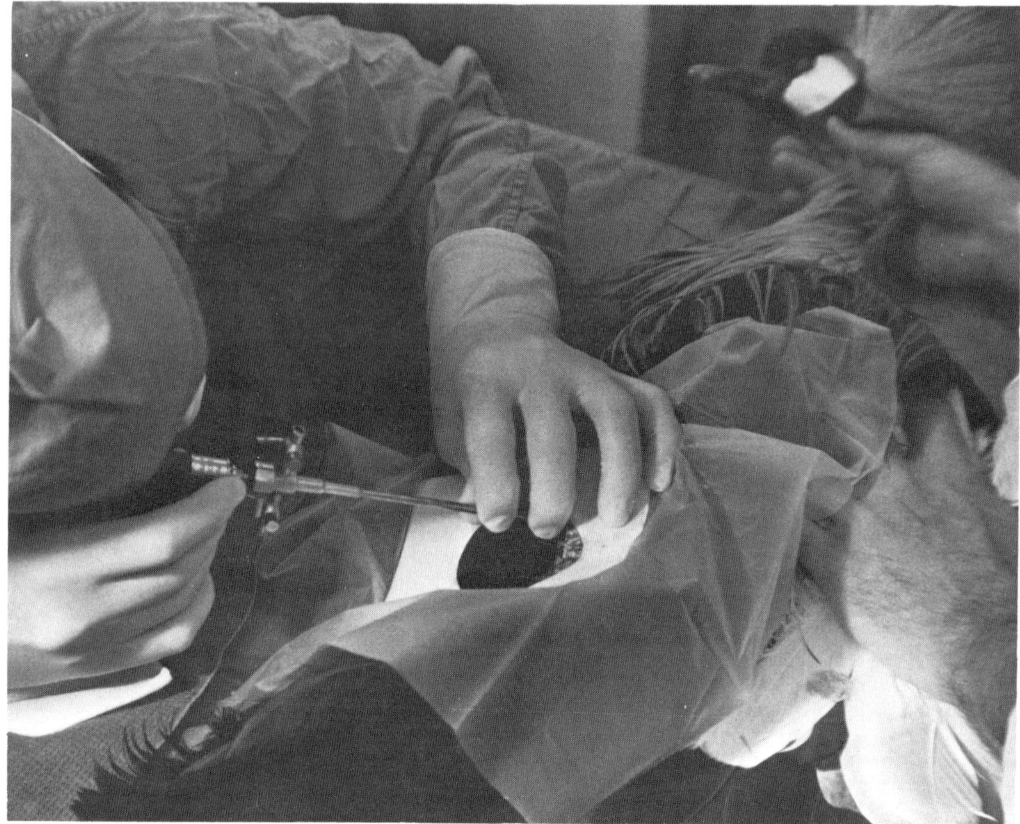

**Figure 11.6**   Laparoscopic visualization of the abdominal contents.

and 8; Pl. 11, Fig. 1), kidney (Pl. 11, Figs. 1 and 2), adrenals (Pl. 11, Fig. 2), stomach, spleen (Pl. 11, Fig. 3), and intestines are visualized.

## EXAMINATION OF THE REPRODUCTIVE ORGANS

To determine the sex of a bird, the laparoscope is inserted into the left abdominal air sac. The gonad is located in the anterior-dorsal aspect of this air sac at the anterior pole of the left kidney. A triad is formed by the adrenal gland, gonad, and anterior pole of the left kidney. The testicle is elliptical to cyclindrical in shape with blood vessels transversing its smooth surface (Pl. 10, Fig. 7). The testes can be partly or totally pigmented (Pl. 11, Fig. 2) and vary in size, depending on the bird's age and stage of the reproductive cycle. Avian testes are paired and, although the left is observed easily, manipulation is required to view the right testicle through the air sac when the endoscope is inserted via the left side.

The ovary of an adult bird has grapelike clusters of prominent follicles and is not a problem to identify (Pl. 10, Fig. 8). These follicles are not present in the immature female which may represent a problem for the novice in differentiating the immature ovary from the testicle. This can be resolved by examining the shape and vascularity of the gonad. The immature ovary (Pl. 11, Fig. 4) is more flat, has a fine granular surface, and lacks the surface vascularity evident in the more rounded, smooth surfaced testicle. In these immature birds the operator can also determine the presence of a second gonad through the membrane in the right abdominal air sac. Detection of another gonad would confirm the sex as male.

The ovary may also be partially or totally pigmented. Size of this organ will vary according to seasonality. It should be noted that because of its anatomical positioning, the left adrenal is often hidden from view in birds with an enlarged active ovary.

In birds lacking external dimorphism, laparoscopic sexing has become a routine procedure at the National Zoological Park. Gonadal inspection is performed in newly received birds still in quarantine. In addition, most birds hatched at our zoo are sexed prior to placement in exhibit or propagation areas. This procedure has allowed early definitive sexing of all birds and has eliminated the inadvertent pairing of the same sexed individuals or the support of birds of the "wrong" sex until sexual dimorphism occurs in later life. As a result, a specific number of birds of known sex are obtained and established in breeding pairs at an early age, thus enhancing propagation potential and yield.

## USE IN AVIAN MEDICINE

In addition to sex determination, laparoscopy has its place as a diagnostic tool in avian medicine. Most abdominal organs can be directly observed for indications of gross alterations in appearance. A number of pathological or abnormal conditions have been diagnosed in birds in our laboratory, including cardiomegaly or pericarditis, hepatic, splenic, or renal amyloidosis, and accumulation of uric acid (gout) in the kidney. Visible granuloma indicative of avian tuberculosis has been observed in the liver (Pl. 11, Fig. 5) and spleen. Aspergillosis, as well as air sacculitis, has also been diagnosed by viewing the air sac or lung.

## TERMINATION OF THE EXAMINATION AND POSTOPERATIVE CARE

Following the examination, the cannula and laparoscope are removed from the cavity. Suturing the incision is the choice of the operator. The author often finds that suturing the incision site is unnecessary, since when the bird regains its normal standing position, the skin incision is nonaligned with the separated muscle fibers. Consequently, herniation does not occur. Incision repair is usually indicated following use of the 5 mm in diameter laparoscope. In this circumstance, 3-0 absorbable suture is used to close the skin tissue only. If a sterile field has been maintained, topical antibacterial ointment or prophylactic antibiotic administration is unnecessary. The bird is removed to a warm, dark, quiet environment to minimize postoperative problems. In some longlegged species, such as cranes, transient, stormy recovery from ketamine hydrochloride anesthesia may occur when the bird attempts to stand prematurely. In such cases, the operator or an assistant should manually hold the bird (usually 10 to 30 minutes) until it is capable of standing. Birds experiencing a difficult recovery can be further protected by utilizing a stockinet to confine the bird's wings and minimize flapping and selfinduced trauma. The restraining stockinet must not be so tight as to restrict chest movement, thus impairing respiration. The bird can be fed and watered as soon as recovery from anesthesia is complete.

## General Considerations

## RESULTS AND COMPLICATIONS

Since 1976, our laboratory has performed over 250 laparoscopic examinations encompassing representative birds from 12 families. Most birds have been subjected to a single laparoscopy; but two individuals in one research study each underwent 12 examinations over a 90 day interval with no complications. Overall, mortality rate has been less than 2%, and these deaths occurred when the laparoscope was used in clinical diagnoses of chronically ill birds. Thus, laparoscopy has proven to be a safe, rapid, and effective method of direct visualization of the abdominal cavity contents.

Certain complications may arise for which the beginning avian laparoscopist should be aware. A common problem occurs in achieving the proper plane of anesthesia. There is often a tendency to handle the bird and initiate the examination prior to the bird reaching the surgical plane of anesthesia. The result is usually similar to that observed in a bird examined under manual restraint only—a struggling patient that can inflict self abuse or damage to the endoscope. Conversely, if the anesthetic plane is too advanced, death occurs as a result of cardiac arrest and respiratory failure. Early recognition of potential anesthetic problems and the knowledge and availability of prompt, supportive measures is critical. Results are most successful when: (1) an adequate postanesthetic administration interval is allowed prior to initiating the examination; (2) if an excessive anesthesia plane is suspected, assisted ventilation is begun immediately. In the latter case, the operator must remember that once cardiac arrest occurs, the bird is dead due to the anatomical incapability of performing external cardiac resuscitative massage.

Internal anatomy varies considerably with different species of birds. The operator should expect the possibility of additional orientation time to locate the specific organs in a species not previously examined by laparoscopy. If possible, anatomical information should be studied prior to performing laparoscopy either by a search of the literature or by dissection of cadavers.

Visualization problems, as in other species, exist in birds and can be attributed to several factors, including improper positioning which disrupts anatomical relationships, hemorrhage, overdistention of the stomach, and obesity. The two most significant hindrances are improper positioning and bleeding, both of which can be eliminated through experience and improved technique. An enlarged gastrointestinal tract can be prevented with proper preoperative fasting. Often obesity will result in a difficult or impossible examination, depending on the amount and location of the deposited fat. This problem is most prevalent in captive raptors which have excessive internal fat, particularly on and around the air sacs. There is little to be done to resolve this problem. A Verres needle (see Chapter 3) can be inserted adjacent to the laparoscope and used to manipulate fat deposits away from the visual field and target organ in some instances.

Inadvertent puncture of an abdominal structure can occur. If the liver is traumatized and hemorrhaging, the examination is terminated and the bird monitored closely during recovery. In incidents in which the trauma is minor, the bird generally survives. Perforation of the stomach or intestine necessitates laparotomy to surgically repair the wounded area. These animals should also receive systemic antibiotics. Occasionally during initial trocar insertion through the air sac, a hematoma is induced on the adjacent kidney or liver tissue. In a healthy bird, such occurrences are usually insignificant and should cause no alarm.

Following most laparoscopies, minor postoperative emphysema can be observed at the insertion site. This is usually inconsequential and subsides within 48 hours. If severe distention of the skin in this area is encountered, the trapped air can be evacuated by aspiration with a needle and syringe. A topical antibacterial ointment should then be applied to this site daily for the next two or three days.

## LAPAROSCOPIC PHOTOGRAPHY

Photography during laparoscopy provides an excellent method of documenting various disease conditions and the anatomical variations inherent among species. Sequential changes occurring because of a disease process or as a result of endoscopic manipulation can be recorded and compared to results obtained in subsequent examinations.

Still photography through a 2.0 to 2.7 mm in diameter laparoscope can be performed (Fig. 11.7) but is often very difficult even with a light source providing 1000 watts of illumination. This type of photography is further complicated by the normally rapid respiration rate of avian species which results in uncontrollable organ movement within

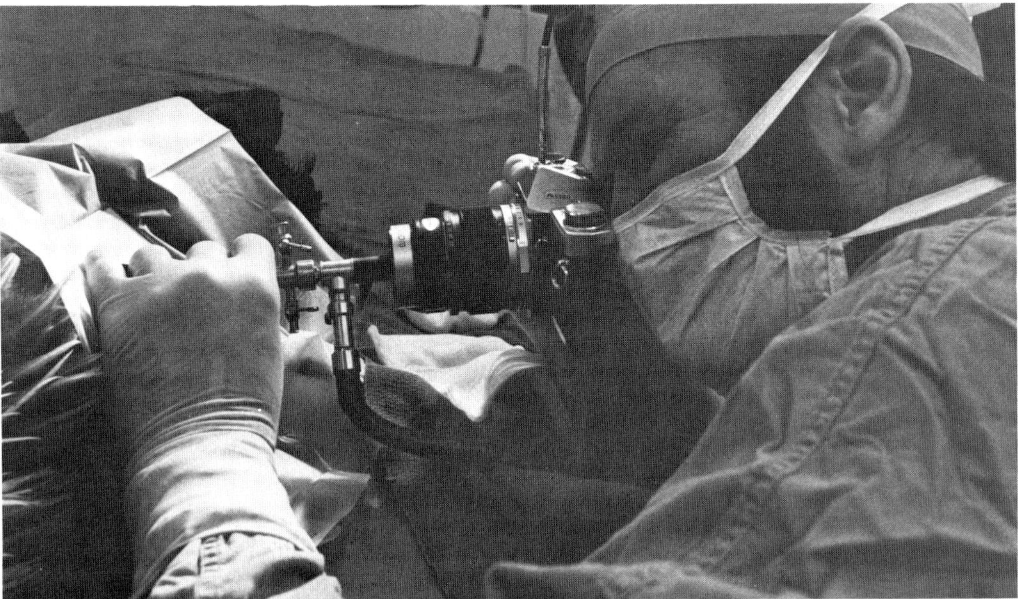

**Figure 11.7** The SLR camera attached to the eyepiece of the endoscope, allowing laparoscopic photography.

the cavity. Average quality photographs occasionally can be achieved in the bird by the experienced operator using this size endoscope, a correct plane of anesthesia and slow shutter speeds (¼th to ¹⁄₁₅th of a second). Less film waste and higher quality photographs are obtained when the 5 mm in diameter laparoscope is employed. Camera exposure time with this instrument generally varies from ¹⁄₆₀th to ¹⁄₁₅th of a second. Quality of the resulting photograph is directly related to the amount of intraabdominal illumination and the operator's capability of minimizing camera—laparoscope movement during the picture taking process. Further investigation is required to determine the additional advantage of electronic flash systems in obtaining photographs using the smaller diameter endoscope.

In our laboratory, the 5 mm in diameter laparoscope has been utilized in conjunction with a color television camera and videotape recorder to document the capabilities of avian laparoscopy (Fig. 11.8). The previous chapter has discussed the details of this equipment. Videotape quality in birds has been very good and these have been found extremely useful for teaching purposes.

## LAPAROSCOPIC RECORDS

A record of each laparoscopic examination is essential. The following basic information requires documentation: species of bird, weight, anesthetic used and result, site of laparoscope insertion, description of organs visualized, anatomical variations, complications, and listing and description of photographs taken. This information is particularly valuable in a research or veterinary medical organization in which a great number of laparoscopies are performed in a wide variety of species.

## REPTILIAN LAPAROSCOPY

### Animal Preparation

Aseptic procedures and instrumentation for laparoscopy in reptiles is essentially the same as that required in birds. Differences in procedure occur with respect to anesthesia

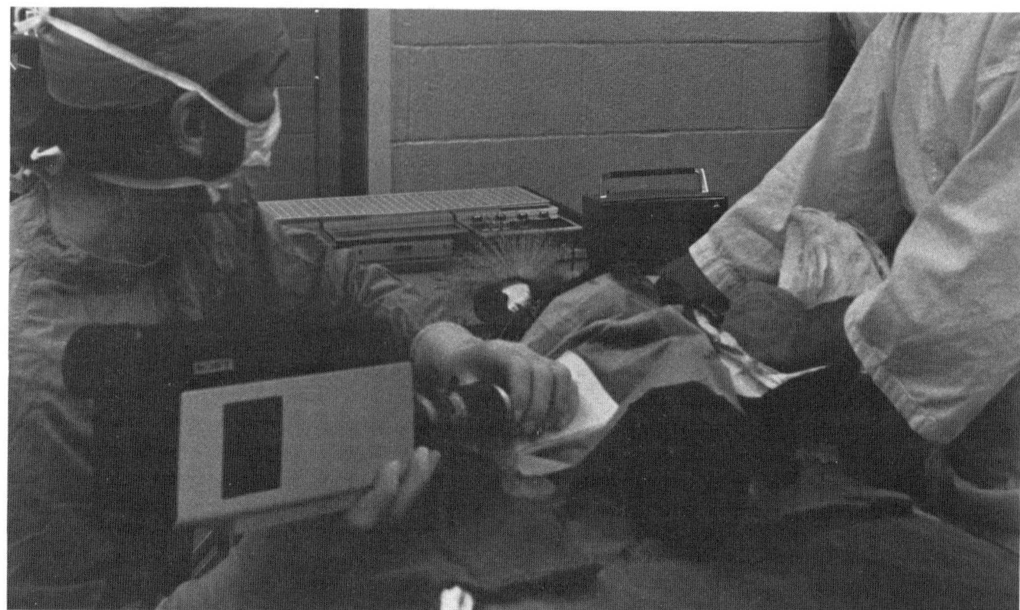

**Figure 11.8**  A portable color television camera attached to the endoscope, allowing videotape recording of abdominal observations.

and method and site of laparoscope insertion. In general, adequate intraabdominal space is normally available for viewing in both snakes and turtles. When visualization is difficult, minor intermittent insufflation may be desirable. In turtles only slight insufflation is recommended because the shell is not expandable. The viewing area in snakes is within the air sac which is the posterior extension of the lung; hence, insufflated air is safely exhaled.

Snakes are placed in a Plexiglas tube and anesthetized by administering halothane (3.5 to 5.0%) and a nitrous oxide-oxygen (ratio, 2:1) combination. A surgical plane is achieved in most animals after an induction period of 12 to 20 minutes in this environment. For the examination, the snake is removed from the tube, transferred to the surgical area and the head of the snake masked for maintenance anesthesia (Fig. 11.9). Surgical anesthesia is difficult to obtain in turtles without administering massive dosages of anesthetic drugs and thus, producing prolonged recovery periods. Therefore, the author recommends the intramuscular injection of ketamine hydrochloride (100 mg/ kg body weight, including shell) supplemented by local anesthesia at the laparoscope insertion site. The injection of ketamine hydrochloride produces basal anesthesia with partial relaxation within 15 to 30 minutes which allows the turtle to be placed on its back and the site of insertion infiltrated with the local anesthetic. For the latter 0.2 to 0.5 ml of lidocaine hydrochloride (2% solution, Wolins Pharmacal Corp.) is employed. Using this anesthesia procedure, the animal will exhibit some random limb movement which can be controlled by an assistant during the examination.

### Laparoscopic Procedure

The mechanics of laparoscope insertion are similar to that described previously for other species. In snakes, the site of insertion is dictated by the area to be examined. Because of the elongated body, the relative positions of internal organs must be understood prior to instrument insertion. This information can be obtained from previous experience or perusal of pertinent anatomical literature. Insertion of the trocar-

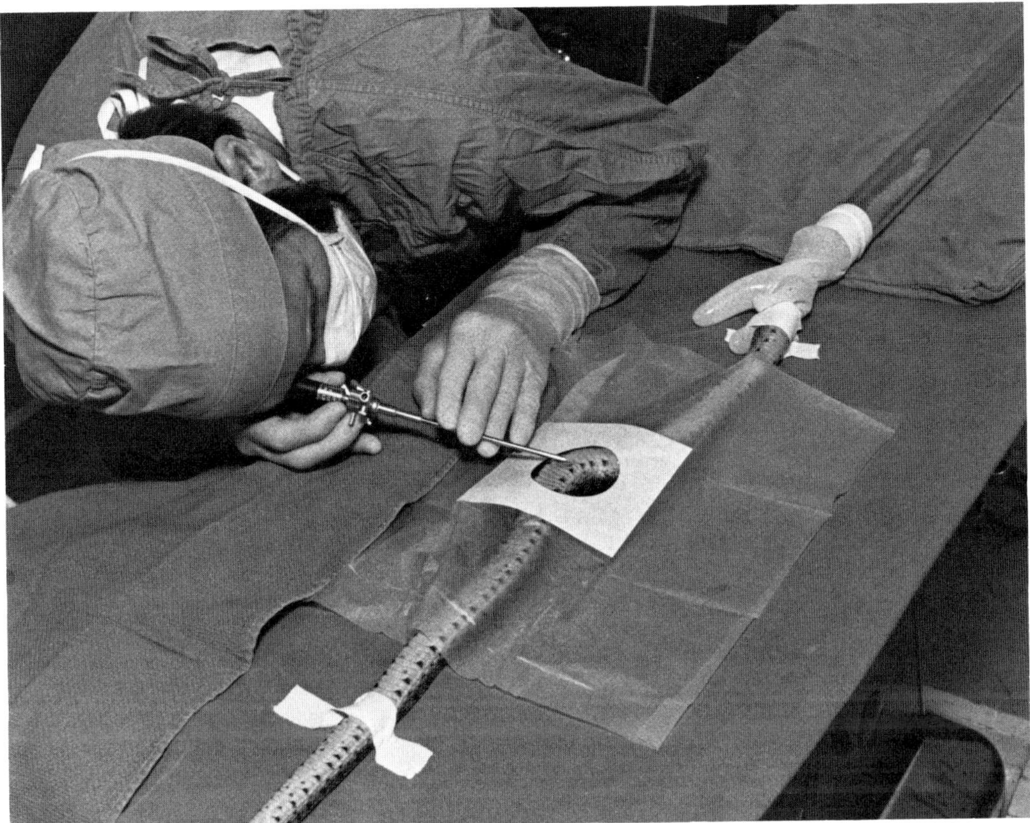

**Figure 11.9**   Site of laparoscope insertion for internal observation in the snake.

cannula is aided by a small incision (5 to 10 mm in length) made ventrally between the scales near the ventral middle (Fig. 11.9). Insertion directly through the ventral midline should be avoided due to a series of blood vessels. An alternative site is to insert the trocar-cannula assembly just lateral to the elongated ventral scales. After the trocar is removed and the telescope inserted (Fig. 11.9), viewing is aided by the retraction of the laparoscope slightly within the cannula to increase the potential viewing space. Because of the elongated body of the snake, the operator may find it necessary to repeat the insertion procedure at a second site to complete or extend a specific examination.

The site of trocar-cannula entry in the turtle is lateral to either rear leg (Fig. 11.10). For most general diagnostic examinations, the operator must use care and controlled insertion since the sac like lung of the turtle is capable of being punctured. An assistant extends the leg and the operator palpates to locate the lateral fossa. This site is surgically prepared, infiltrated with the local anesthetic and following a suitable time interval, the skin incision is made and the trocar-cannula inserted into the coelomic cavity. Following endoscope insertion (Fig. 11.11), the heart, lung (Pl. 11, Figs. 6 and 7), intestines, liver (Pl. 11, Fig. 7), bladder, and gonads (Pl. 11, Fig. 8) may be observed.

At the completion of the examination in both snakes and turtles, the cannula is withdrawn and the puncture site examined. Depending on size and the choice of the operator, it may be desirable to repair the wound using 3-0 absorbable suture. The reptile is placed in a warm area and allowed to recover. Generally, no antibiotics or further postoperative care is necessary.

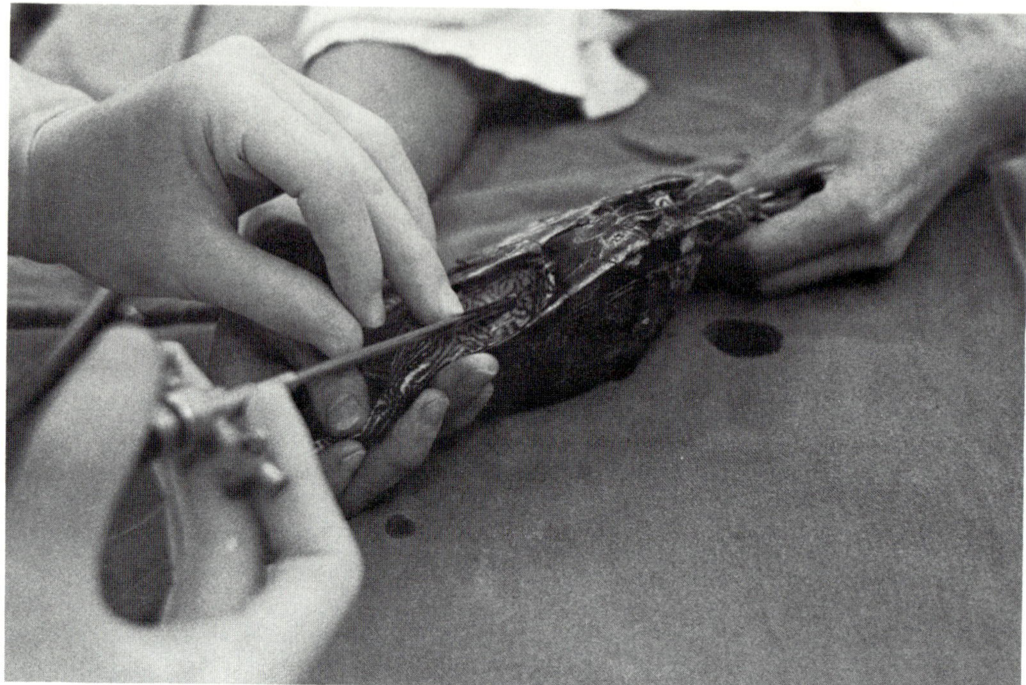

**Figure 11.10**   In the turtle the trocar-cannula is inserted lateral to either rear leg.

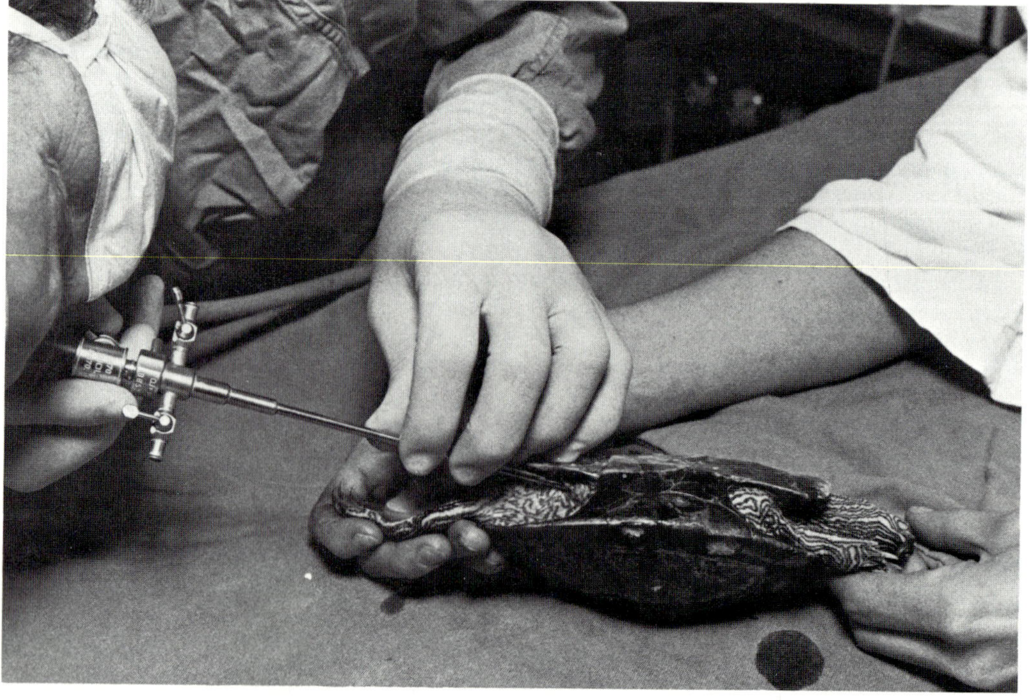

**Figure 11.11**   Viewing into the coelomic cavity of the turtle.

## CONCLUSION

In comparison to other major animal groups, avian and reptilian laparoscopy is in its infancy. Laparoscopy in birds, initially born as a management tool for sex determination, has developed as an important diagnostic adjunct in avian medicine. In the future, laparoscopy may likely evolve into an ideal research technique for documenting alterations in organ function, such as gonadal responses to exogenous hormone therapy or varying environmental stimuli. The imaginative and constructive development of this tool in both birds and reptiles is still in progress and a need certainly exists for further refinement and experimentation in various basic and ancillary techniques.

**References**

Berthold, von, Peter. (1969) Ein Hilfsmittel zur Geschlechtsbestimmung und zur Beobachtung des Gonadenzyklus. *Der Zoologische Garten* 37:271–279.

Bush, M., Kennedy, S., Wildt, D. E., and Seager, S. W. J. (1978a) Sexing birds by laparoscopy. *Int. Zoo Yearb.* 18:197–199.

Bush, M., Wildt, D. E., Kennedy, S., and Seager, S. W. J. (1978b) Laparoscopy in zoological medicine. *J. Am. Vet. Med. Assoc.* 173:1081–1087.

Harrison, G. J. (1978) Endoscopic examination of avian gonadal tissue. *Vet. Med. Small Anim. Clin.* 73:479–484.

Ingram, K. A. (1977) Laparotomy technique to determine sex of psittacine birds. *Proc. Annu. Meet. A.A.Z.V.* pp. 40–42.

# CHAPTER 12

# Laparoscopic Instrumentation

## Richard M. Harrison, Ph.D., and David E. Wildt, Ph.D.

### INTRODUCTION

Discussion in Chapter 2 emphasized that endoscopes and their accessories require proper care for prolonged and effective use. The first section of this chapter is concerned with describing some precautions and instrument handling procedures and reemphasizing some of the suggestions made by various authors throughout the text.

The variation in instrumentation available for the potential laparoscopist is illustrated by a quick comparative analysis of the various instruments described in each chapter. Each author has made recommendations on the optimum size instruments for each representative species. The beginning operator must now make a personal judgment on the number and type of instruments to utilize in his own laboratory. It is strongly suggested that the potential buyer of laparoscopy equipment comparatively examine instrumentation from at least two and possibly three different manufacturers. It is the general policy of most companies to send a representative directly to the customer's laboratory or clinic. In most instances, demonstration equipment will be available for the potential operator to evaluate or even utilize in an *in vivo* examination. The latter section of this chapter is designed to familiarize the reader with four major endoscopy companies in the United States which offer equipment suitable for animal laparoscopy.

### PHYSICAL HANDLING

#### Laparoscope

Of all instrumentation, the laparoscope itself is the most handled and, because of its obvious importance to the examination and expense, deserves optimal care. The metal housing of the telescope provides protection during routine use. This instrument is surprisingly resistant to damage when handled properly. The greatest danger comes from inadvertent bending of a small diameter endoscope or dropping or striking *any* size endoscope against a hard surface.

The operator should be aware of more subtle problems which can occur with routine use. Some chemicals used as surgical disinfectants can damage the immersed telescope when exposed for long periods of time. Best results are obtained when the laparoscope is exposed to the disinfectant for the required period immediately prior to the examination, and immediately following laparoscopy the instrument is washed in warm water and dried.

Often a common handling mistake occurs during examination of the animal. The operator should not support the inserted laparoscope by the barrel of the instrument, rather by the laparoscopic cannula. Holding the inserted telescope near the eyepiece produces a fulcrum effect. Bending, albeit slight, can occur, resulting in glass fiber breakage and perhaps dislodging of an internal lens. This problem is more acute with the smaller diameter endoscope.

### Light Cables

The only other instrument component that requires additional discussion on handling is the light cable. It should always be remembered that the critical light and image transmission elements of both the laparoscope and light cable consist of glass. Early constructed light cables were covered with a protective metal sheathing which was reasonably flexible. More recently cables have been manufactured to be lighter in weight and more flexible; hence, a rubber instead of metal sheathing is commonly used. The light cable should never be bent or stored in a tight loop or angled position. The internal thin glass fibers will break, reducing light transmission. Similar breaks may be caused by stepping on the cable during the examination or dropping on a hard surface.

Light transmission through the cable can be simply evaluated. One end of the free cable is directed toward a bright light and the glass covering the other end of the cable examined. Darkened areas of the glass indicate the loss of light transfer due to broken glass fibers. If the damage appears extensive, cable replacement will likely be necessary.

## SURGICAL PREPARATION OF INSTRUMENTS

Three methods of sterilization or disinfection are used for laparoscopes: steam autoclaving; gas (ethylene oxide) sterilization; and liquid chemical disinfection.

### Autoclaving

All laparoscopes are *not* autoclavable. To autoclave a laparoscope not specifically designed for this procedure is to court disaster. The extreme heat and pressure associated with autoclaving probably have some deteriorating effects on any instrument not made of all metal or all glass construction. Most experienced laparoscopists who utilize autoclavable laparoscopes autoclave them periodically but not between each examination. Generally, chemical disinfectants are used between serial laparoscopies.

### Gas Sterilization

Gas sterilization is an effective and safe procedure for the laparoscope and accessory instruments. The disadvantage to this method is the time required. Most experts suggest 24 hours aeration after the sterilization before instrument use. This presents a problem to the operator with access to a single set of instruments and the need to perform multiple examinations on a single day. Again, many individuals find that periodic gas sterilization during periods of reduced instrument use is preferable with liquid chemical disinfection used routinely between examinations.

### Chemical Disinfection

The most common method of surgically preparing laparoscopic instruments prior to an examination is by immersion in a disinfectant solution. A survey of services in which a large number of human laparoscopies were performed daily indicated that instrument immersion for 10 minutes in activated dialdehyde (Cidex, Arbrook, Inc.) was sufficient to prevent infection (Taylor, 1973). Other solutions used and reported in this survey included: benzalkonium chloride (Zephiran, Winthrop Laboratories, 10 to 20 minutes), 10% formalin solution (12 minutes), Detergicide™ (15 minutes), and Lehn-Fink germicidal solution (30 minutes). Our results indicate that Amerase (Vestal Laboratories, 10 minutes) and chlorhexidine (Nolvasan-S, Fort Dodge Laboratories, 20 minutes) are satisfactory. A recent report found that soaking laparoscopes in fresh glutaraldehyde solution for 15 minutes provided clinically safe disinfection (Corson *et al.*, 1978). Regardless of the solution used, most laparoscopists suggest rinsing the instruments with sterile water prior to use.

## CLEANING OF INSTRUMENTS

Following laparoscopy the telescope, cannula, trocar, and Verres needle should be washed in warm water and dried prior to storage. The telescope and trocar present no problems and require no special attention with respect to thorough cleaning. The trumpet valve on the cannula should be depressed and the cannula flushed with water and periodically disassembled for a thorough cleaning. The trumpet valve should be cleaned well and lubricated before reassembly. Various components will require alignment for proper reassembly. Test tube brushes are effective for cleaning the insides of the cannula. The Verres needle can and should be disassembled for cleaning on a routine basis. Tissue and blood should be flushed from the internal lumen after each examination to prevent needle blockage. A large (20 or 35 ml) syringe containing water can be attached to the hub of the Verres needle and used for flushing. A pipe cleaner can be used to clean the lumen.

Metal instruments, with the exception of the telescope, can be dried in a laboratory oven before storage. Although some instruments can be dried with towels or gauze sponges, oven drying is preferred for the Verres needle and cannula(e). The oven should be regulated to approximately 50°C, a temperature that will dry without causing deterioration of rubber gaskets or plastic parts.

## STORAGE OF LAPAROSCOPIC INSTRUMENTS

The optimal method of storing the laparoscope, fiber optic cable, trocar, cannula, and accessory instruments is in a foam lined carrying case (Fig. 3.34). Such cases, which are available from most dealers, will prevent contact between instruments during storage and transportation, and are considered a wise investment. Laparoscopists performing all examinations in a central surgical area will find that shallow padded drawers with suitable dividers are quite satisfactory. Cases or drawers should be of sufficient size so that the light cable can be stored without being tightly bent. If possible the laparoscopic instrumentation should be stored in a locked area to prevent damage from those inexperienced in the proper handling of such equipment.

## PNEUMOPERITONEUM DEVICE

The automatic pneumoperitoneum device requires minimal attention. As discussed in Chapter 3, this apparatus is attached to an external gas source (tank) by means of a combination yoke-cable. After filling the internal tank of the pneumoperitoneum device from the external tank, the regulatory valve on the latter is closed. This prevents maintaining constant pressure on the yoke and cable fittings and reduces the possibility of creating a gas leak from a chronic weakening in the gas transfer cable. In addition, when laparoscopy is completed for the day, the internal tank is drained to eliminate all gaseous pressure.

## LIGHT SOURCE

Because of the high wattage lamp(s), the light source generates a tremendous amount of heat. A great portion of this energy is dissipated by an internal fan. Therefore, it is critical that the light source be positioned so that the air intake for the fan is not blocked. At the end of the laparoscopy examination, the light source unit should be cooled by shutting off the lamp but allowing the fan to operate for several minutes.

Other care procedures may be less obvious but are also important. Lamp bulbs will require periodic exchanging. The bulbs should be handled carefully, avoiding finger-printing the bulb or the reflecting mirrors which will reduce light intensity. Some high wattage bulbs are encased or partially surrounded by their own reflector. The latter may become pitted with use, decreasing illumination and necessitating replacement, even though the bulb remains working. Finally, as with most electrical devices, the light source will contain fuses. It is wise to have several additional fuses kept with the light source in case of fuse failure during a laparoscopy examination.

## AVAILABLE INSTRUMENTATION

The remainder of this chapter consists of illustrations and discussion of specific laparoscopic instrumentation useful for animal laparoscopy. Four manufacturing companies are represented and the instruments and most of the text provided were selected by the respective companies and edited by the authors. Specific instruments are identified by numbers and/or letter sequence and are the current catalogue identification numbers for each company. A listing of the manufacturers' current addresses and telephone numbers is found at the end of the chapter.

## EDER INSTRUMENT COMPANY, INC.

The Eder Instrument Company, Inc. is a United States manufacturer of medical optics and accessories for laparoscopy. The laparoscopes come in a wide variety of lengths, diameters, and angles of vision. Diameters range from 3 to 10 mm and lengths up to 122 cm. The angles of vision range from direct forward to retrograde. All laparoscopes are compatible for use with 35 mm SLR, movie, and closed circuit television cameras. Operative laparoscopes are also available with built in channels for insertion of operative instruments such as probes, cautery forceps, or aspirating tubes.

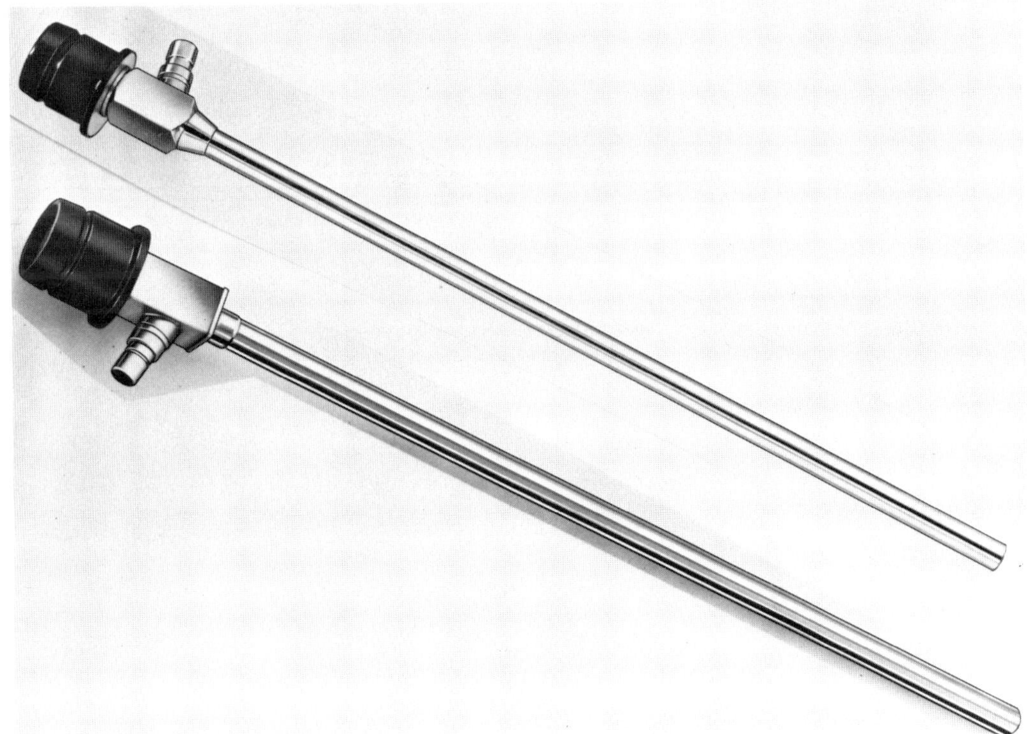

**Figure 12.1**   Standard 8 and 10 mm in diameter laparoscopes.

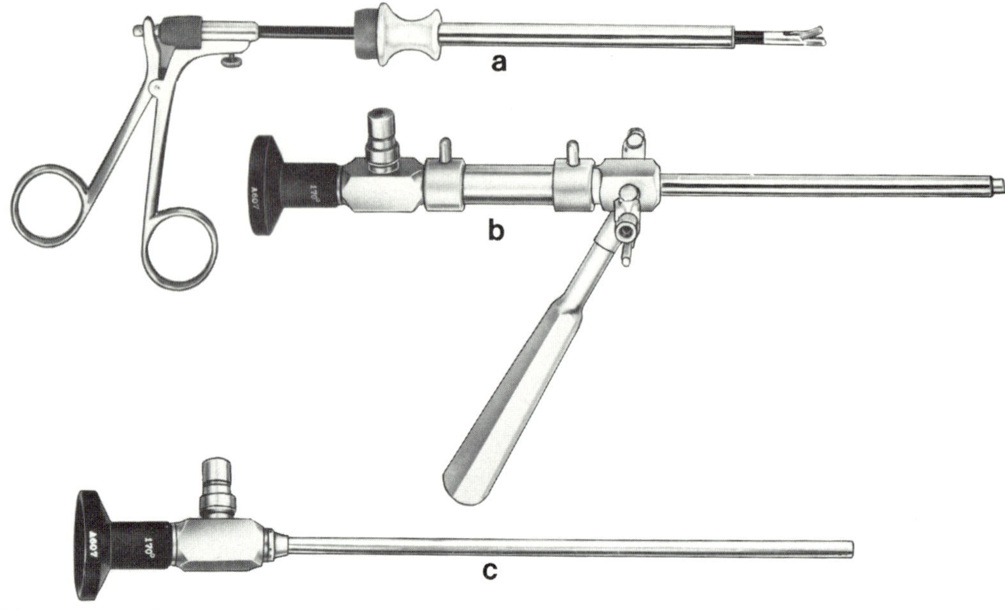

**Figure 12.2** **(a)** Scissors inserted through a cannula for use with two puncture operating technique. **(b)** Laparoscope, available in 3 or 5 mm diameter, inserted through cannula. Handle on cannula aids in stabilization; twin cannula ports are for irrigation during arthroscopy. **(c)** Small laparoscope without cannula.

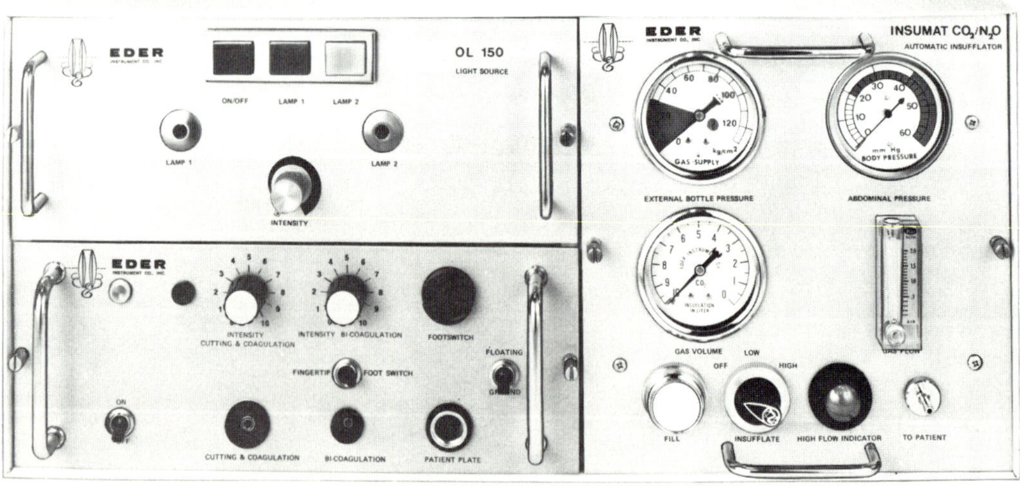

**Figure 12.3** The TOTALAP system, including insufflator, electrosurgical unit, and light source.

The TOTALAP is a self contained modular system that includes a $CO_2$ or $N_2O$ insufflator, Martin cold current electrosurgical unit, and a 150 watt dual outlet light source. The construction of this unit allows easy serviceability since each sectional unit may be removed by simply loosening two screws. The insufflator will operate on either

CO$_2$ or N$_2$O without adjustment. Special valves are incorporated to insure safety in both filling the inner tank and in insufflating the peritoneal cavity. The electrosurgical unit is a 120 watt, cold current system with automatic tissue compensation. A separate outlet is provided for use with a bipolar forceps. The light source features two outlets for either simultaneous or individual use. A rheostat, located between the outlets, regulates the intensity of both bulbs.

Accessory instruments are required to assist in insufflating the peritoneal cavity, manipulating internal organs, obtaining tissue samples, and electrocoagulating tissue. These and other specialized instruments are presented in Figure 12.4.

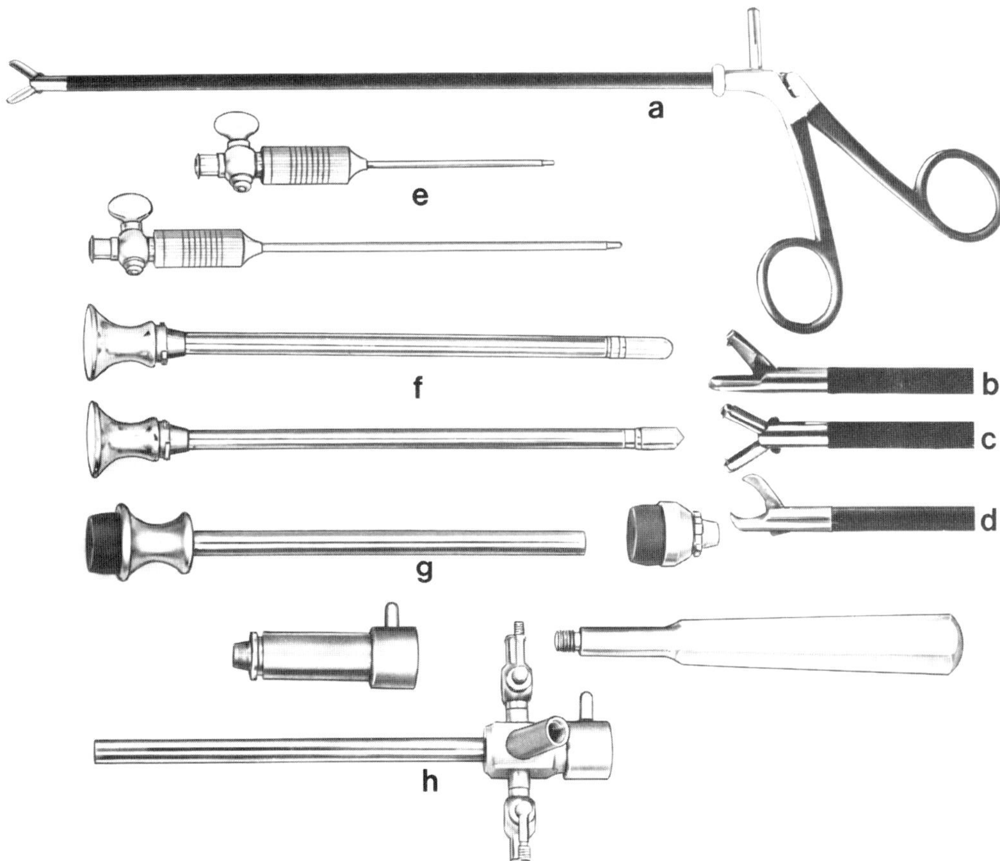

**Figure 12.4** **(a)** Grasping forceps, blunt jaws; **(b)** Biopsy forceps; **(c)** Grasping forceps, with teeth; **(d)** Scissors. These four instruments all come with insulated handles for electrocoagulation; **(e)** Verres needles, available in 4, 5, and 6 inch working lengths; **(f)** Blunt (above) and pyramidal (below) trocars; **(g)** Stainless steel cannula, available with fiberglass barrel; **(h)** Cannula, with proximal extension (above, left) and attachable handle (above, right). Twin ports on cannula provide for irrigation during arthroscopic examination.

The light source is a critical part of the laparoscopist's instrumentation. The Eder OL-1000 projector (Fig. 12.5a) contains a 150 watt lamp for diagnostic work and a 1000 watt photographic lamp that can be used for documentation with color slides or cinematography. A slide movement activates either lamp. The OL-150 projector (Fig. 12.5b) contains two 150 watt lamps. Either or both lamps can be used at one time. Both lamps have adjustable intensity with a control knob located between the two outlets. Both the OL-1000 and OL-150 provide backup lighting should one lamp burn out during an examination. The fiber light transmitting cable (Fig. 12.5c) may be either autoclaved, gas sterilized, or chemically disinfected. It is available in either 5 or 6.5 mm diameters.

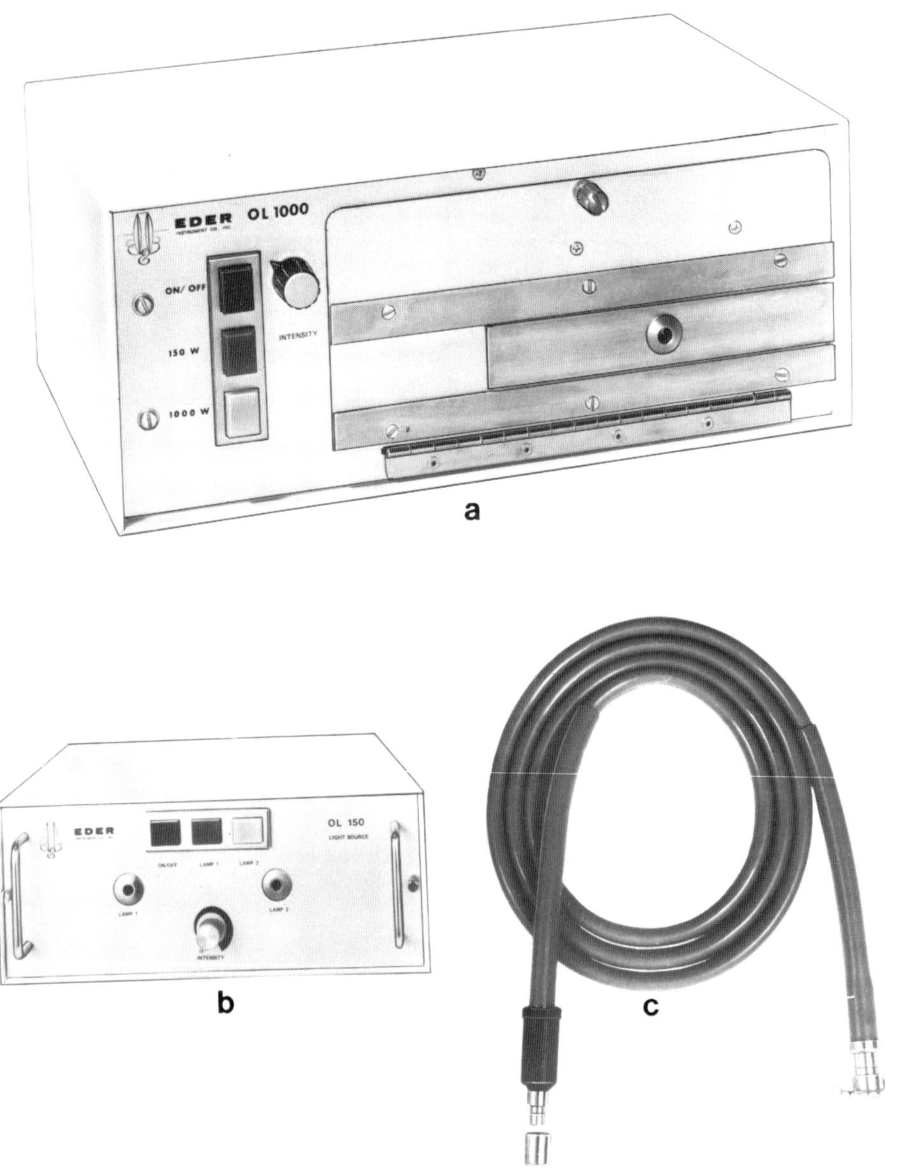


**Figure 12.5**   Light sources and transmission cable. **(a)** The OL-1000 projector. **(b)** The OL-150 projector. **(c)** Fiber light transmission cable.

Photography through the laparoscope has been possible by using special distal flash laparoscopes or by having extremely bright light transmitted from a projector through a light cable to the laparoscope itself. As described in Chapter 2, light is lost as it passes through the system in relation to the distance travelled and number of junctions required. Eder provides a means to circumvent part of this loss with a miniaturized battery powered strobe light for endoscopic photography (Fig. 12.6). This portable, lightweight mini-flash unit attaches to the hot shoe of the camera and directly to the endoscope. The light cable from the projector attaches to the strobe to provide light for focusing. The unit is supplied with a recharger and provides 60 to 80 flashes per charge.

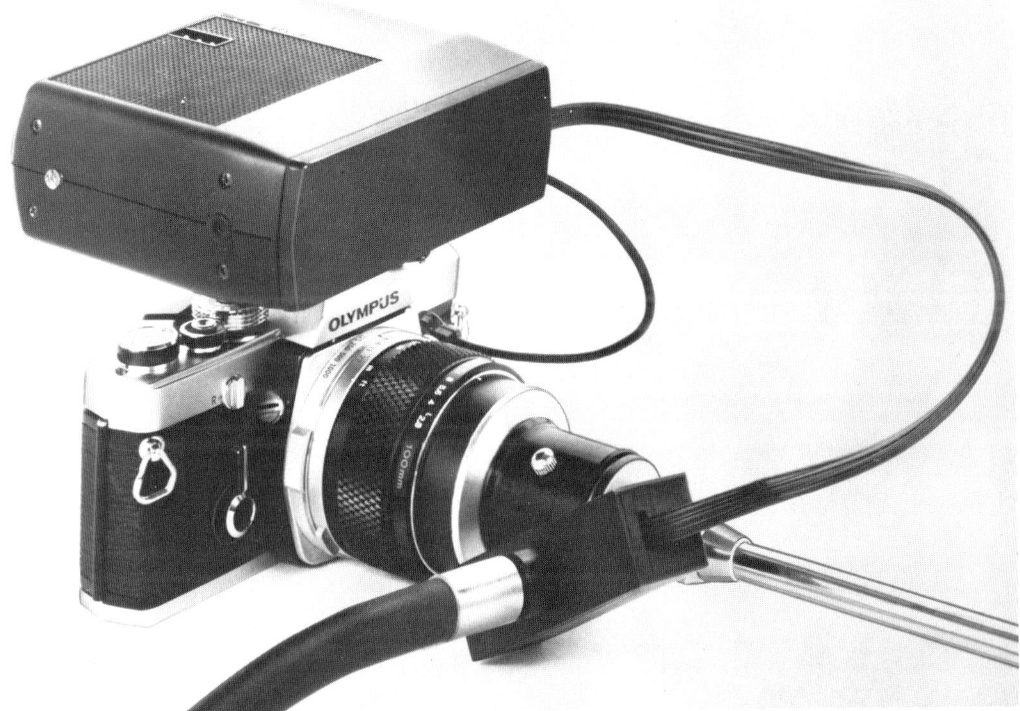

**Figure 12.6**  Mini-flash, battery powered strobe light for endoscopic photography. Ni-Cad battery pack has five year expected life.

Hysteroscopes are designed for visualization of the uterine lumen. The Cohen-Eder hysteroscope (Fig. 12.7a) is of single unit construction. It has two channels for flushing and expansion of the uterine cavity and one channel for 3 mm rigid or flexible biopsy, coagulation, or tubal occlusive devices.

Teaching attachments allow two individuals to view through the laparoscope at one time. The L shaped design gives greater mobility than the out of date Y shape and virtually eliminates interference.

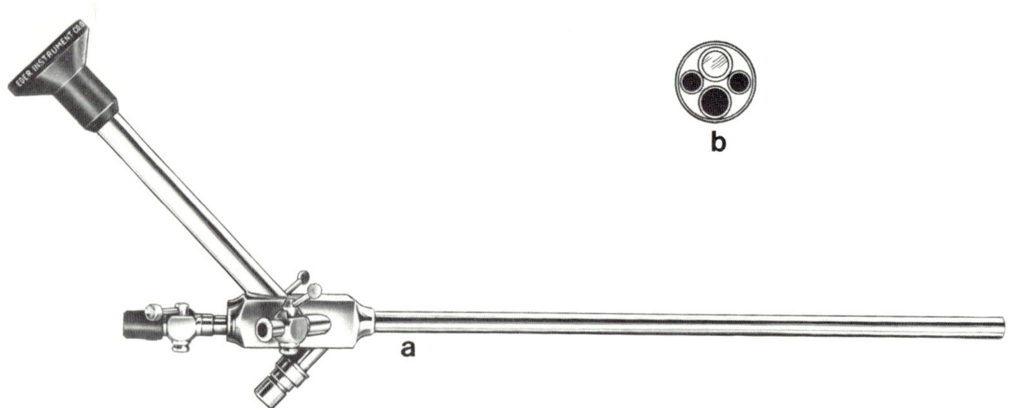

**Figure 12.7** **(a)** The Cohen-Eder hysteroscope incorporates a photographic HELIO optic with fiber illumination. **(b)** Distal tip of hysteroscope showing optic (upper), two flow channels, and 3 mm instrument channel (lower).

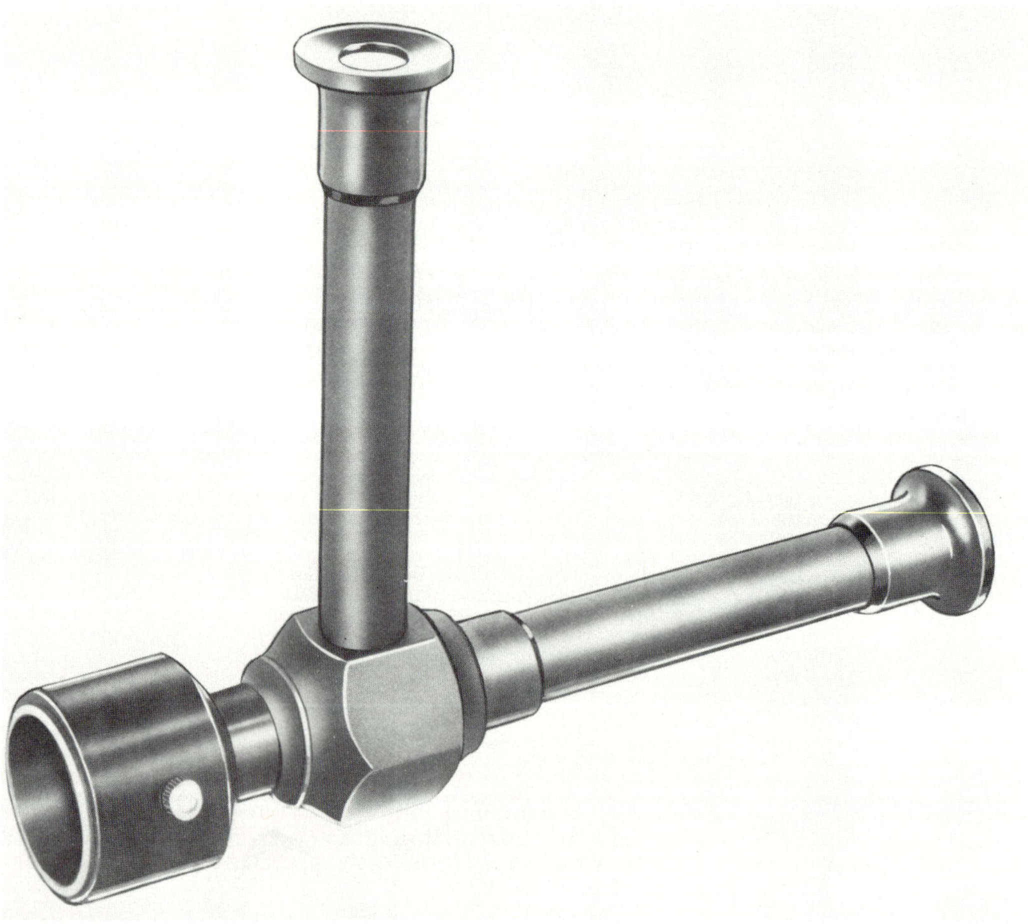

**Figure 12.8** Teaching attachments incorporate HELIO optic to provide a bright image and same field of vision to both observers.

## KARL STORZ ENDOSCOPY-AMERICA, INC.

The laparoscopes of Karl Storz Endoscopy-America, Inc. all use the Hopkins rod-lens optical system, providing a wide field of vision. Instruments come in a wide range of sizes and viewing angles and may be either double puncture or operating types.

Trocars and cannulae are required for insertion of both telescopes and accessory instruments when a two puncture technique is used. All cannulae contain valves to prevent loss of insufflated gas and those below are 5.5 mm in diameter except for the insulated cannula, 26172 CJ, which is 6.5 mm in diameter.

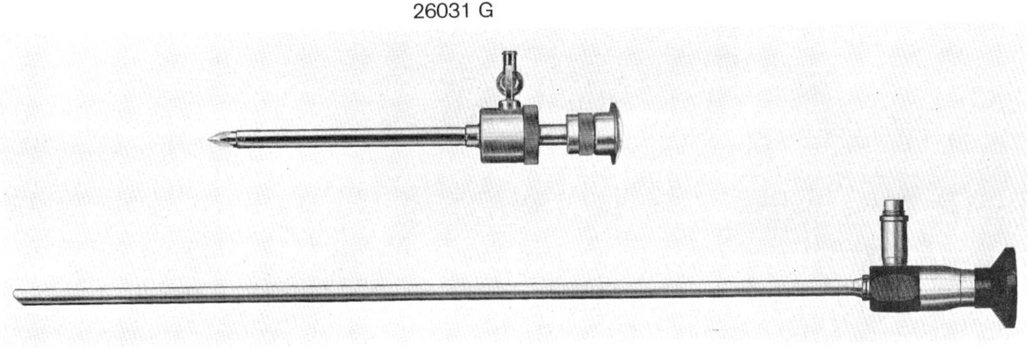


**Figure 12.9**  26031 B. A forward-oblique (30° viewing angle) telescope, 6.5 mm in diameter. 26031 G. Pyramidal trocar with cannula, for above laparoscope. Cannula has internal valve and side arm stopcock, 7.0 mm in diameter.

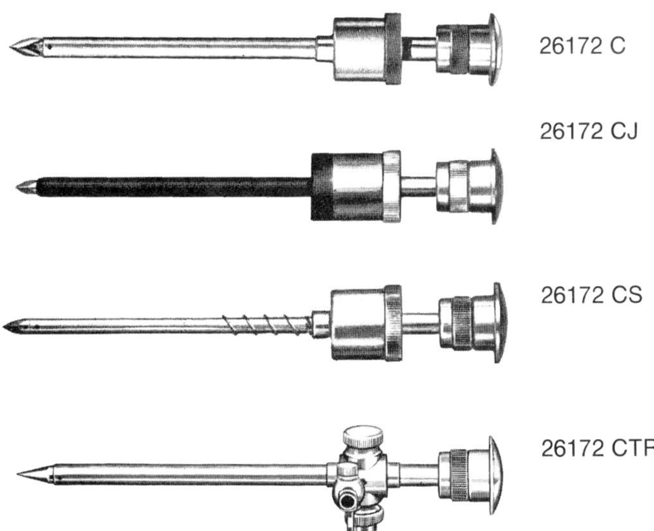


**Figure 12.10**  Trocar-cannula units for second puncture. 26172 C. Cannula with pyramidal tip trocar; 26172 CJ. Insulated cannula, used with operating instruments having high frequency current; 26172 CS. Havlicek trocar with spiral cannula; 26172 CTR. Conical tip trocar in cannula with trumpet valve.

Operating instruments inserted through a second puncture cannula may be used for grasping, cutting, coagulation, aspiration, or biopsy of tissue. The following unipolar coagulation instruments (Fig. 12.11) have insulated stems and handles and are available in a wide variety of types. Other second puncture operating instruments available without electrocoagulation capacity include: 26173 DB. Biopsy forceps; 26175 DH. Biopsy punch forceps; 26173 EH. Scissors; 26175 P,R. Injection, puncture needle, Luer-lock; 26175 T. Palpation probe.

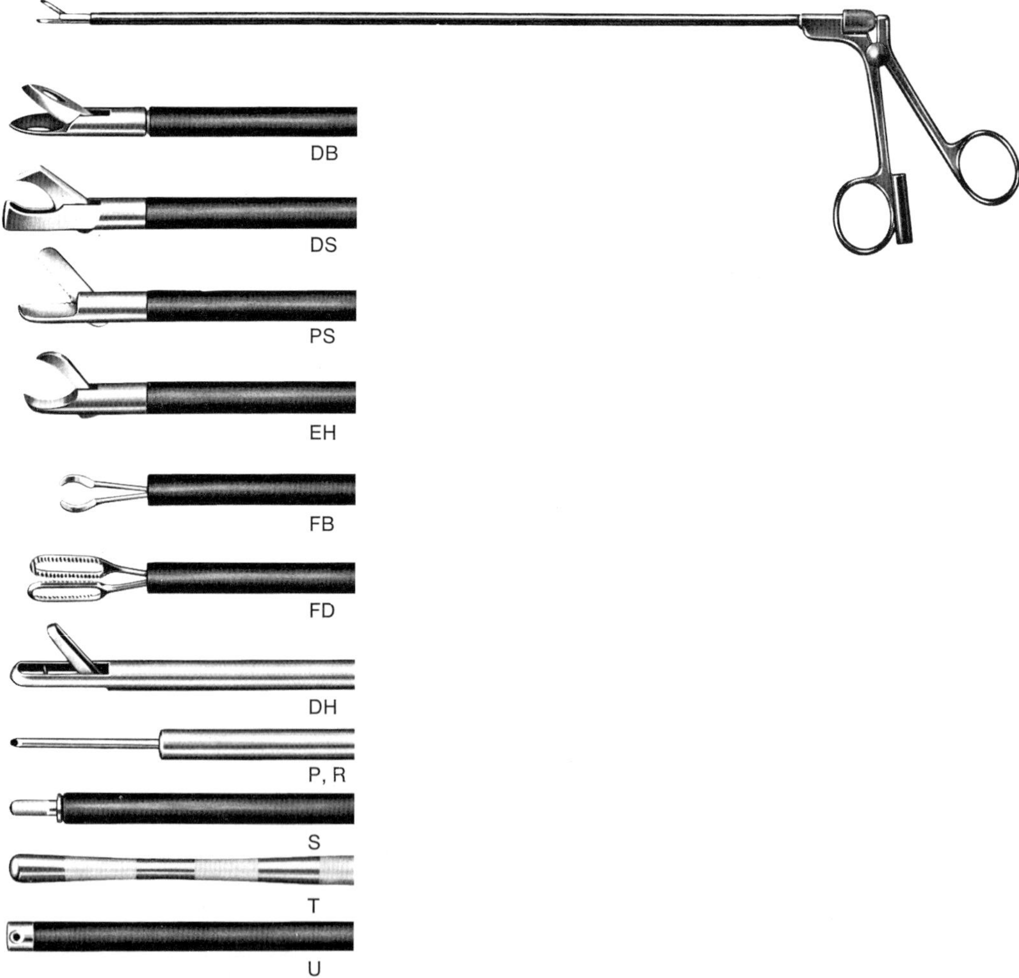


**Figure 12.11**   Second puncture instruments. 26175 DB. Biopsy forceps; 26175 DS. Frangenheim biopsy forceps; 26175 PS. Scissors with teeth; 26175 EH. Scissors; 26175 FB. Semm grasping forceps; 26175 FD. Atraumatic grasping forceps; 26175 S. Coagulation electrode; 26175 U. Cannula with trumpet valve for suction and coagulation.

Bipolar coagulation provides several advantages: there are no patient plates (no skin burn hazard), the field of coagulation is limited to the contact area of the electrodes, and the voltage and current required are low. The operating instruments pictured below can be inserted through the second puncture cannulae shown earlier.

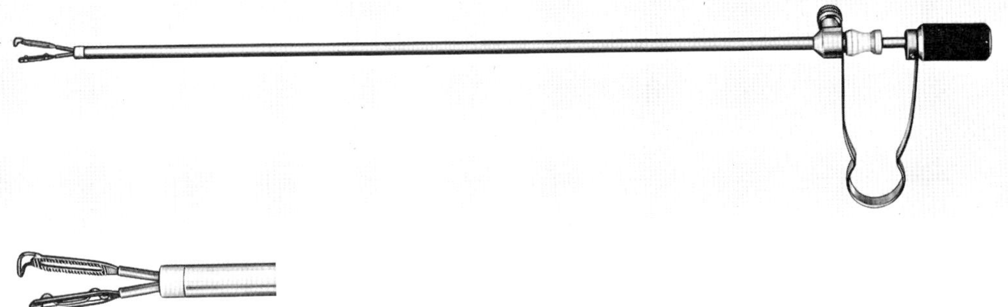

**Figure 12.12**    26176 FB. Bipolar grasping forceps.

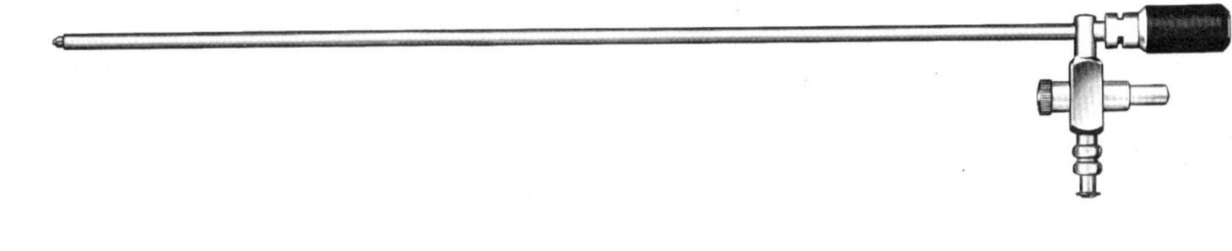

**Figure 12.13**    26176 UB. Bipolar suction-coagulator with trumpet valve.

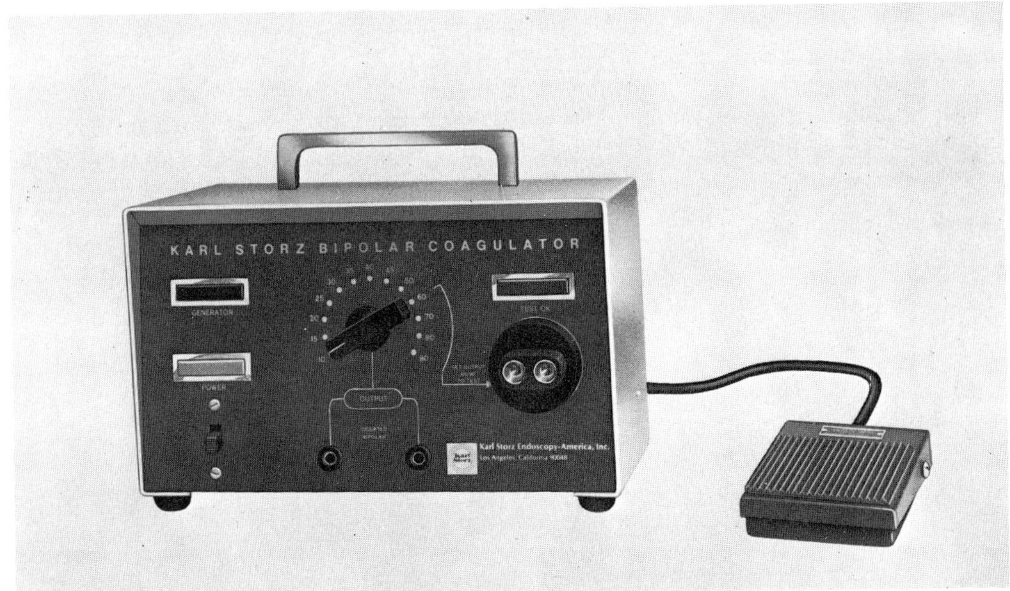



**Figure 12.14**    For use with bipolar coagulation instruments: 26020 XA. Bipolar coagulator, 115 V AC, 60 HZ; 26020 XB. Same but with 220 V AC 50 Hz.

Operating laparoscopes are designed with an instrument channel through which instruments can be inserted to obtain biopsies, sever adhesions, coagulate tissues, or manipulate structures. Only one puncture is required for the procedure. Operating laparoscopes described below (Fig. 12.15) require the 12 mm in diameter trocar-cannula for the puncture.

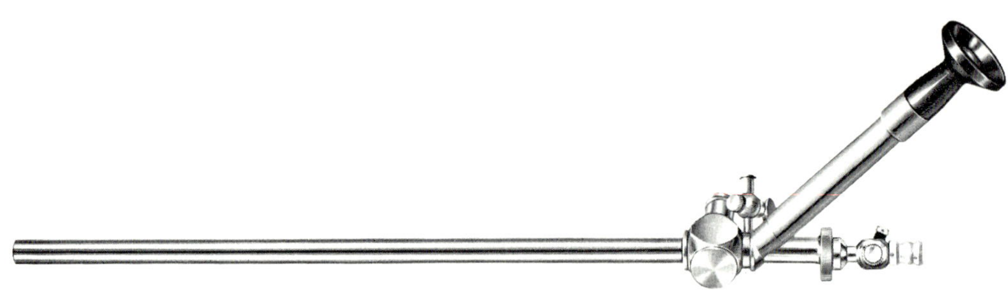


**Figure 12.15**  26038 A. Hopkins lens, straightforward operating telescope, 0°, wide angle, 10 mm in diameter. Fiber optic light transmission incorporated. Has a 6 mm instrument channel for rigid operating instruments and for use of ring applicator for tubal sterilization. Also available as 26039 A with 5 mm instrument channel for rigid operating instruments. Specially designed for photography, cinematography, and television.

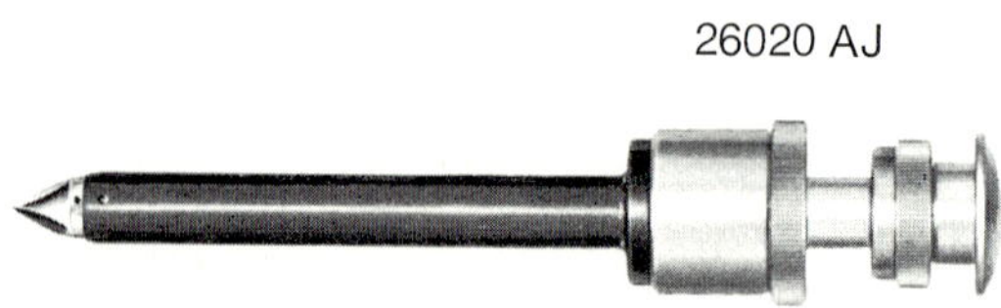


**Figure 12.16**  26020 AJ. Pyramidal trocar with 12 mm O.D. insulated cannula with valve. Also available as 26020 A, a pyramidal trocar with 11 mm O.D. noninsulated cannula with valve.

The smaller "pediatric" laparoscopes and operating instruments provided by Karl Storz Endoscopy-America, Inc. are of the size used by investigators in earlier chapters of this text for examination of cats, dogs, monkeys, rabbits, and large birds. Small laparoscopes can also be used in larger animals with proper precautions.

Operating instruments may be introduced through a second cannula. These instruments are presented in Figure 12.18. Other instruments include: 26183 UB. Bipolar suction-coagulator with trumpet valve; 26180 P. Luer-lock injection needle; 26180 T. Palpation probe.

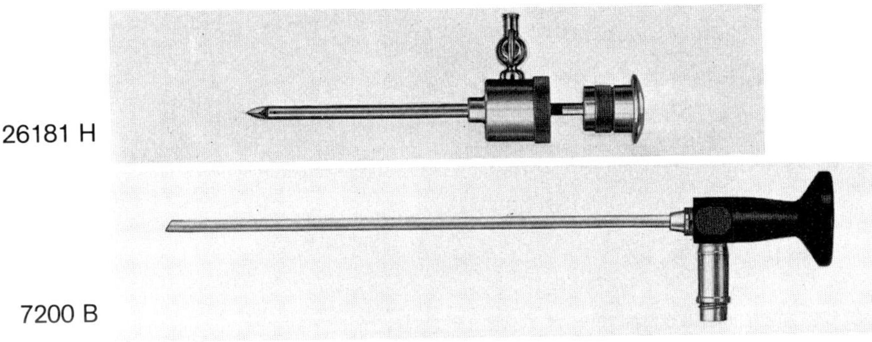


**Figure 12.17**  7200 B. Hopkins lens, forward-oblique telescope, 30°, 4 mm in diameter. With fiber optic light transmission incorporated. 26181 H. Trocar-cannula with valve and stopcock, cannula 4.5 mm in diameter, without insulation.

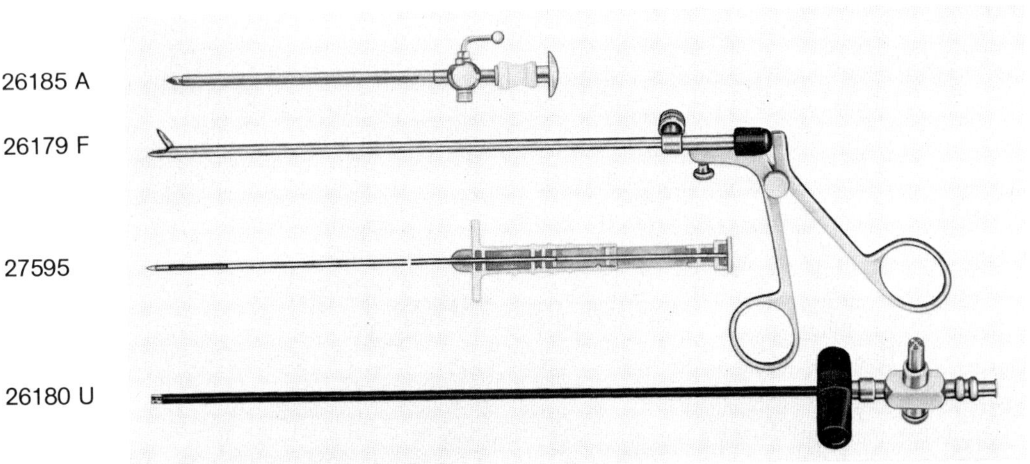


**Figure 12.18**  26185A. Trocar and cannula with stopcock, 4 mm in diameter; 26179 F. Biopsy forceps with "rinse through" device to facilitate thorough cleaning after liver biopsy; 27595. TRU-CUT liver biopsy needle; 26180 U. Insulated cannula and palpation probe, with trumpet valve, for suction and coagulation.

A most critical piece of equipment for the laparoscopist is the light source. Each laparoscopist needs to evaluate his needs prior to the purchase of the source. Large units are necessary to provide the amount of light required for television or cinematography but are not as portable as the smaller units. The following range of light sources from Karl Storz should meet the needs of all laparoscopists. All of these units are fully approved under UL Specification 544 for hospital use.

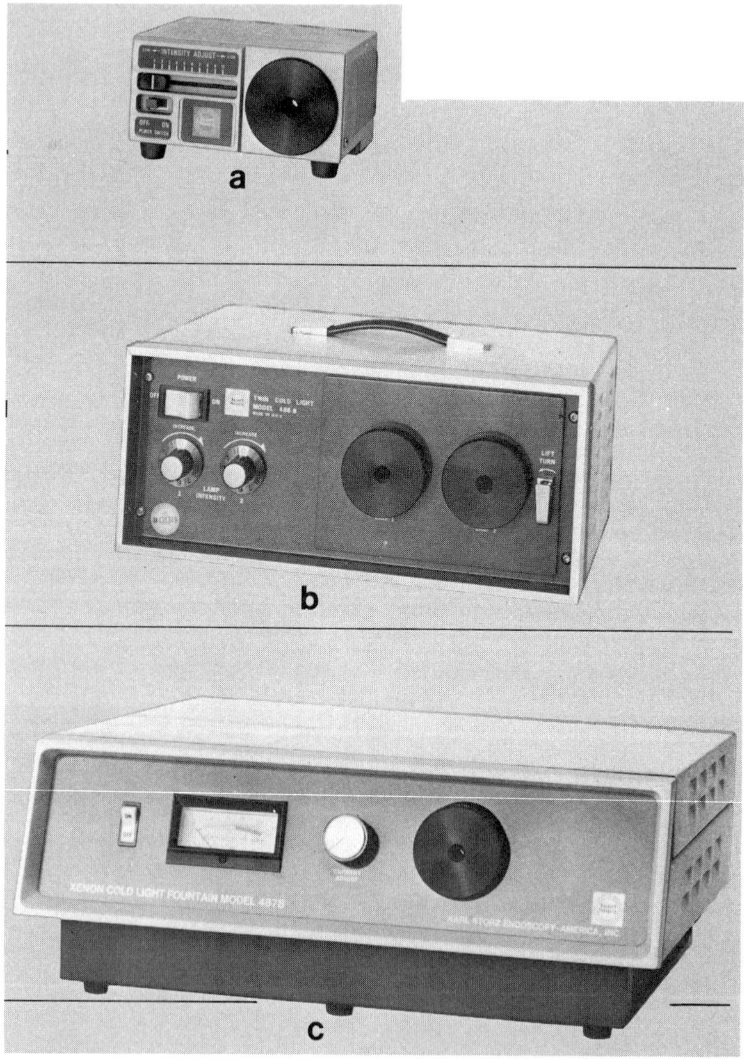

**Figure 12.19**   (a) 481 C. Cold Light Fountain, Miniature, single 150 watt halogen lamp; height, 8.25 cm; depth, 13.0 cm; width, 15.8 cm; weight 3.2 kg. (b) 483 C. Cold Light Fountain, Universal, with two 150 watt halogen lamps and dual controls for two instruments simultaneously; height, 20.3 cm; depth, 25.0 cm; width, 35.5 cm; weight, 10.0 kg. (c) 487 C. Cold Light Fountain, Xenon, "Instant Sunlight," 6000 Kelvin (approx.), 300 watts, for routine examination or documentation by photography, filming, and television; height, 19.0 cm; depth, 44.0 cm; width, 48.0 cm; weight, 24.0 kg.

The above light sources accept standard fiber optic cables and bifurcated cables for simultaneous double light transmission. Adapters are available to accept most existing instrumentation and accessories.

Automatic equipment to establish a pneumoperitoneum is essential for the safety of some patients. Ease in maintaining a proper level of pneumoperitoneum is also provided and allows the laparoscopist more freedom for his observations. The main equipment required is the pneumoperitoneum apparatus. The Semm apparatus (Fig. 12.20) features continuous and controlled flow into the abdominal cavity; preadjusted intraabdominal pressure; dial-indicator for intraabdominal pressure and flow-volume; visual indicator (flow meter) for gas inflow; immediate observation (indicator-dial) of sudden changes of intraabdominal pressure (e.g., adhesions); and automatic regulation (refill) of intraabdominal pressure during the procedure.

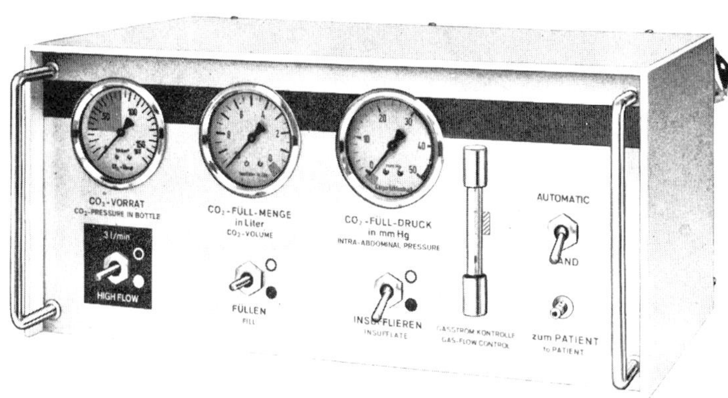


**Figure 12.20**   26020 S. Semm Pneumoperitoneum Apparatus, fully automatic. Related equipment includes: 26020 V. $CO_2$ cylinder, 1000 cm³; 26020 ST. Stand with casters for 26020 V.

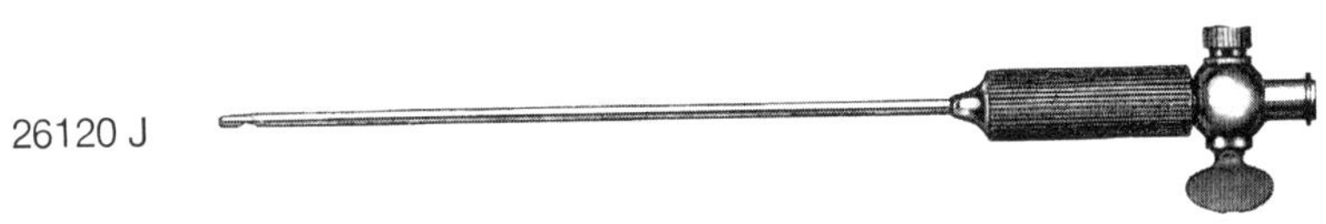


**Figure 12.21**   26120 J. Verres needle with spring loaded blunt stylet, with Luer-lock hub, 100 mm in length; also available as 26120 JL. 120 mm in length and 26120 JK. 70 mm in length.

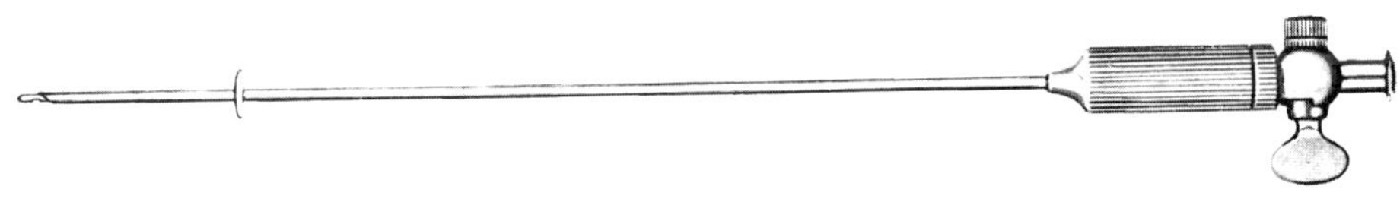

**Figure 12.22**   26120 JF. Verres needle for Douglas puncture.

## Accessory Attachments

### TEACHING ATTACHMENTS

It is frequently advantageous for two individuals to observe through a single laparoscope simultaneously. Consultation on diagnoses, teaching, and demonstrations are all simplified when teaching attachments are available. The instrument below can be attached to the eyepiece of any rigid or flexible endoscope; it provides simultaneous observation by the operator and an observer, and it can be used with any standard light source.

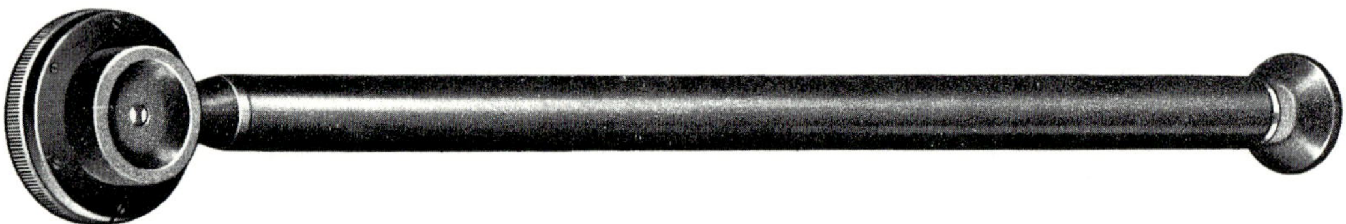

**Figure 12.23**   29015. Rigid teaching attachment, straight; also available as 29015 A. Right angle observer eyepiece.

### CAMERA ATTACHMENT

Proper connection of the endoscope to a photographic, film, or television camera is essential. The system below provides this connection or for the simultaneous observation by the operator and an observer (Fig. 12.24).

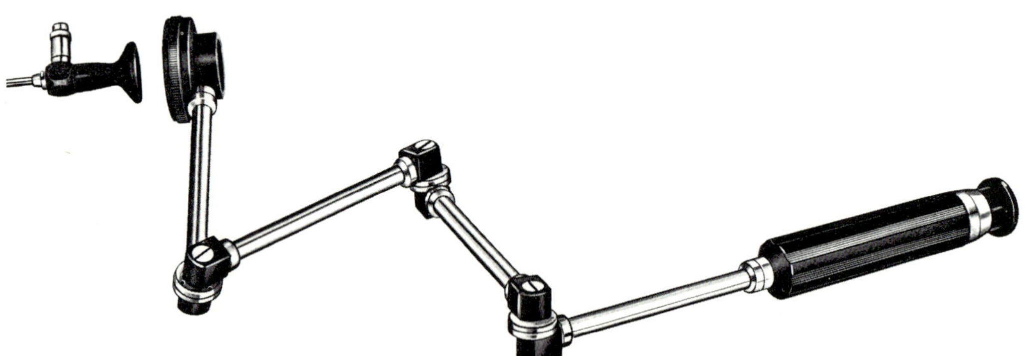

**Figure 12.24**   29020 A. Wittmoser articulated optical arm, with Hopkins lens system; attaches to all Hopkins lens telescopes.

# RICHARD WOLF MEDICAL INSTRUMENT CORP.

## Aviary Instrumentation

The first instruments presented below have the greatest application for use in avian laparoscopy. The determination of sex and diagnosis of internal injury or illness are simplified by use of the small diameter endoscopes.

The basic instrument for accomplishing an endoscopic examination in small birds for aviary medicine is the small diameter telescope (Fig. 12.25). The telescope is inserted with the aid of a trocar-cannula unit (Fig. 12.26). With small birds the use of a cannula is not always necessary since it increases the puncture diameter. Care must be taken to protect the telescope when the cannula is not in use.

The light projector (Figs. 12.27 and 12.28) provides the required illumination for all diagnostic or operative procedures. The light is transmitted from the projector through the telescope by a fiber optic system.

The 5 mm in diameter telescope may be used in larger birds. A telescope of this diameter is available in several lengths and viewing angles. This diameter instrument (Fig. 12.29) will also permit photography when connected to a special photo light source.

The Verres needle (Fig. 12.30), used for insufflation in mammals, and the tactile probe (Fig. 12.37d and h) may be used to manipulate internal organs for closer endoscopic examination.

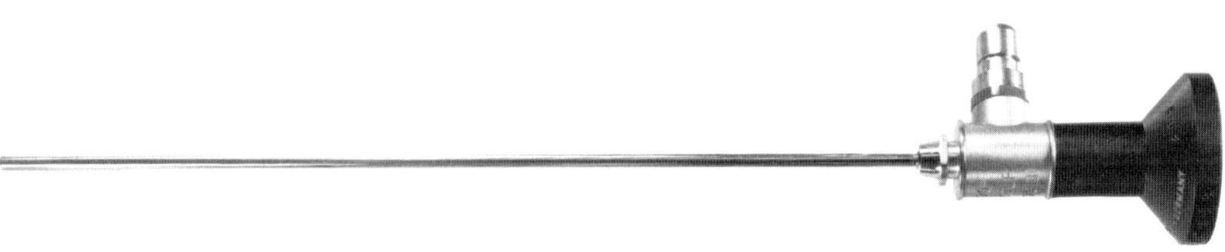

**Figure 12.25**   8670.31. 170°, 2.7 mm LUMINA-SL telescope, 2.7 mm in diameter with special wide angle viewing.

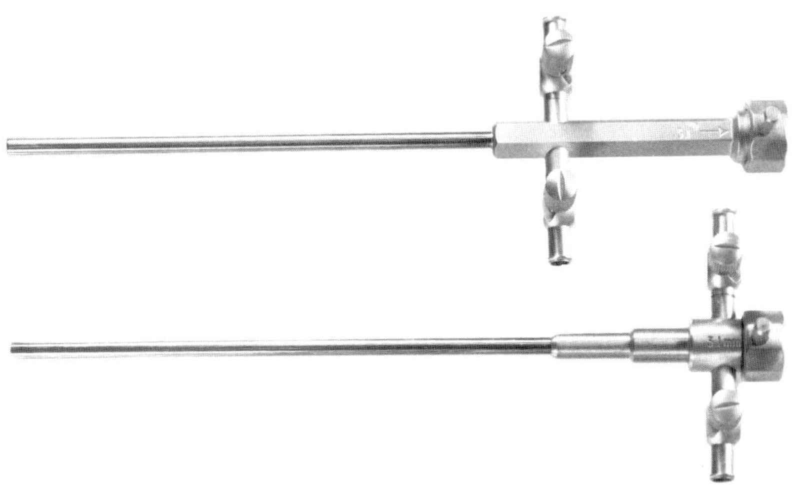

**Figure 12.26**   8852.04. 3.4 mm in diameter cannula for use with 8670.31 telescope.

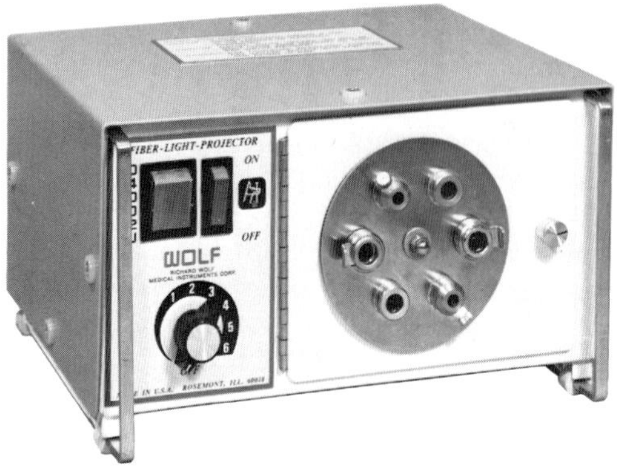

**Figure 12.27** D-4002 U Light projector containing two 150 watt lamps.

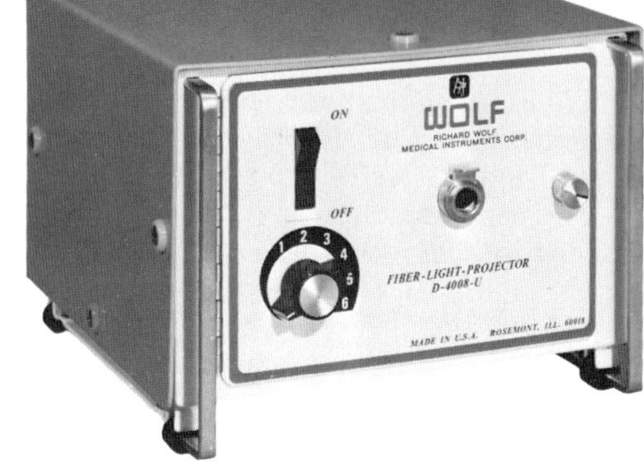

**Figure 12.28** 4008 U Light projector containing a single 150 watt lamp.

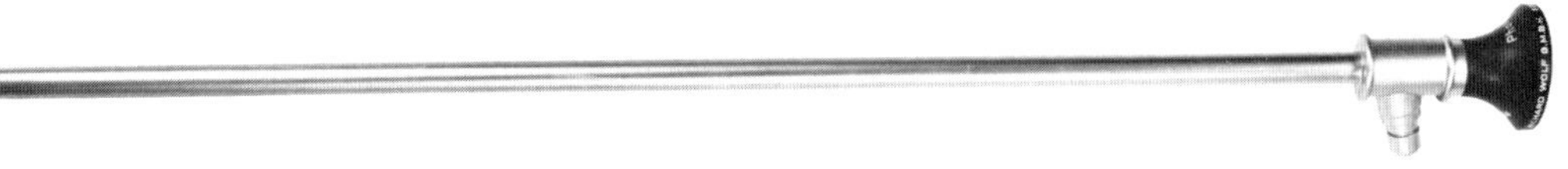

**Figure 12.29** 4935 H. 180° telescope with LUMINA optics.

**Figure 12.30** Verres needle for establishing the pneumoperitoneum, standard 120 mm length.

## Mammalian Laparoscopic Instrumentation

Endoscopy in mammals opens up an exciting and dynamic new area for the veterinarian or biomedical researcher. The potentials for diagnostic and operative procedures are just beginning to be explored. If the capability of photographic documentation is included, the uses become almost unlimited.

The standard laparoscopic telescopes (Fig. 12.31) as well as those discussed in aviary medicine may be used for mammalian endoscopy. The important point is to choose the telescope with regard to animal size unless photographic documentation is a major consideration. The standard 5 mm in diameter laparoscope offers the greatest versatility for diagnostic and operative procedures and when some photography is desired. If photography is the principal choice, a larger 8 or 10 mm in diameter telescope should be used. (Refer to the photography instrument section.)

The telescope is inserted with the aid of a trocar-cannula unit (Fig. 12.32) of a size compatible with that of the telescope.

The Verres needle, used as a probe in aviary medicine, is also used to insufflate the peritoneal cavity of mammals. This expands the internal working space and permits introduction of the trocar-cannula and telescope with a greatly reduced risk of puncturing an organ. The Automatic $CO_2$ Insufflator (Fig. 12.33) is connected to the Verres needle by a Silastic hose. Initially, manual control will insufflate the cavity to the desired level. When the proper level is reached, the switch is set to automatic and the insufflation level will be maintained.

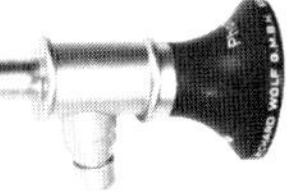

**Figure 12.31** 8932.40 or 8934.40. 8 or 10 mm in diameter, respectively, 180° telescope with LUMINA optics.

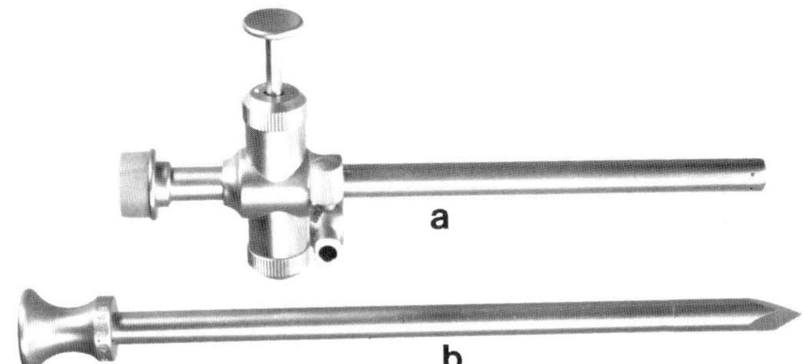

**Figure 12.32 (a)** 934 BF.10. Trocar cannula with trumpet valve. **(b)** 8934.12. Trocar with pyramidal tip.

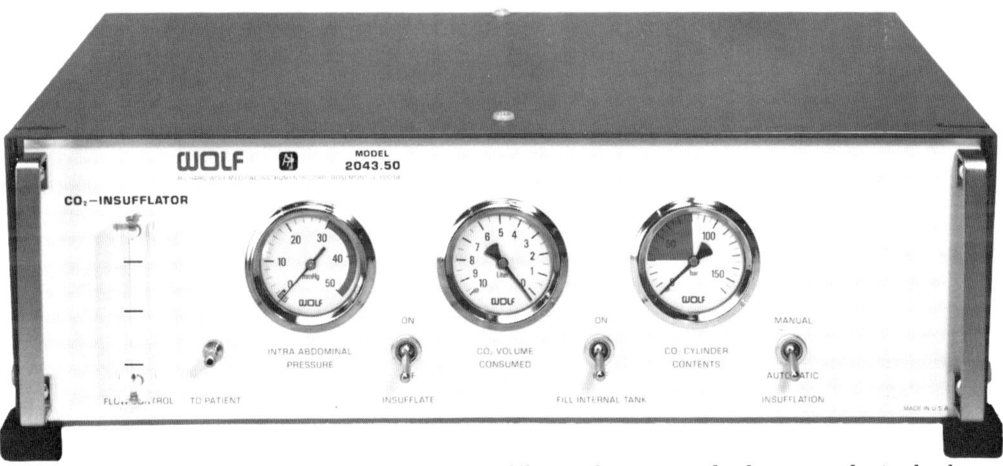

**Figure 12.33** 2043.50. $CO_2$ Automatic Insufflator, featuring the latest technical advancements. Snap lock toggle switches eliminate wear on moving parts for longer service and greater dependability. Dial gauges provide continued monitoring during a procedure. The unit is adaptable for use with a size D or E supply bottle and may be ordered with a $CO_2$ or $N_2O$ pin indexed yoke.

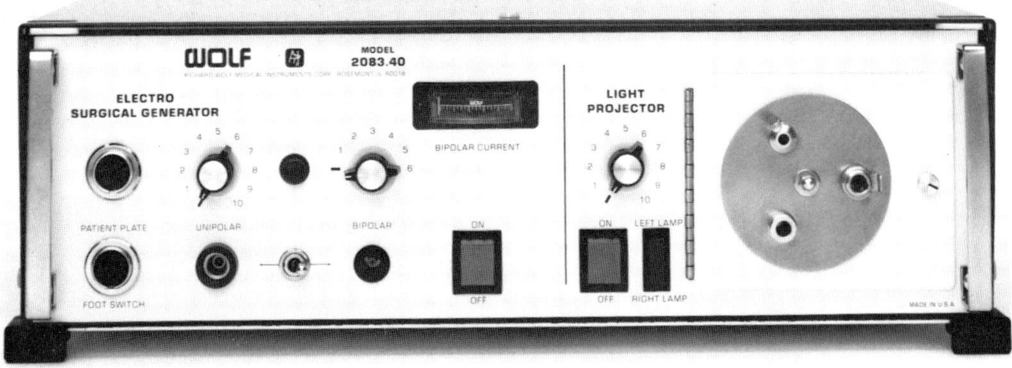

**Figure 12.34** 2083.40. Electrosurgical unit with bipolar ammeter and fiber light projector.

In mammalian laparoscopy, operative techniques may often be facilitated by an electrosurgical unit. The unit presented (Fig. 12.34) combines a standard light source with a cautery unit in one compact unit. Other units not in combination are shown in the "stackable piggy-back system."

The combination unit combines a standard 100 watt electrosurgical generator with the 50 watt bipolar generator and exclusive bipolar ammeter and multiport dial-a-light projector. The versatility of this combination is unsurpassed, creating the ultimate electrosurgical unit. The unit is complete with all connecting cables, ground plate, and foot switch.

The following instrumentation is designed for use in operative endoscopic procedures. The instruments shown are available in both 3 and 5 mm diameters, 32 cm length, with the exception of the bipolar forceps which are available in the 5 mm diameter only.

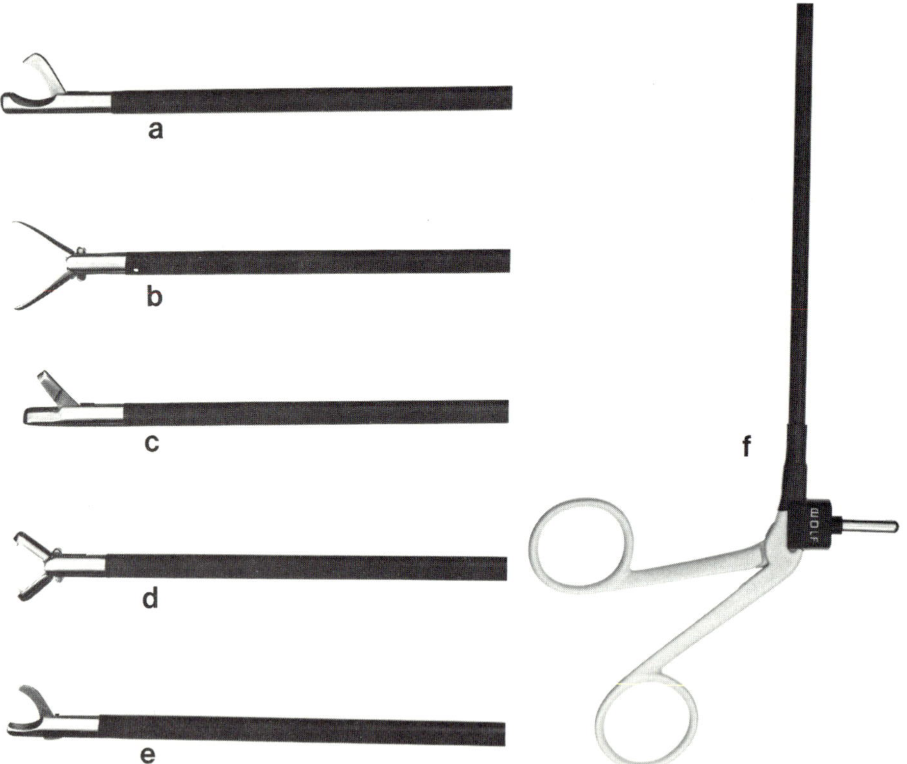

**Figure 12.35** **(a)** 8383.13. Frangenheim hook coagulation forceps; **(b)** 8383.03. Grasping forceps; **(c)** 8383.12. Biopsy forceps; **(d)** 8383.10. Ovarian biopsy forceps; **(e)** 8383.02. Hook scissors; **(f)** Insulated handle.

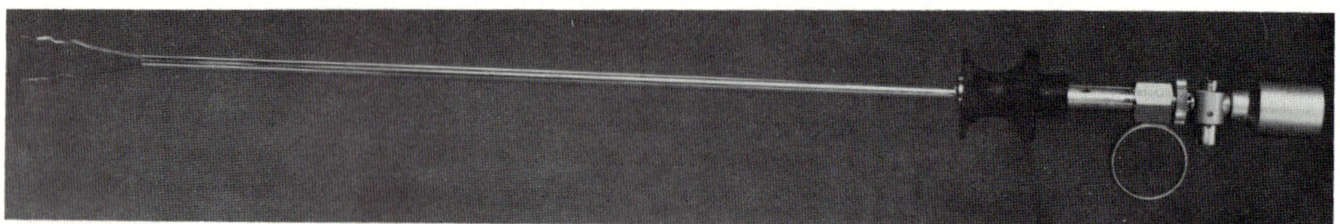

**Figure 12.36** 8383.21. Kleppinger bipolar forceps. Also available in a 45 cm length (8384.21).

Instruments for two puncture techniques are presented below. These instruments are inserted through a 3 mm in diameter trocar-cannula.

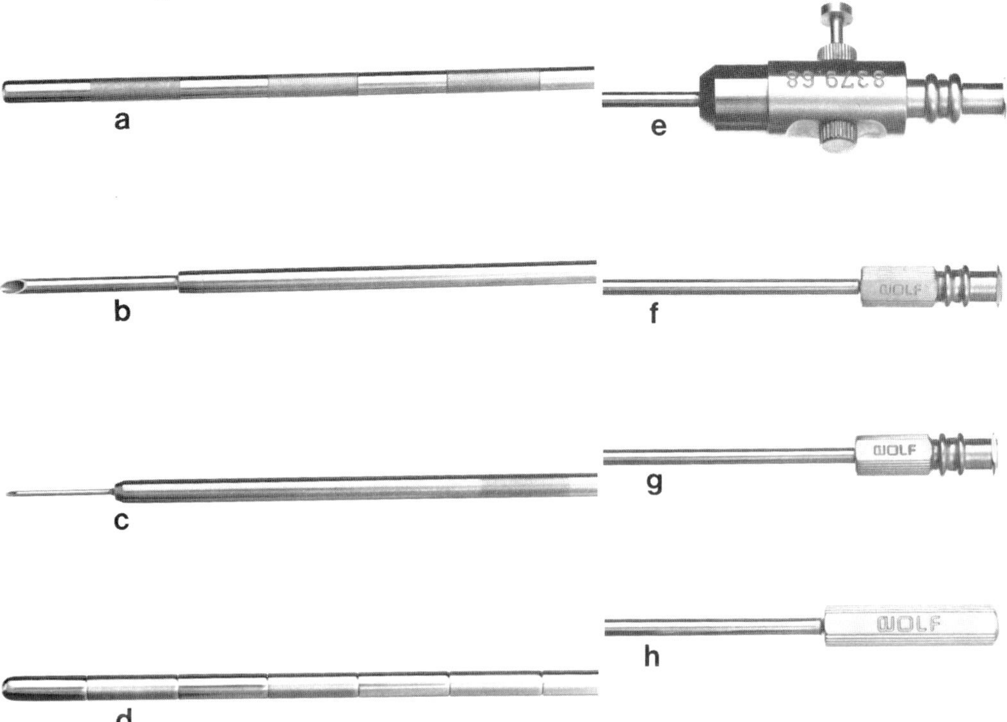

**Figure 12.37**   **(a)** 8379.68. Calibrated aspiration tube; **(b)** 8379.65. Injection and puncture needle, 1.8 mm in diameter (15 G); **(c)** 8379.60. Anesthesia needle, 0.7 mm in diameter (22 G); **(d)** 8379.66. Calibrated tactile probe; **(e–h)** External ends of the instruments to the left.

### Special Wolf Instrumentation

The newest addition to the Richard Wolf line of special endoscopes is the "mini-scope." This 2.7 mm endoscope is available with viewing angles of 170 or 100° and is inserted through a trocar-cannula 3.7 mm in diameter. The trocar-cannula is a redesign of the Verres cannula and as such may be used for the initial puncture and insufflation. The obturator is then removed and the "mini-scope" inserted for examination.

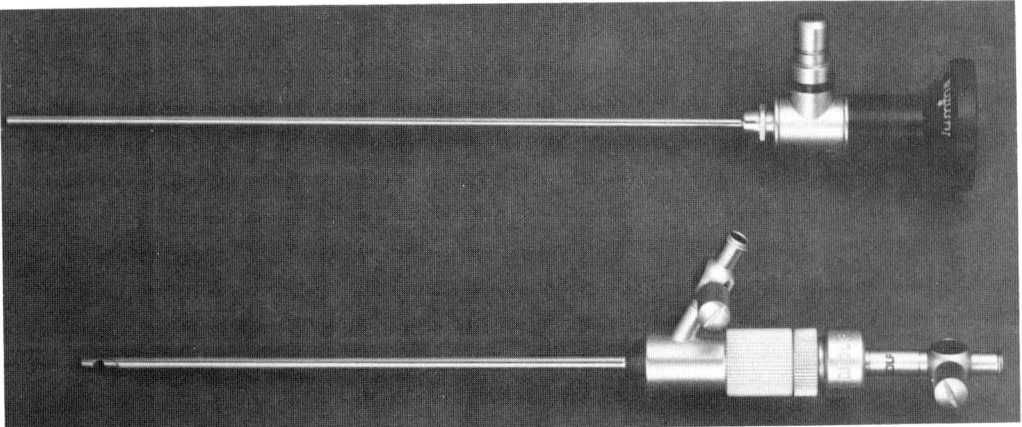

**Figure 12.38**   Mini-Scope and special trocar-cannula for insertion.

The Hulka Clip Applicator and Hulka Clip for tubal ligation are exclusive instruments with Richard Wolf. The Hulka Clip is a mechanical device for occluding the oviduct, thus eliminating the need for electrocautery.

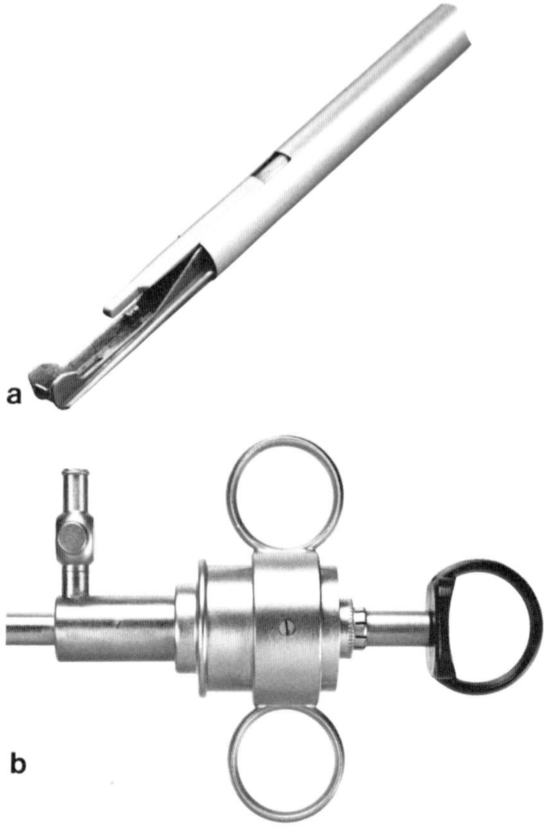

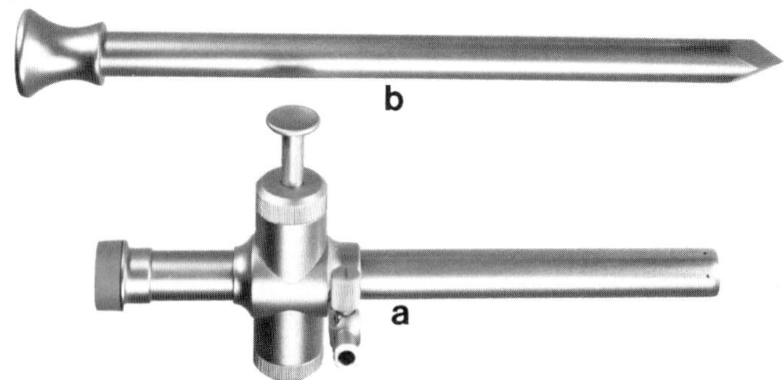

**Figure 12.39**  E8387.85. Hulka Clip forceps for second puncture, 7 mm in diameter. **(a)** Details of applicator tip. **(b)** Handle of applicator, also available in syringe type upon request.

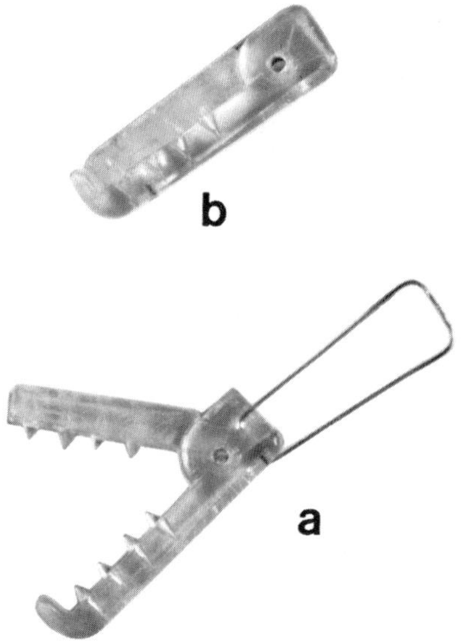

**Figure 12.40**  E4986.90. Hulka Clip with two jaws of inert plastic (Lexan) pressed together with a gold plated stainless steel spring (two per package). **(a)** Spring loaded clip with jaws in open position. **(b)** Clip with jaws closed and locked by spring.

**Figure 12.41**  E8933.01. **(a)** 7 mm in diameter metal trocar cannula with piston valve. **(b)** Trocar for above cannula, with pyramidal point.

## Piggy-Back System

Complete laparoscopy is facilitated in most animal species with the use of a "stackable piggy-back system." It incorporates the insufflator, light source, and electrosurgical units into one laparoscopy system. The combined system allows the convenience of a modular unit with the versatility and serviceability of an individual unit.

The versatility of this system eliminates equipment not needed while allowing maximum utilization of space and serviceability. The piggy-back units are designed for stacking, and each unit is held firmly in place by a slot and rubber foot lock arrangement. The units can be stacked four high but each may be removed for service or transport to another room as may be required.

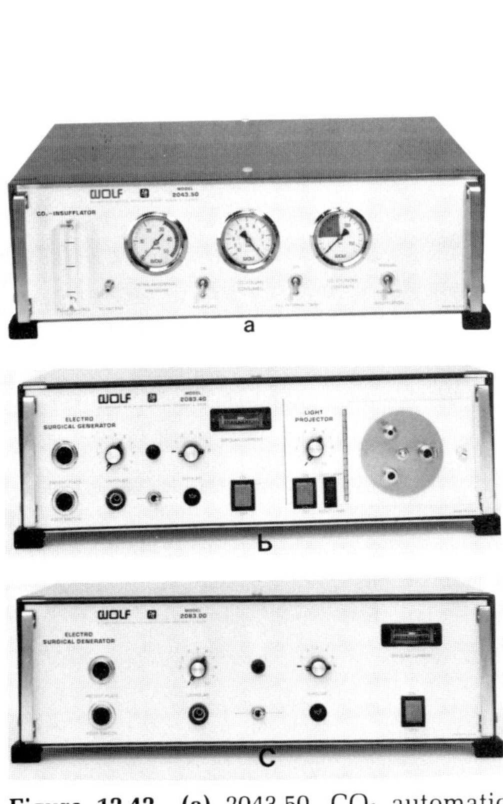

**Figure 12.42** **(a)** 2043.50. $CO_2$ automatic insufflator; **(b)** 2083.40. Electrosurgical combination with bipolar ammeter; **(c)** 2083.00. Electrosurgical generator with bipolar ammeter. Available units include: 2078.40. Bipolar combination with ammeter; 5000.40. Heavy duty light projector.

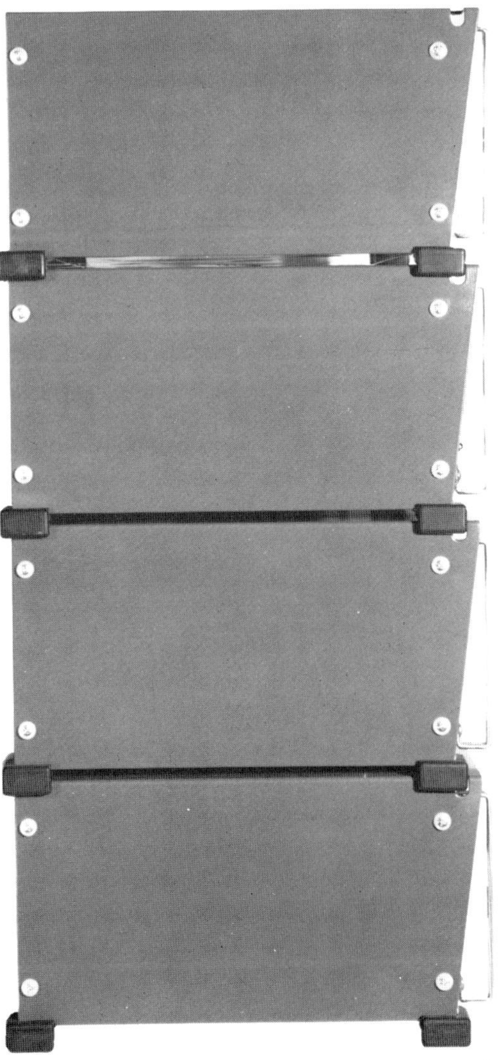

**Figure 12.43**   Side view of 4 units stacked.

## Photography

Various types of photographic units can be utilized. The proximal generators are specifically designed for slide documentation and provide best quality results for professional presentations. The Cine-Arc unit is most versatile and will provide illumination for production of slides, cinematography, and television video.

The system of transmitting the light for observation as well as the electronic flash through the one cable makes it possible to take photographs with the small diameter telescopes. The second light outlet permits simultaneous lighting of another instrument. Both diagnostic lights have a variable intensity control. The proximal flash has a three stage intensity control for photographic applications.

The above projector gives the operator immediate photo documentation ability for cinematographic, television, or still camera procedures. The 5000.40 features the Marc 300/16 A lamp with an efficiency of 50 lumens per watt advantage in photography. In addition to greater illumination efficiency, a dimmer system has been added to permit reduction of illumination to standby or increasing lamp output to maximum. An ammeter indicates current flow. It is not necessary to turn the Marc lamp off if a delay is expected. The lamp may be dimmed and then returned to full illumination by a simple turn of the dial. Cooling and reignition periods are not required and life expectancy of the lamp is increased.

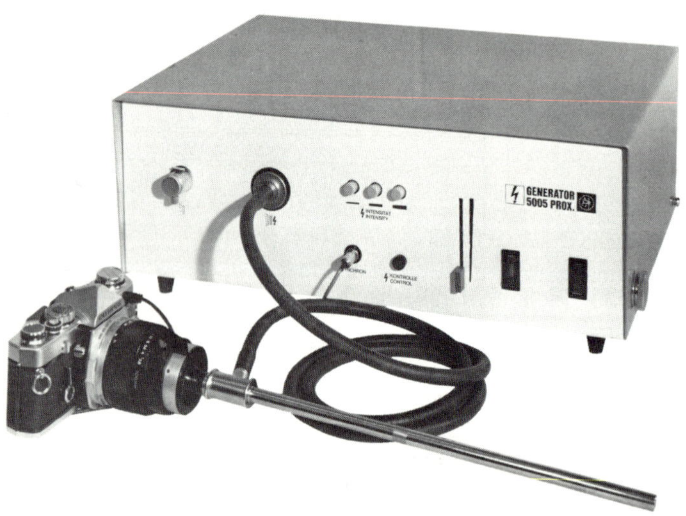

**Figure 12.44** 5005. Proximal fiber light flash generator, with Olympus 35 mm SLR camera, and integrated fiber bundle 10 mm in diameter telescope.

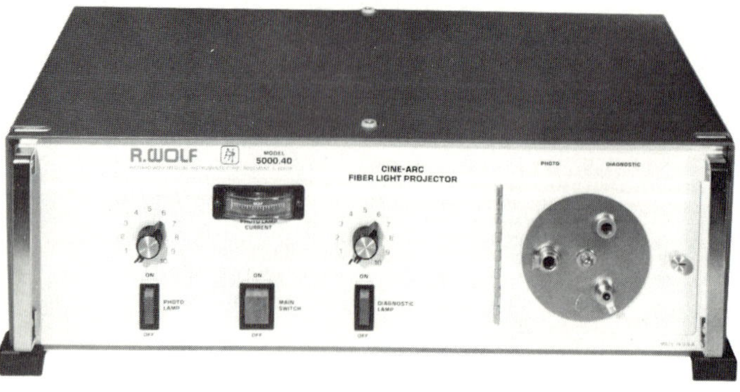

**Figure 12.45** —5000.40. Cine-Arc fiber light projector.

## DYONICS, INC.

The Needlescope[R] is the ultimate in laparoscopic instrumentation, an endoscope in a hypodermic needle. It affords the benefits of internal visualization with an absolute minimum of trauma. The self sealing puncture wound does not require suture and will not herniate. The small cannulae and trocars penetrate with an ease and control that provide a significant margin of safety when compared to larger instruments. In several reported cases of bowel perforation no morbidity resulted. The instrument's length places the operator's face well away from the point of entry as well as providing precision control and a comfortable grip.

The ease and convenience of this superbly engineered instrument is causing a revolution in diagnostic and operative endoscopy. In human clinical medicine most procedures using the Needlescope[R] are performed under local anesthesia in examination rooms and many are routinely done in wards. In laparoscopy, pneumoperitoneum is minimal with greatly decreased procedural and postprocedural discomfort. For many it is the preferred instrument when adhesions are probable. In arthroscopy many joints too small to be penetrated by larger endoscopes are easily visualized.

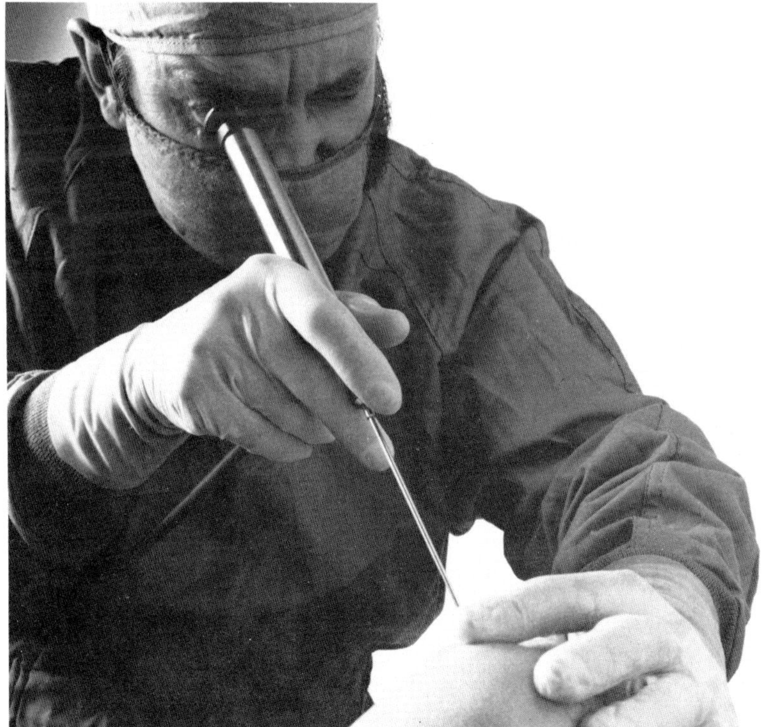

**Figure 12.46**  Needlescope[R] in use during arthroscopy of the knee.

### Cope Biopsy System

One of the many ancillary instruments developed for use with the Needlescope[R] is the Cope Biopsy System, developed with C. Cope, M.D., Albert Einstein Hospital. It allows easy and safe biopsy of tissue under direct visualization in laparoscopy or thoracoscopy. The added confidence in the resulting pathology report is substantial.

The biopsy instrument, which passes down the cannula alongside the endoscope and appears directly in the center of the area visualized, may be a liver core aspiration needle (Fig. 12.48) or a microcupped biopsy instrument (Fig. 12.49). The simplicity, quickness, and ease of the procedure saves both doctor and patient time.

### Dual Viewing Aid and Camera Adapters

Designed specifically for use with the Needlescope[R] (but adaptable to a number of other endoscopes) a compact dual visualizer (Fig. 12.50) allows the operator and a coviewer to see exactly the same field simultaneously without loss of resolution. This device is invaluable in teaching and consultive work.

A complete line of camera adapters gives suitable formats for 35 mm slides, 8 or 16 mm movies and videocameras (Fig. 12.51).

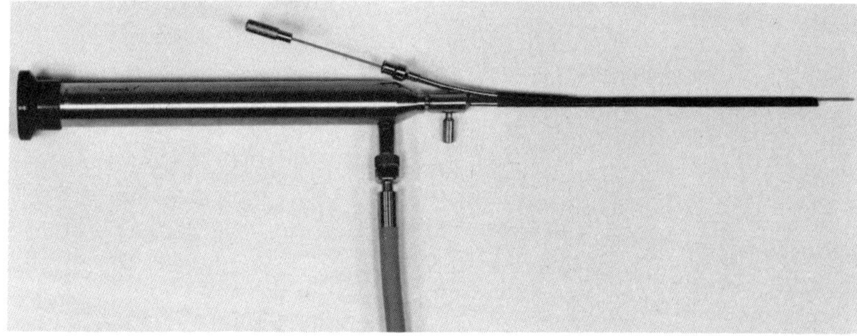

**Figure 12.47**   Needlescope[R] with Cope Biopsy System.

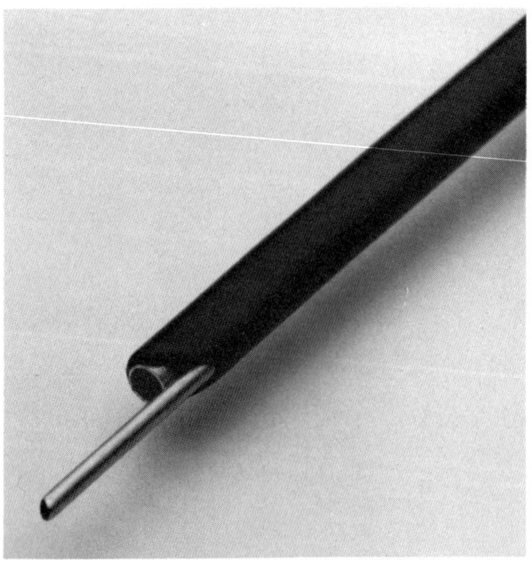

**Figure 12.48**   Liver core aspiration needle.

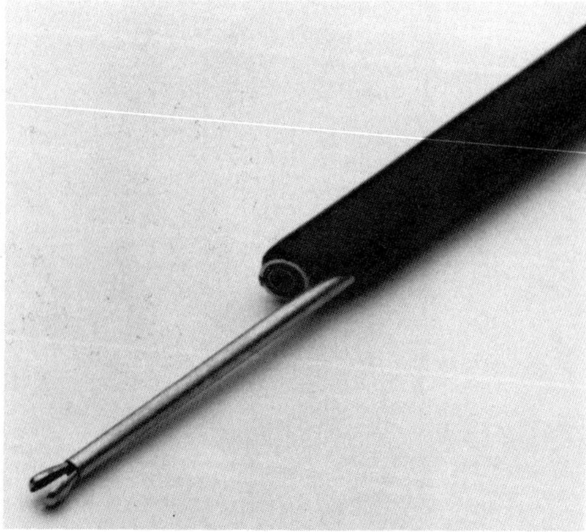

**Figure 12.49**   Microcupped biopsy instrument.

## Fiber Optic Illuminators

The Dyonics Model 450 Fiber Optic Illuminator (Fig. 12.52a) provides a variable brightness, high intensity, cool light which is conveyed directly to the distal tip of the Needlescope[R]. It contains a reserve lamp which is ready for immediate use. A built in meter allows lamp voltage regulation for maximizing lamp life.

The Dyonics Model 500 Fiber Optic Illuminator (Fig. 12.52b) provides a cool, high intensity, enriched mercury-vapor light source of daylight quality for photography and videotaping, or a tungsten-halogen lamp for routine viewing.

A bifurcated light guide (Fig. 12.52c) may be used with any of these illuminators to provide ancillary illumination through a halo light (a special cannula with an integral light guide) or a light wand, which may be used through a separate cannula to provide a very high level of illumination for transillumination of tissue or for photography or videocamera.

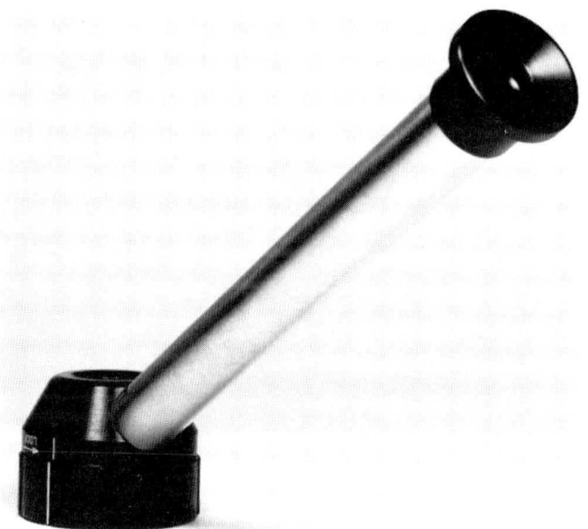

**Figure 12.50** Dual visualizer for simultaneous viewing by two persons.

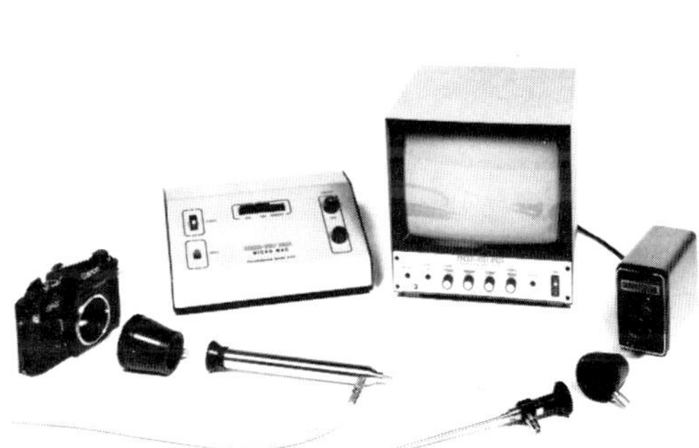

**Figure 12.51** Needlescope[R] with cameras and adapters.

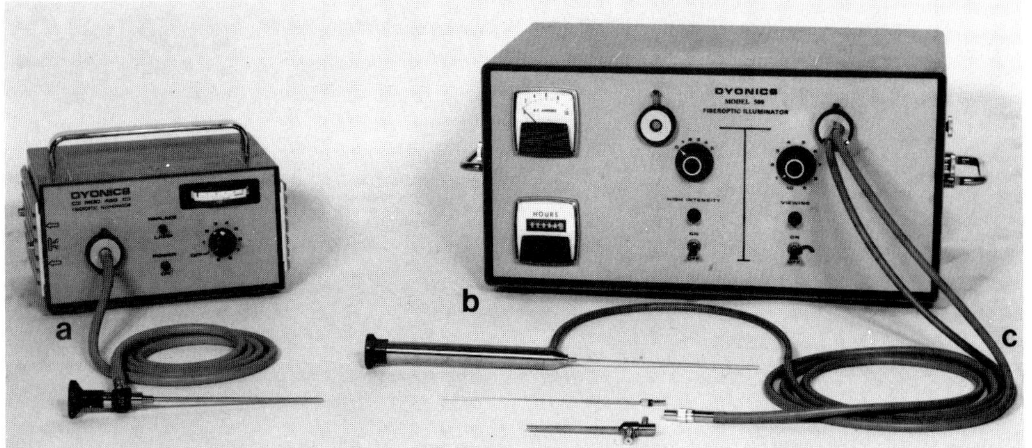

**Figure 12.52** Dyonics model 450 Fiber Optic Illuminator.

## Dyonics Endoscope Systems

Although endoscopic procedures are normally considered to be diagnostic, Dyonics, as a matter of policy, is developing a line of surgical instruments which allow operative procedures through cannulae, thus avoiding major surgery. Figure 12.53 demonstrates a complete surgical system.

One remarkable surgical instrument is the electrically powered Intraarticular Shaver™ (Fig. 12.54). With this instrument patellar chondrectomy and synovectomies can be performed through three simple punctures. A meniscal cutter attachment is available (Fig. 12.55) and partial meniscectomies can be carried out in selected patients on the same basis.

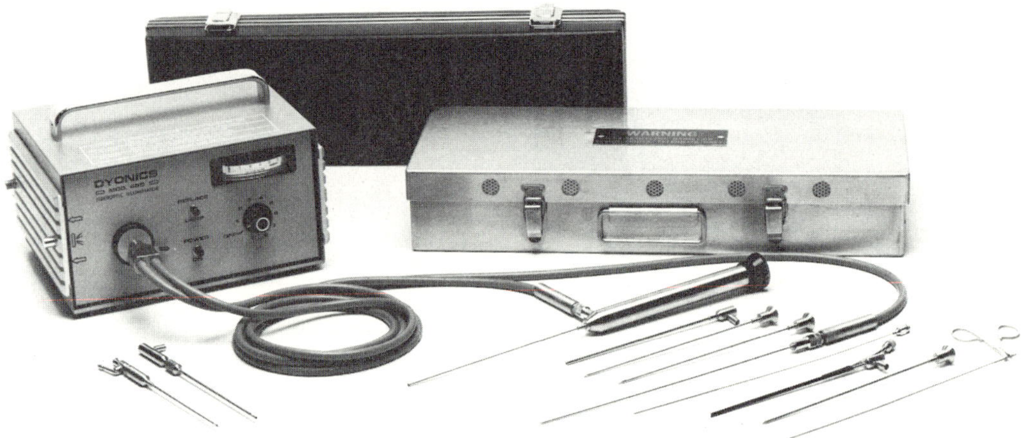

**Figure 12.53**  Complete surgical system for use with the Needlescope.

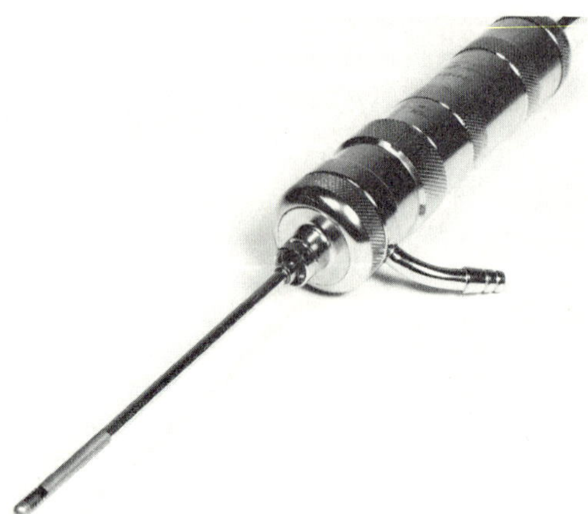

**Figure 12.54**  Intraarticular Shave™.

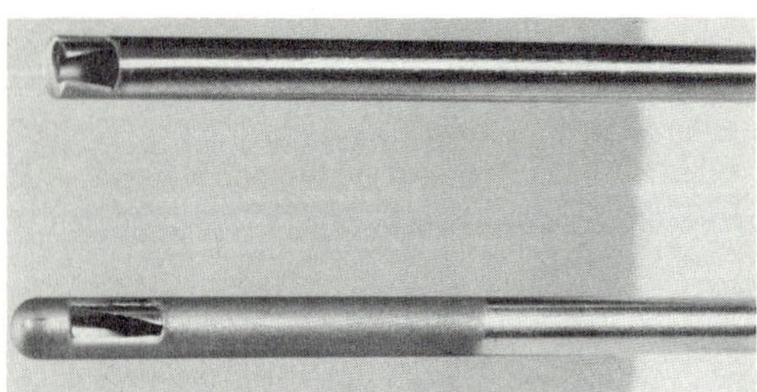

**Figure 12.55**  Meniscal cutter attachments.

Additional information concerning instruments previously presented, possible modifications, and current prices can be obtained from the various manufacturers:

Eder Instrument Company, Inc.
5115 North Ravenwood Avenue
Chicago, Illinois 60640
(312) 769-1944

Karl Storz Endoscopy-America, Inc.
658 South San Vicente Boulevard
Los Angeles, California 90048
(800) 421-0837

Richard Wolf Medical Instruments Corp.
7046 Lyndon Avenue
Rosemont, Illinois 60018
(312) 298-3150

Dyonics, Inc.
71 Pine Street
Woburn, Massachusetts 01801
(617) 935-5900
(Bibliography on Needlescope[R], reprints, and literature available.)

### References


Corson, S. L., Block, S., Mintz, C., Dole, M., and Wainwright, A. (1978) Sterilization of laparoscopes—is soaking sufficient? *Fertil. Steril.* 30:753.

Taylor, D. L. (1973) Sterilization of laparoscopic instruments by soaking. *Obstet. Gynecol. Letters Series* 14:73–77.

# Color Atlas

## CODE FOR BLACK AND WHITE DIAGRAMS

1—abdominal fluid
2—abdominal wall
3—adrenal
4—air sac membrane
5—air sac membrane opening
6—biopsy forceps
7—biopsy needle
8—biopsy site
9—bladder
10—broad ligament
   a. right
11—colon
12—corpus albicans
13—corpus hemorrhagicum
14—corpus luteum
15—diaphragm
16—fat
17—fimbria
18—follicle
   a. after aspiration
19—follicular cyst
20—follicular stigma
21—gallbladder
22—granuloma
23—grasping forceps
24—greater omentum
25—heart
26—hemorrhage
27—Hulka Clip
28—inguinal ring
29—inner rim of laparoscopic cannula
30—kidney
   a. left

31—liver
32—lung
33—mesosalpinx
   a. covering ovary
34—ovarian artery
35—ovarian blood supply
36—ovarian bursa
37—ovary
   a. left
   b. right
38—oviduct
39—ovulation fossa
40—parietal peritoneum
41—probe
42—rectum
43—scissors
44—small intestine
45—spermatic artery-vein
46—spleen
47—stomach
48—testicle
49—tumor
50—uterine horn
   a. left
   b. right
51—uterus
52—vas deferens
   a. left
   b. cauterized section
   c. right
   d. severed ends

* The following color plate figures were reproduced with permission from the following journal articles: Plate 1, Figures 6 and 7; Plate 2, Figure 4: *Anat. Rec.* (1977) 189:443–449. Plate 1, Figure 8; Plate 2, Figures 1 and 2: *In*: Laparoscopic determination of ovarian and uterine morphology. *Current Therapy in Theriogenology* (in press, 1979). Plate 2, Figure 5: *Biol. Reprod.* (1978) 18:561–570. Plate 3, Figures 3 and 6; Plate 4, Figures 2 and 4: *Primates* (1977) 18:261–270. Plate 3, Figures 4, 5 and 7: *Primates* (1974) 15:305–309. Plate 9, Figure 7; Plate 8, Figure 8; Plate 10, Figure 8; Plate 11, Figures 2, 3, 5, 7 and 8: *J. Am. Vet. Med. Assoc.* (1978) 173:1081–1087.

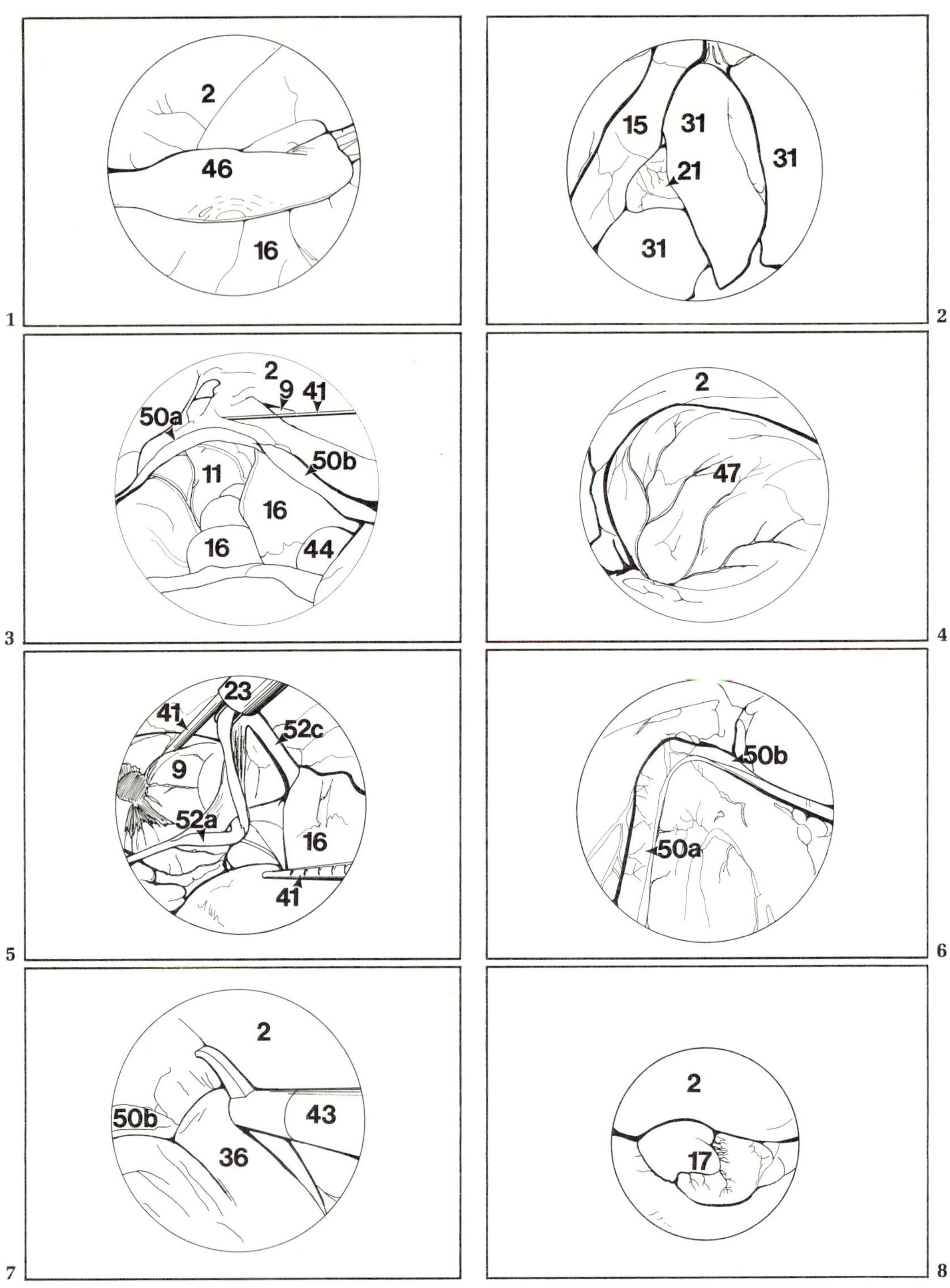

**DIAGRAMS FOR PLATE 1.** **2**—abdominal wall; **9**—bladder; **11**—colon; **15**—diaphragm; **16**—fat; **17**—fimbria; **21**—gallbladder; **23**—grasping forceps; **31**—liver; **36**—ovarian bursa; **41**—probe; **43**—scissors; **44**—small intestine; **46**—spleen; **47**—stomach; **50a**—uterine horn, left; **50b**—uterine horn, right; **52a**—vas deferens, left; **52c**—vas deferens, right.

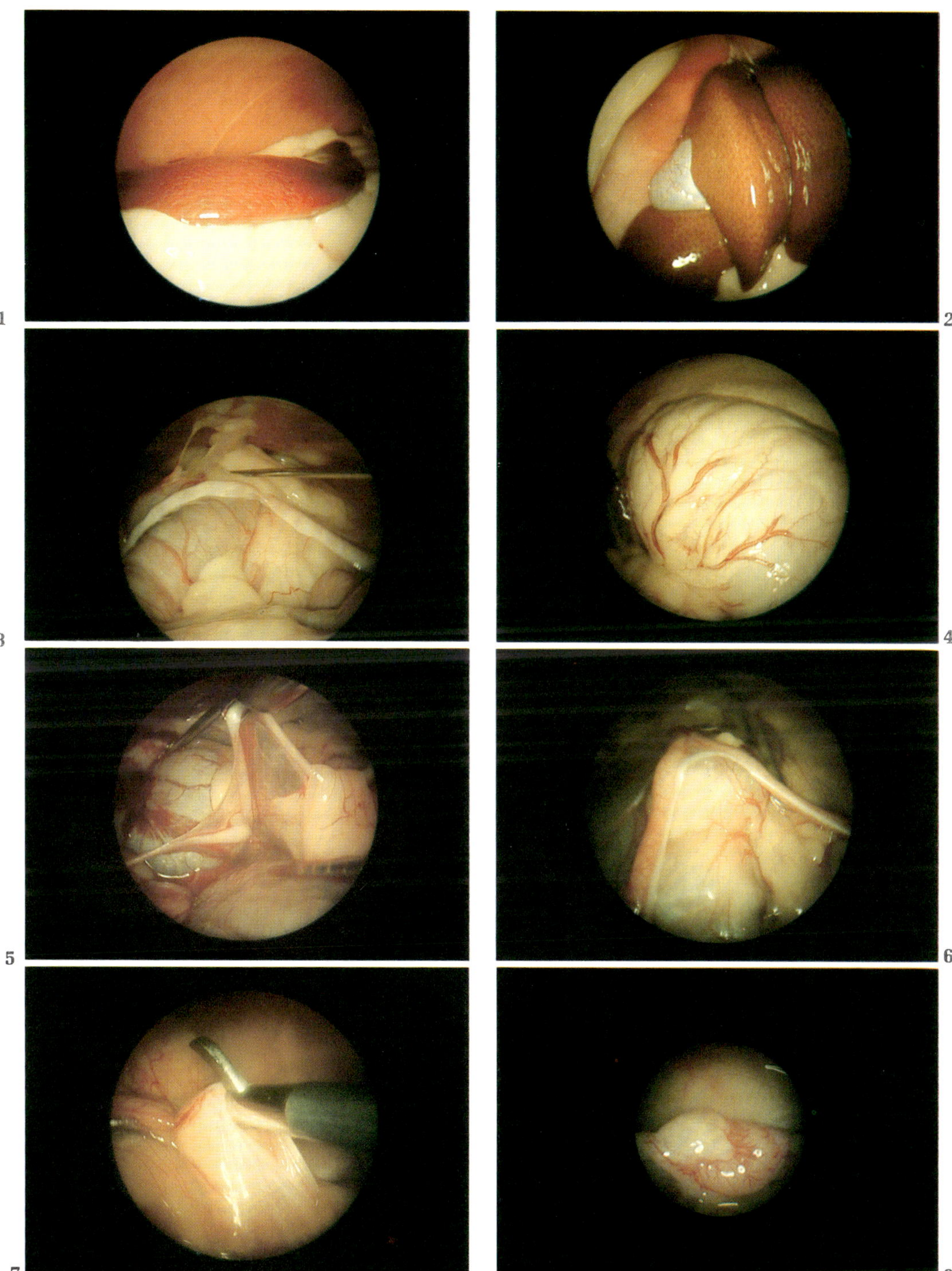

COLOR PLATE 1. **Figure 1.** Spleen of a cat (Chapter 3). **Figure 2.** Liver and gallbladder of a cat (Chapter 3). **Figure 3.** Caudal abdominal cavity of cat, including uterine horns and colon (Chapter 3). **Figure 4.** Ventral surface of the stomach of a cat (Chapter 3). **Figure 5.** Bilateral vas deferens and bladder of a dog (Chapter 3). **Figure 6.** Canine uterine horns (Chapter 3). **Figure 7.** Accessory scissors used to extend the natural ovarian bursa slit of the bitch (Chapter 3). **Figure 8.** Feline (right) ovary covered by transparent ovarian fimbria. Lateral portion of fimbria very vascular (Chapter 3).

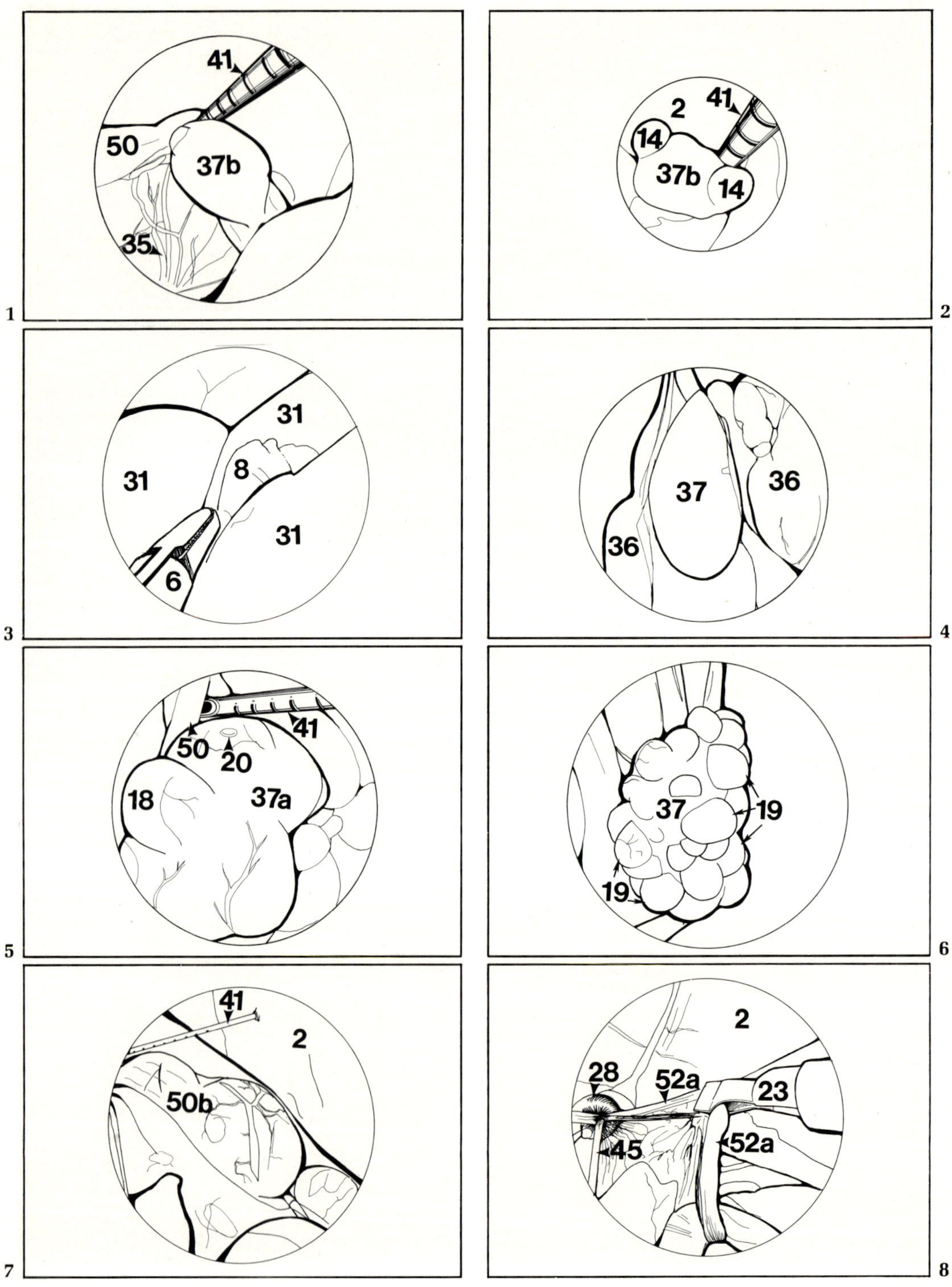



**DIAGRAMS FOR PLATE 2.** **2**—abdominal wall; **6**—biopsy forceps; **8**—biopsy site; **14**—corpus luteum; **18**—follicle; **19**—follicular cyst; **20**—follicular stigma; **23**—grasping forceps; **28**—inguinal ring; **31**—liver; **35**—ovarian blood supply; **36**—ovarian bursa; **37**—ovary; **37a**—ovary, left; **37b**—ovary, right; **41**—probe; **45**—spermatic artery-vein; **50**—uterine horn; **50b**—uterine horn, right; **52a**—vas deferens, left.

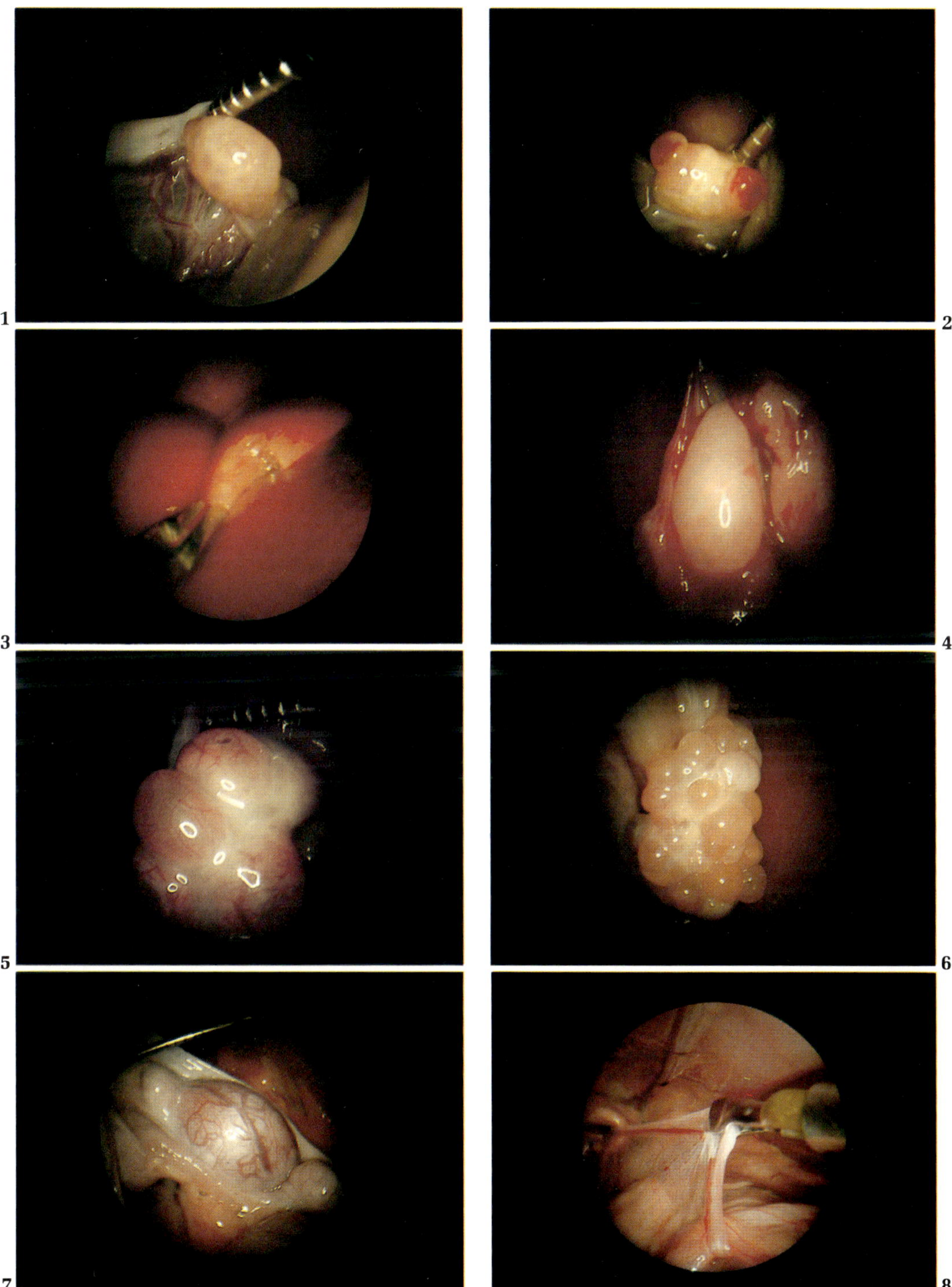

**COLOR PLATE 2. Figure 1.** Verres needle used to elevate the quiescent cat ovary (Chapter 3). **Figure 2.** Corpora lutea in the cat (Chapter 3) **Figure 3.** Canine liver immediately following forceps biopsy (Chapter 3). **Figure 4.** Canine ovary immediately following laparoscopic surgical exposure (Chapter 3). **Figure 5.** Canine ovary containing both follicles and corpora lutea (Chapter 3). **Figure 6.** Canine ovary containing cystic follicles (Chapter 3). **Figure 7.** Segment of highly vascularized gravid uterine horn of a bitch (Chapter 3). **Figure 8.** Grasping the left vas deferens with the bipolar cautery forceps (Chapter 3).

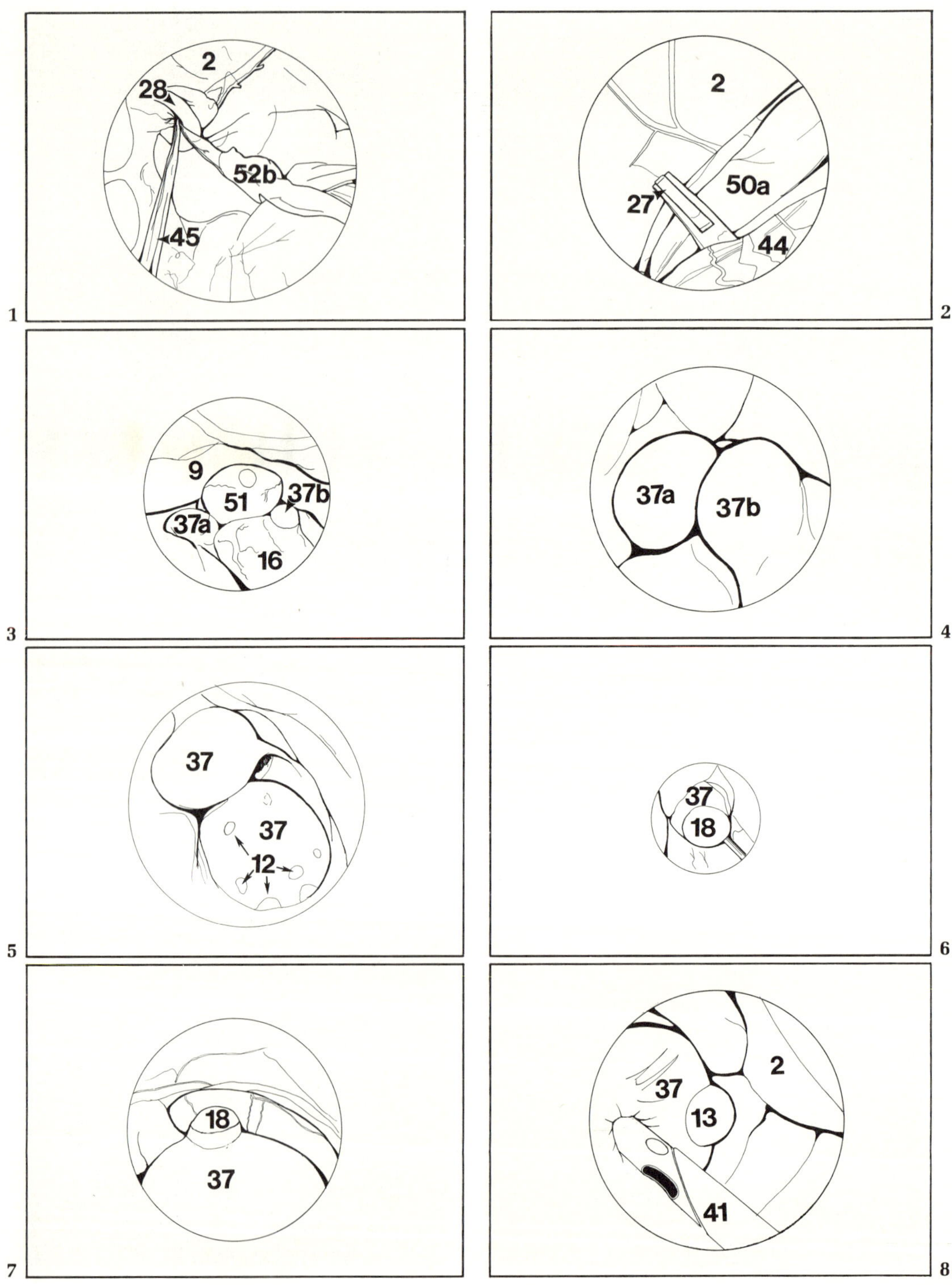

**DIAGRAMS FOR PLATE 3.** **2**—abdominal wall; **9**—bladder; **12**—corpus albicans; **13**—corpus hemorrhagicum; **16**—fat; **18**—follicle; **27**—Hulka Clip; **28**—inguinal ring; **37**—ovary; **37a**—ovary, left; **37b**—ovary, right;
**41**—probe; **44**—small intestine; **45**—spermatic artery-vein; **50a**—uterine horn, left; **51**—uterus; **52b**—vas
deferens, cauterized section.

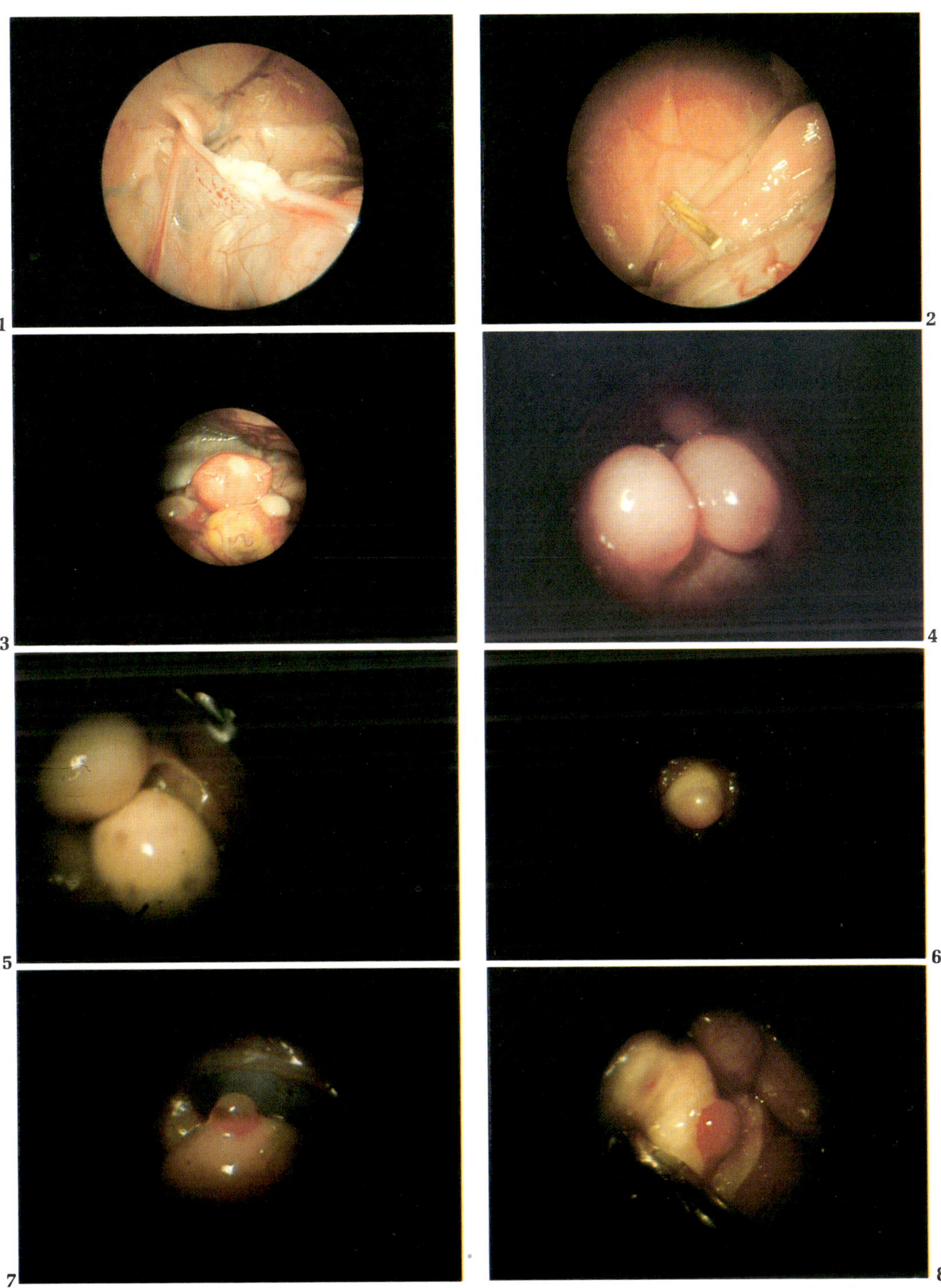

**COLOR PLATE 3. Figure 1.** Cauterized left vas deferens; spermatic artery-vein located laterally (Chapter 3). **Figure 2.** Canine uterine horn occluded with Hulka Clip (Chapter 3). **Figure 3.** Baboon uterus and ovaries (Chapter 4). **Figure 4.** Quiescent squirrel monkey ovaries (Chapter 4). **Figure 5.** Luteal scars on squirrel monkey ovaries (Chapter 4). **Figure 6.** Baboon preovulatory follicle (Chapter 4). **Figure 7.** Early postovulatory squirrel monkey follicle (Chapter 4). **Figure 8.** Corpus hemorrhagicum in the squirrel monkey (Chapter 4).

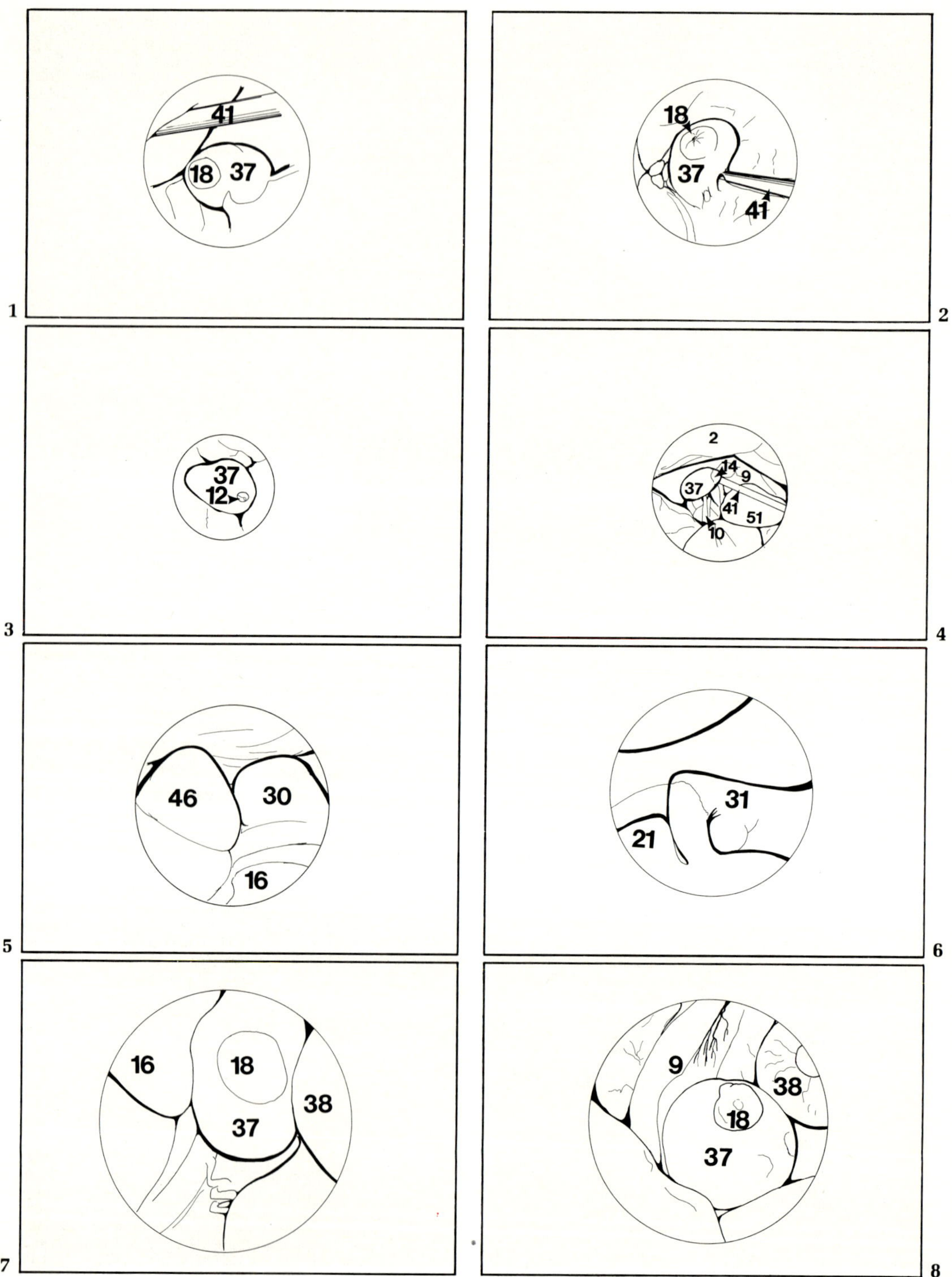

**DIAGRAMS FOR PLATE 4.** **2**—abdominal wall; **9**—bladder; **10**—broad ligament; **12**—corpus albicans; **14**—corpus luteum; **16**—fat; **18**—follicle; **21**—gallbladder; **30**—kidney; **31**—liver; **37**—ovary; **38**—oviduct; **41**—probe; **46**—spleen; **51**—uterus.

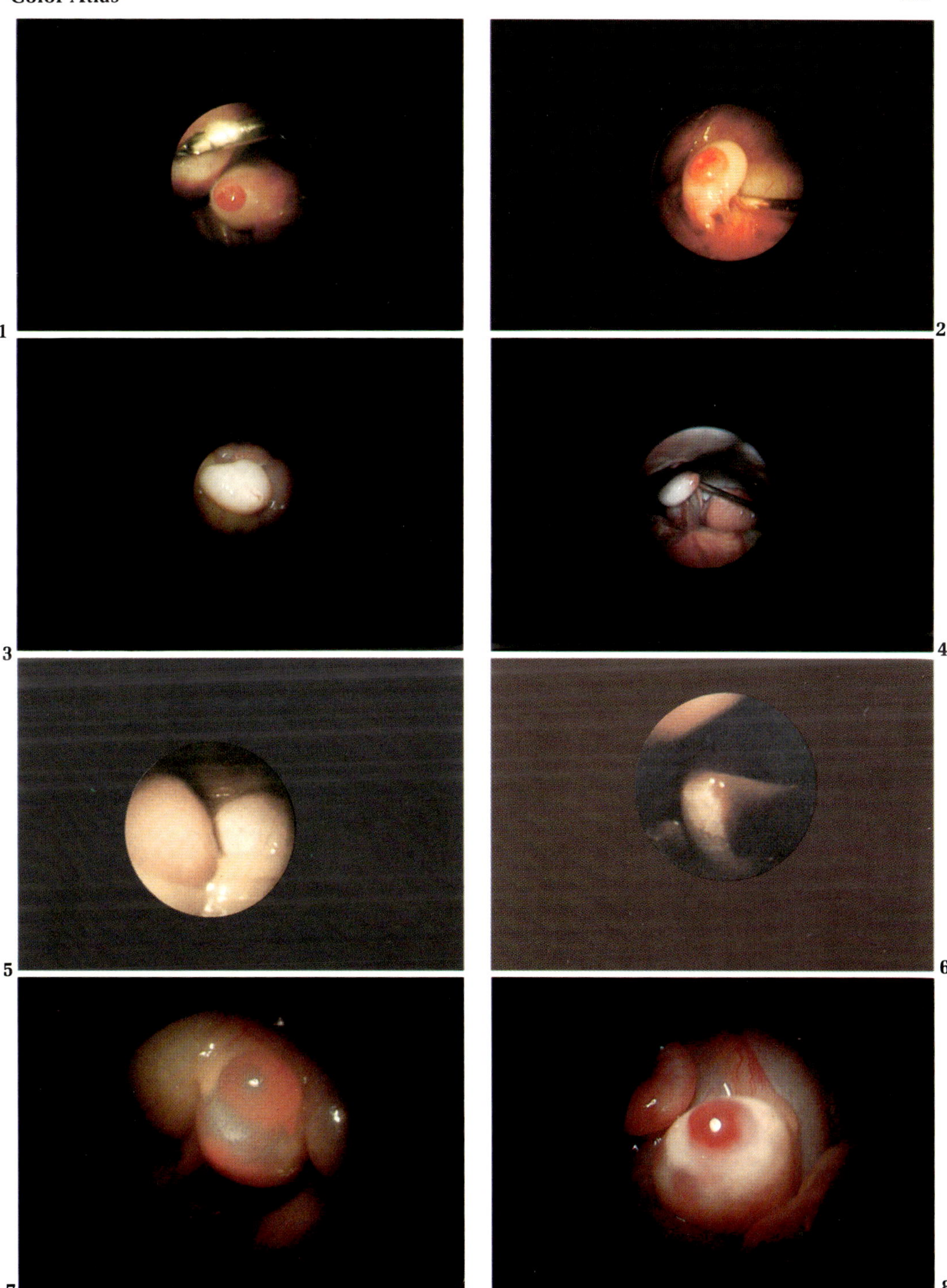

COLOR PLATE 4. **Figure 1.** Early luteinization in a rhesus monkey follicle (Chapter 4). **Figure 2.** Baboon postovulatory follicle cratered and luteinized (Chapter 4). **Figure 3.** Baboon luteal scar (60 days postovulation) (Chapter 4). **Figure 4.** Baboon reproductive tract, including uterus and ovary (Chapter 4). **Figure 5.** Spleen and kidney in *Macaca fascicularis* (Chapter 4). **Figure 6.** Gallbladder and liver in *Macaca fascicularis* (Chapter 4). **Figure 7.** Proestrous sheep ovary containing follicles (progesterone, nondetectable) (Chapter 6). **Figure 8.** Ovine ovary on day of estrus (progesterone, nondetectable) (Chapter 6).

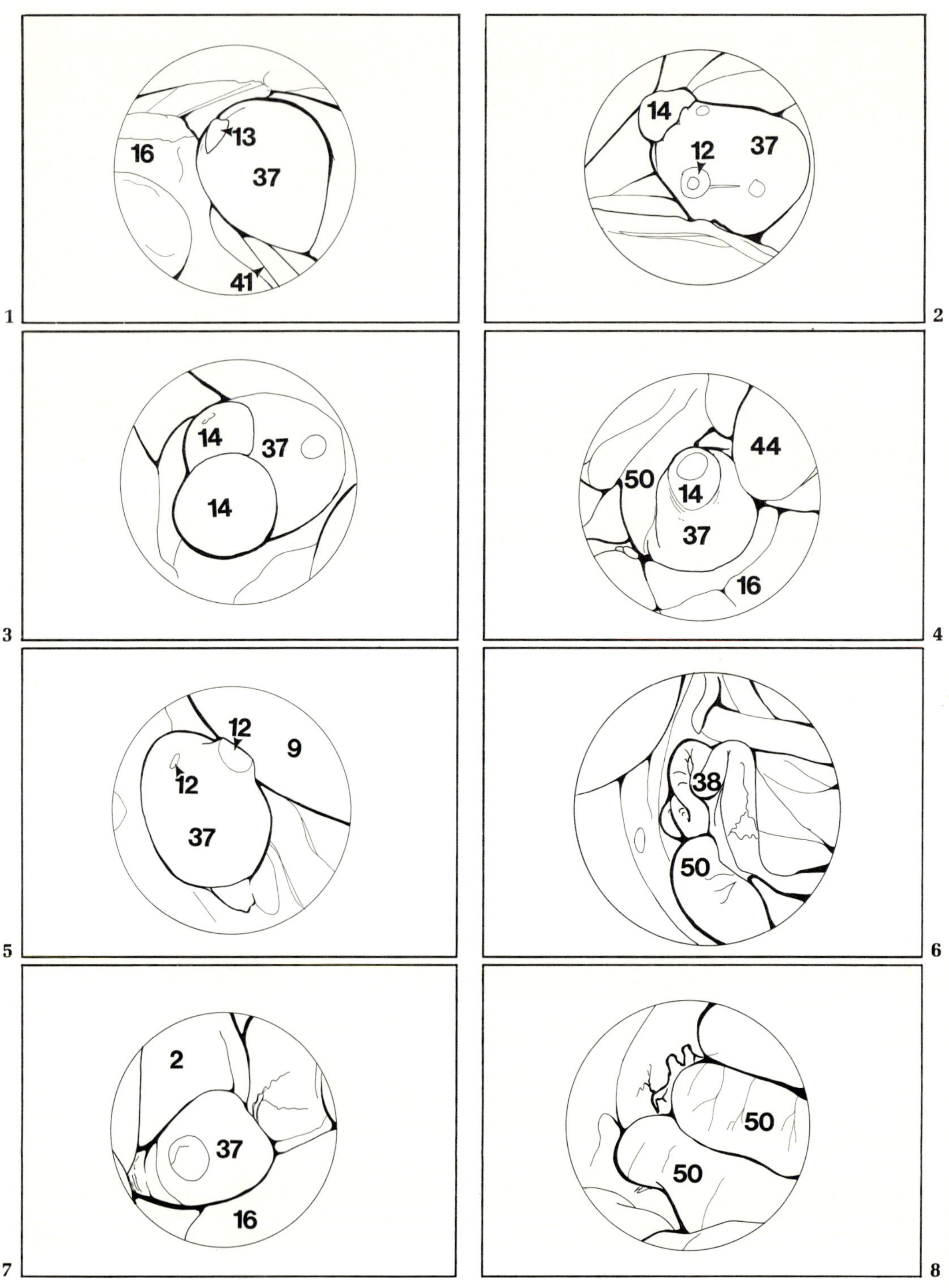

DIAGRAMS FOR PLATE 5.  **2**—abdominal wall; **9**—bladder; **12**—corpus albicans; **13**—corpus hemorrhagicum; **14**—corpus luteum; **16**—fat; **37**—ovary; **38**—oviduct; **41**—probe; **44**—small intestine; **50**—uterine horn.

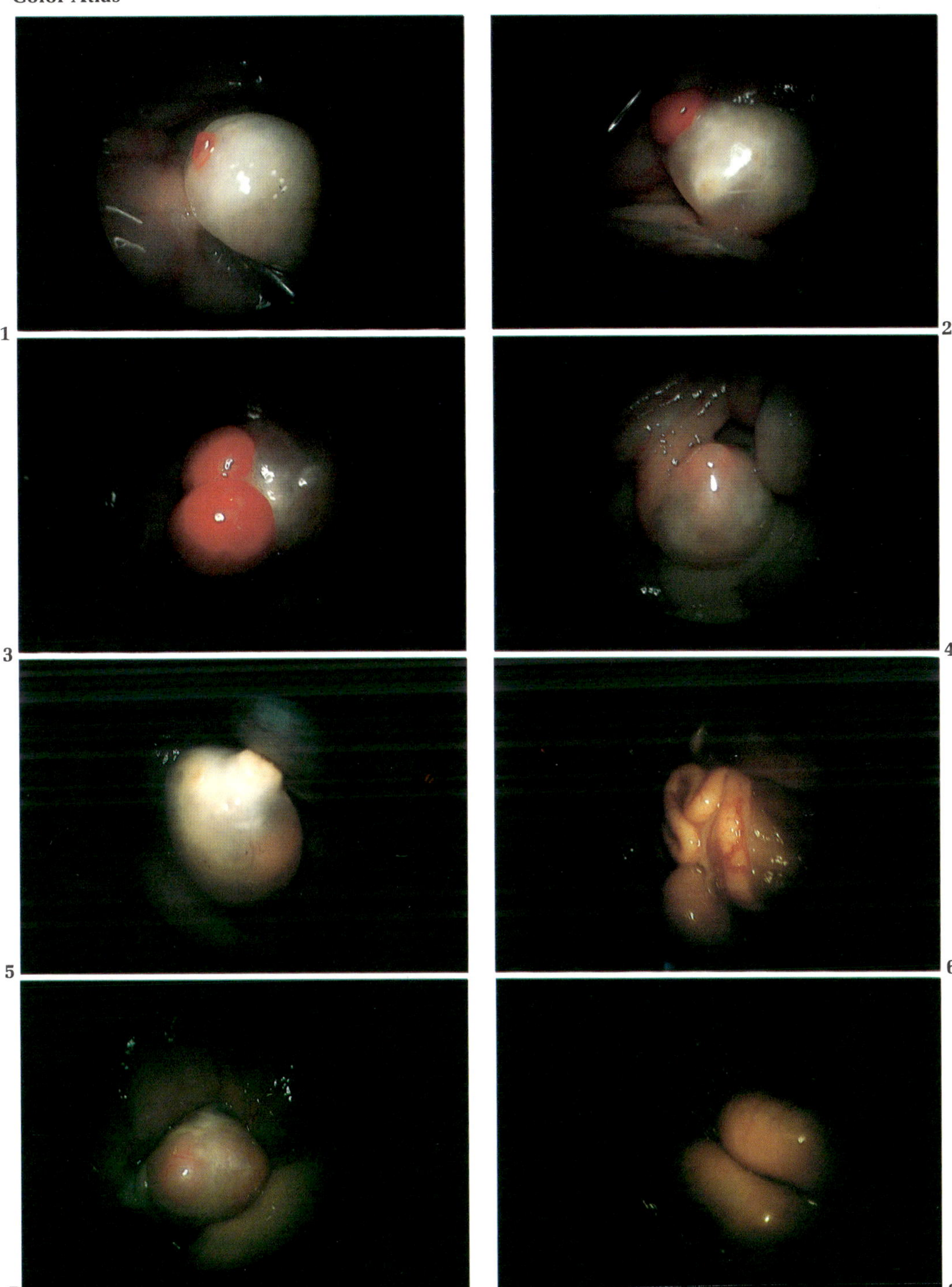

**COLOR PLATE 5. Figure 1.** Ovine ovary one day postovulation (progesterone, <0.1 ng/ml) (Chapter 6). **Figure 2.** Ovine ovary with six day old corpus luteum and luteal scar (progesterone, 0.8 ng/ml) (Chapter 6). **Figure 3.** Ovine ovary with two corpora lutea, six or seven days old (progesterone, 1.8 ng/ml) (Chapter 6). **Figure 4.** Ovine ovary with 12 day old corpus luteum (progesterone, 3.0 ng/ml) (Chapter 6). **Figure 5.** Ovine ovary with 22 day old corpus albicans (Chapter 6). **Figure 6.** Ovine oviduct with blood vessels, tip of a uterine horn (Chapter 6). **Figure 7.** Ovine ovary with corpus luteum, 20th day of pregnancy (progesterone, 1.3 ng/ml) (Chapter 6). **Figure 8.** Ovine nonpregnant uterine horns (Chapter 6).

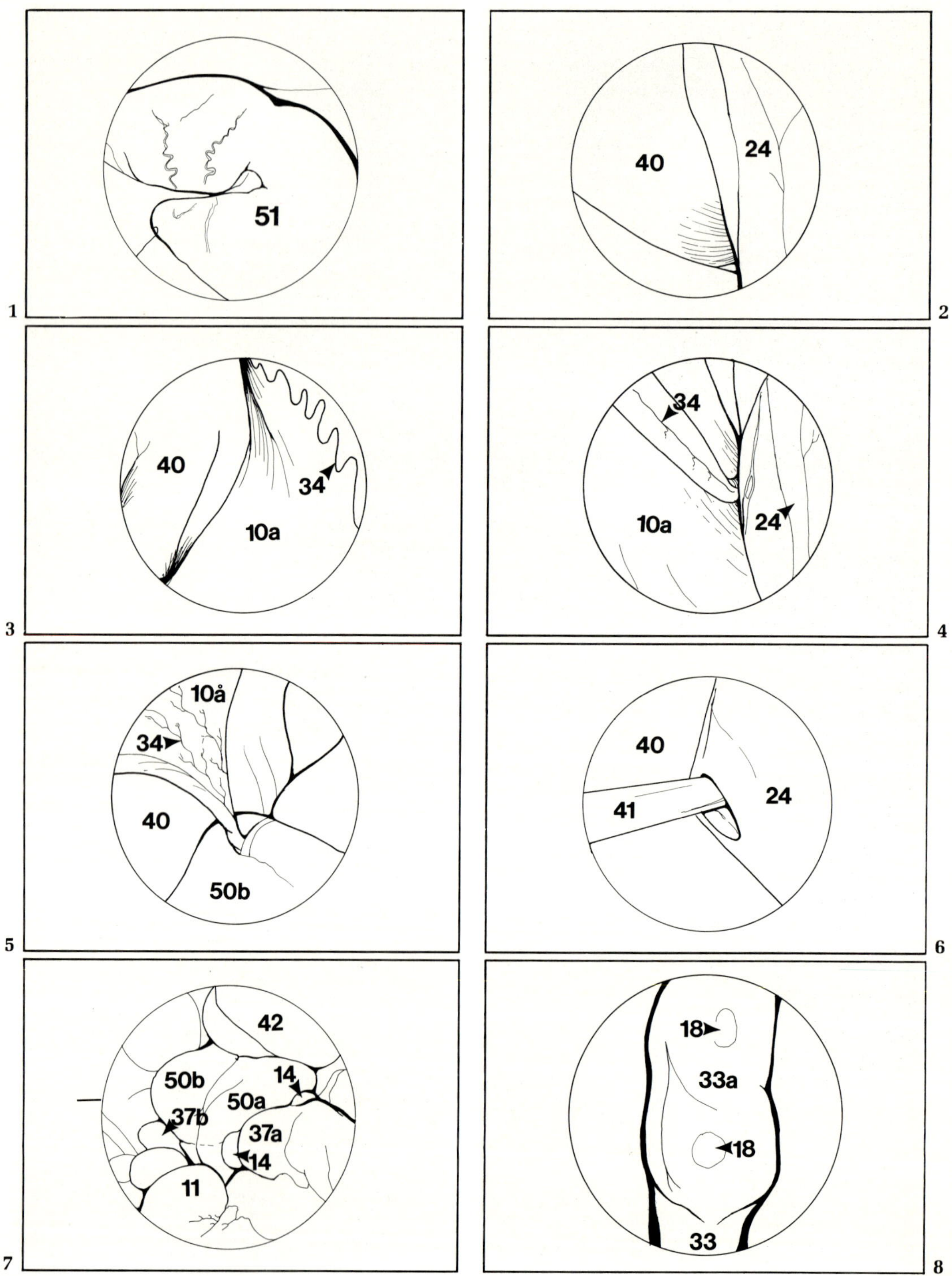


**DIAGRAMS FOR PLATE 6.** **10a**—broad ligament, right; **11**—colon; **14**—corpus luteum; **18**—follicle; **24**—greater omentum; **33**—mesosalpinx; **33a**—mesosalpinx, covering ovary; **34**—ovarian artery; **37a**—ovary, left; **37b**—ovary, right; **40**—parietal peritoneum; **41**—probe; **42**—rectum; **50a**—uterine horn, left; **50b**—uterine horn, right; **51**—uterus.

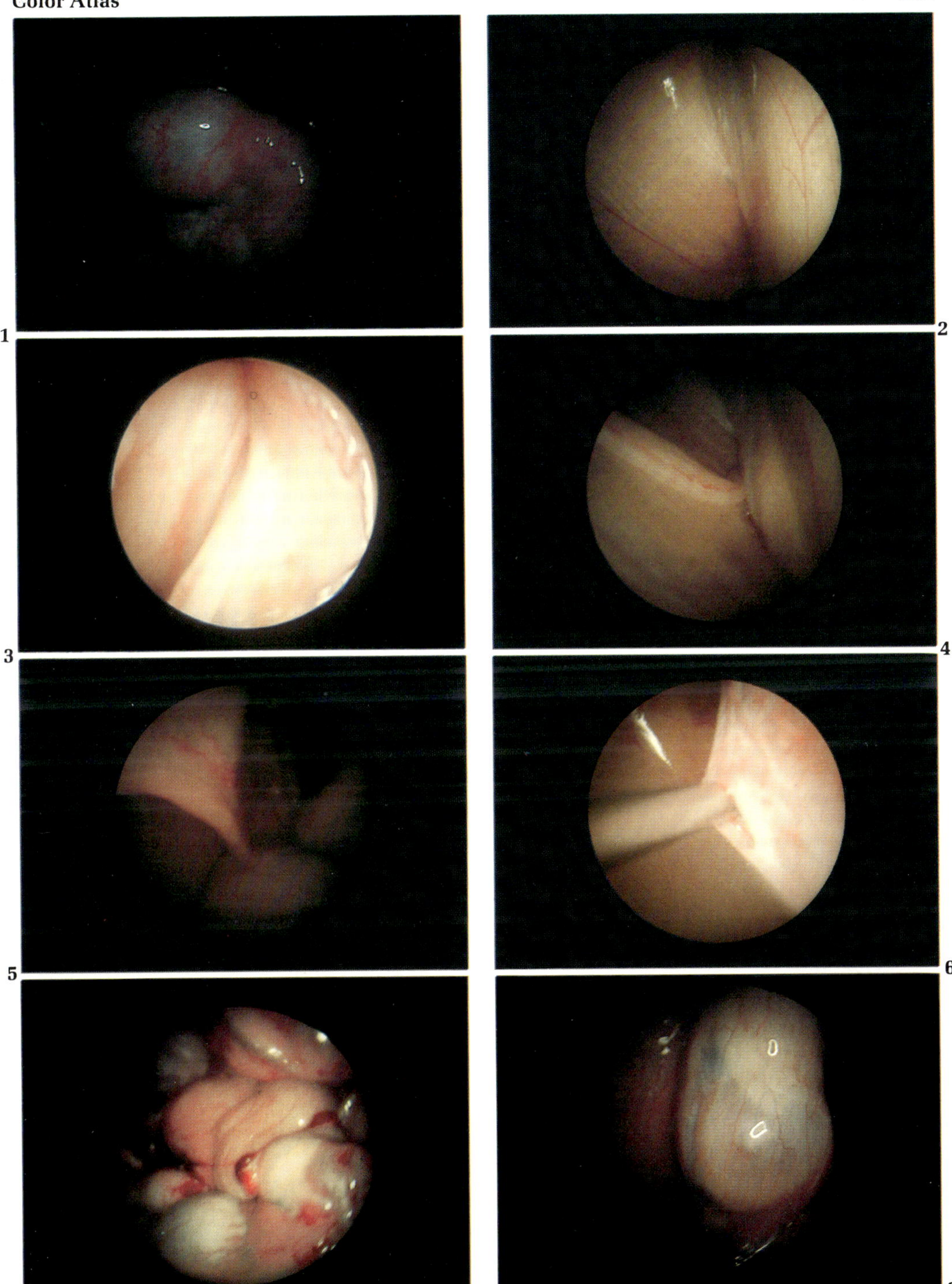

**COLOR PLATE 6. Figure 1.** Ovine pregnant uterus 25 to 30 days of gestation (progesterone, 3.0 ng/ml) (Chapter 6). **Figure 2.** Bovine peritoneal cavity (right approach) bordered by greater omentum and parietal peritoneum (Chapter 8). **Figure 3.** Distal aspect of bovine broad ligament (right approach) (Chapter 8). **Figure 4.** Intermediate aspect of broad ligament (Chapter 8). **Figure 5.** Ventral aspect of broad ligament (Chapter 8). **Figure 6.** Perforation of greater omentum with probe (Chapter 8). **Figure 7.** Bovine reproductive organs following exogenous hormone stimulation (Chapter 8). **Figure 8.** Bovine ovary covered by mesosalpinx (Chapter 8).

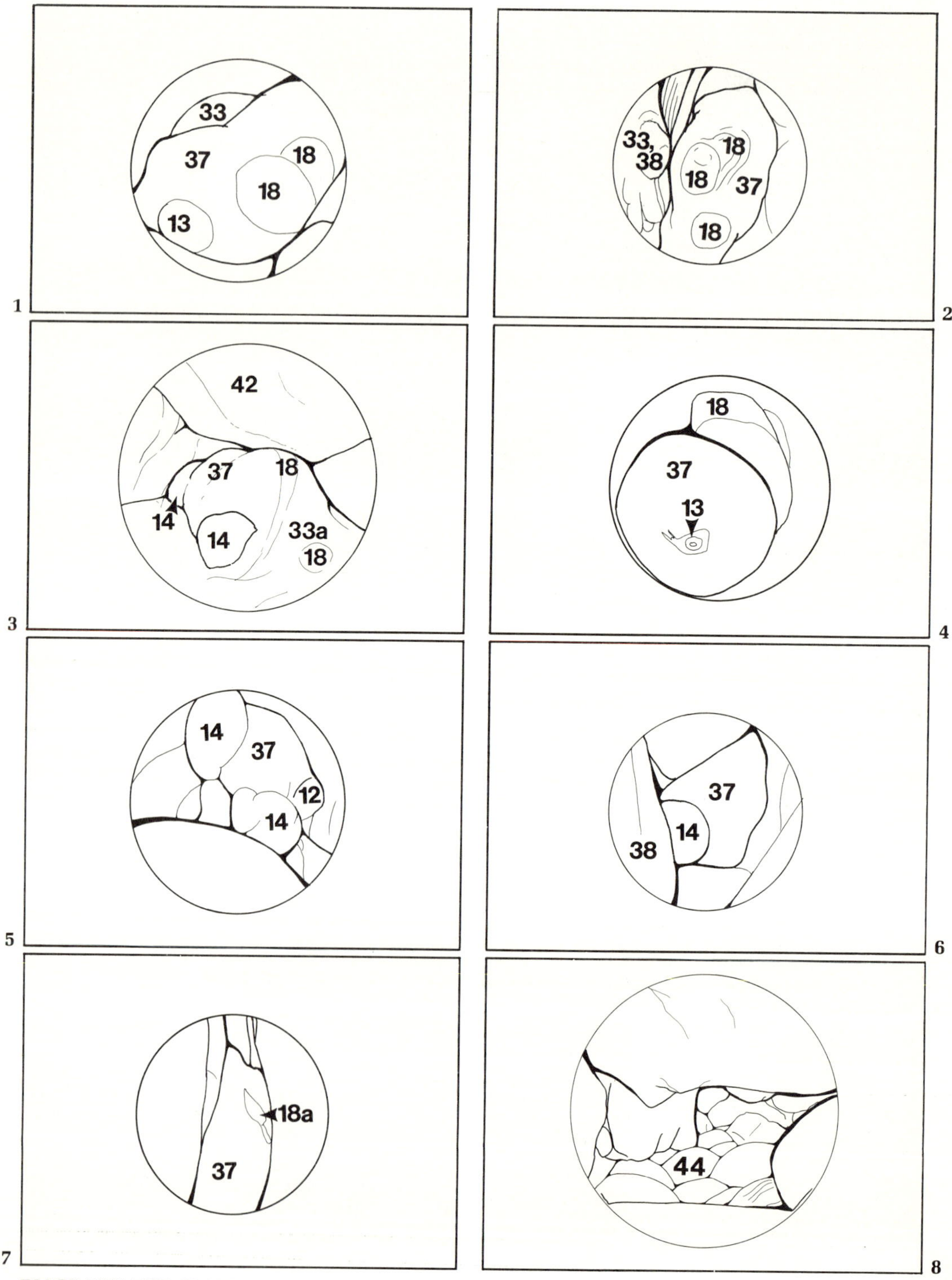



**DIAGRAMS FOR PLATE 7.** **12**—corpus albicans; **13**—corpus hemorrhagicum; **14**—corpus luteum; **18**—follicle; **18a**—follicle, after aspiration; **33**—mesosalpinx; **33a**—mesosalpinx, covering ovary; **37**—ovary; **38**—oviduct; **42**—rectum; **44**—small intestine.

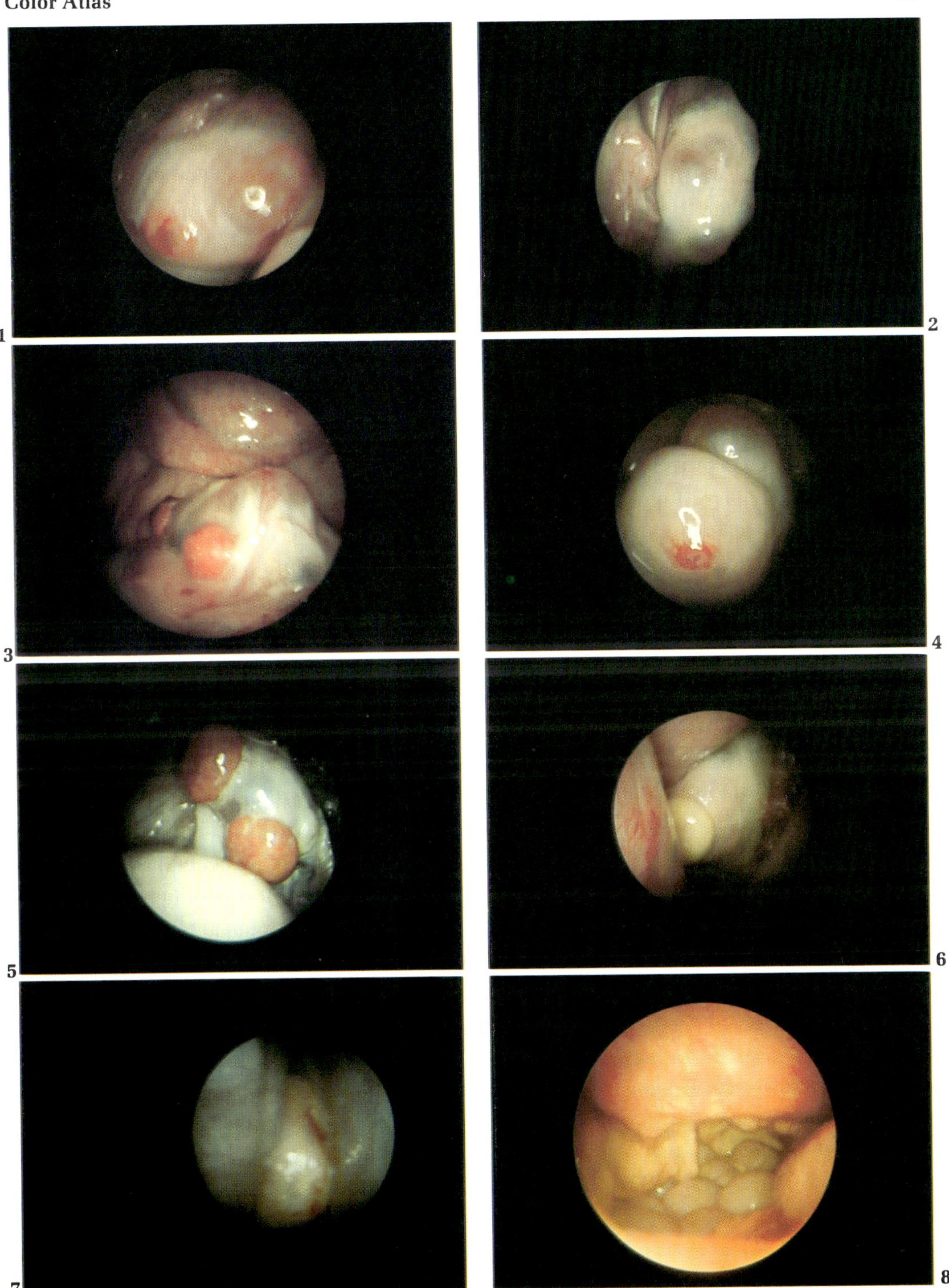

**COLOR PLATE 7. Figure 1.** Follicle and corpus hemorrhagicum on bovine ovary (Chapter 8). **Figure 2.** Bovine oviduct and ovary with follicle (Chapter 8). **Figure 3.** Bovine ovary containing follicles and corpora lutea covered by mesosalpinx (Chapter 8). **Figure 4.** Bovine ovary with corpus hemorrhagicum (Chapter 8). **Figure. 5.** Bovine ovary with two mature corpora lutea (Chapter 8). **Figure 6.** Bovine ovary with regressing corpus luteum (Chapter 8).**Figure 7.** Ovary after collection of bovine oocyte by laparoscopic follicle aspiration (Chapter 8).**Figure 8.** Convoluted small intestine in the horse. (Chapter 9).

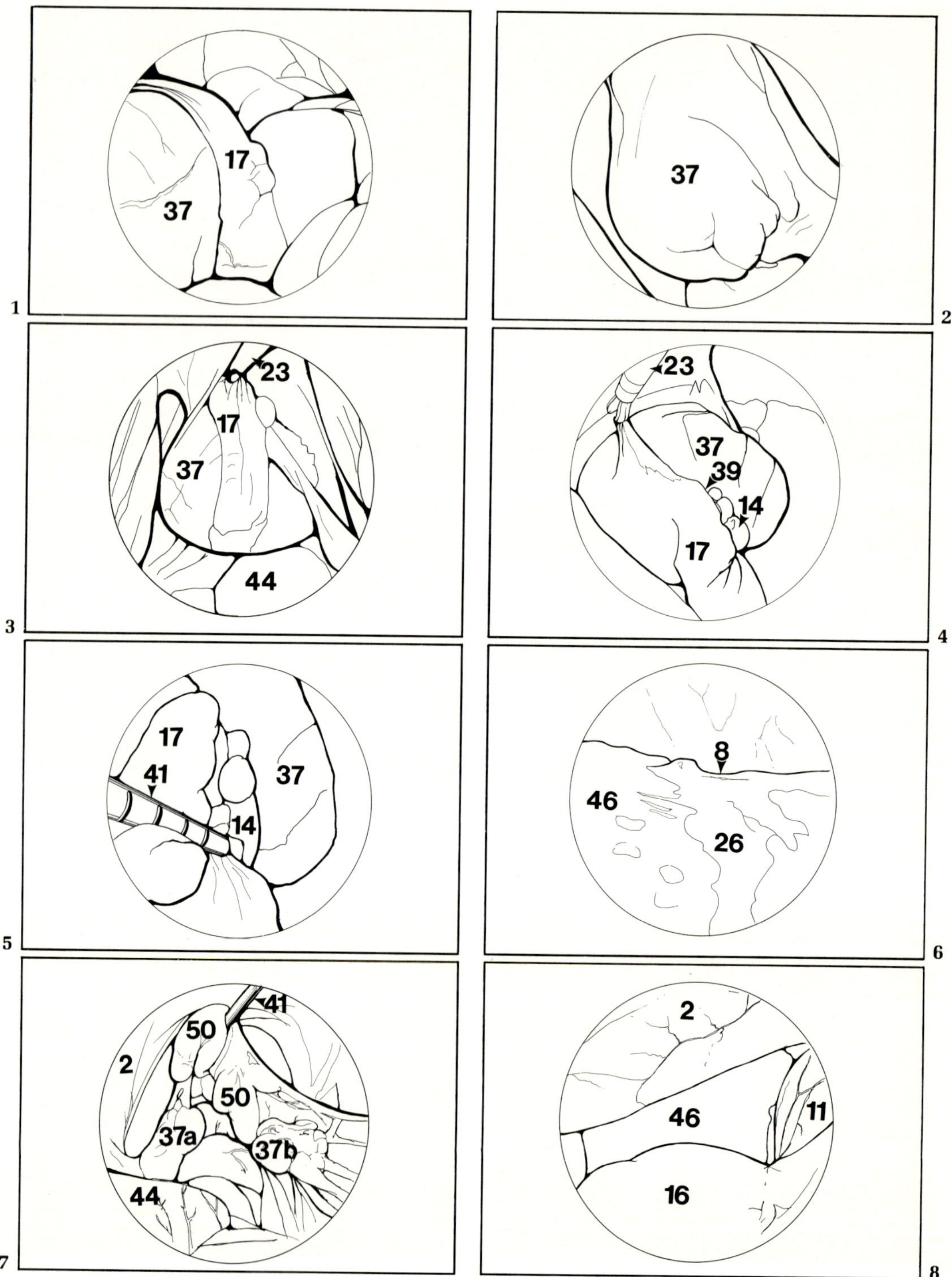

**DIAGRAMS FOR PLATE 8.** **2**—abdominal wall; **8**—biopsy site; **11**—colon; **14**—corpus luteum; **16**—fat; **17**—fimbria; **23**—grasping forceps; **26**—hemorrhage; **37**—ovary; **37a**—ovary, left; **37b**—ovary, right; **39**—ovulation fossa; **41**—probe; **44**—small intestine; **46**—spleen; **50**—uterine horn.

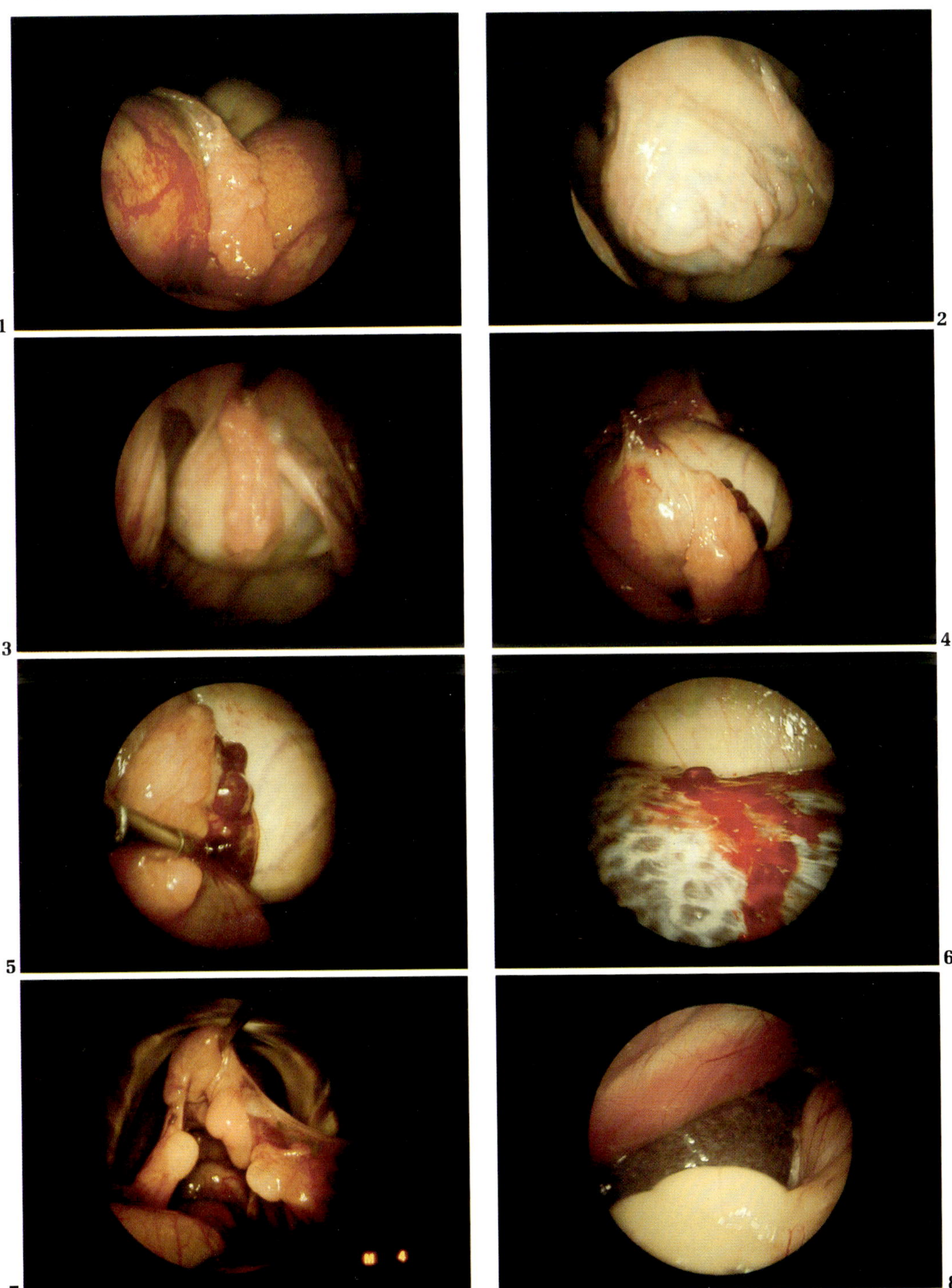

**COLOR PLATE 8. Figure 1.** Fimbria adjacent to equine ovary (Chapter 9). **Figure 2.** Inactive lateral portion of equine ovary (Chapter 9). **Figure 3.** Medial portion of ovary after forceps manipulation (Chapter 9). **Figure 4.** Equine ovary, fimbria, and ovulation fossa containing a corpus luteum (Chapter 9). **Figure 5.** Close-up of equine fimbria and corpus luteum (Chapter 9). **Figure 6.** Equine spleen immediately following biopsy (Chapter 9). **Figure 7.** Uterus and ovaries of a Reeves' muntjac (Chapter 10). **Figure 8.** Spleen of clouded leopard (Chapter 10).

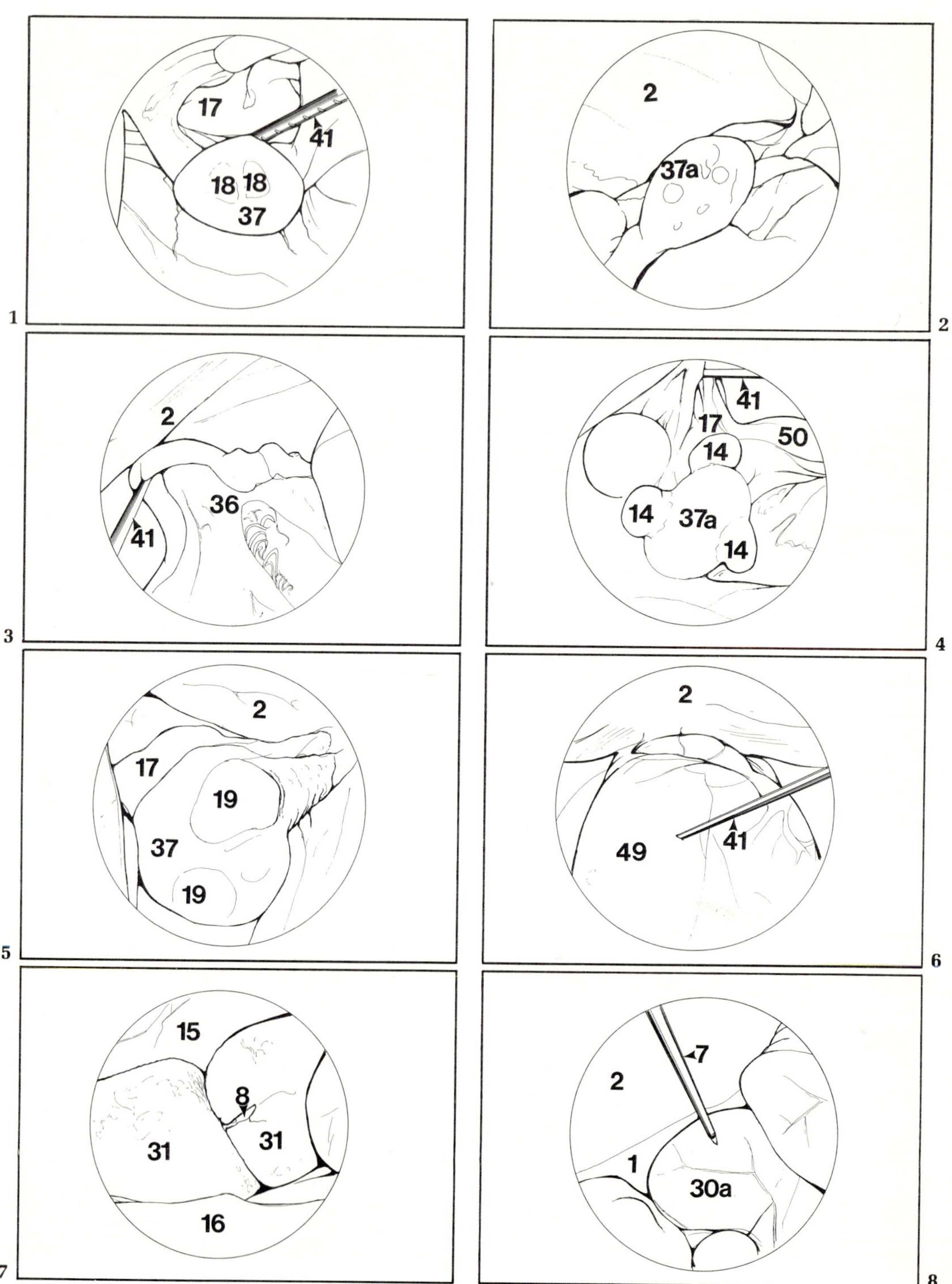

**DIAGRAMS FOR PLATE 9.** **1**—abdominal fluid; **2**—abdominal wall; **7**—biopsy needle; **8**—biopsy site; **14**—corpus luteum; **15**—diaphragm; **16**—fat; **17**—fimbria; **18**—follicle; **19**—follicular cyst; **30a**—kidney, left; **31**—liver; **36**—ovarian bursa; **37**—ovary; **37a**—ovary, left; **41**—probe; **49**—tumor; **50**—uterine horn.

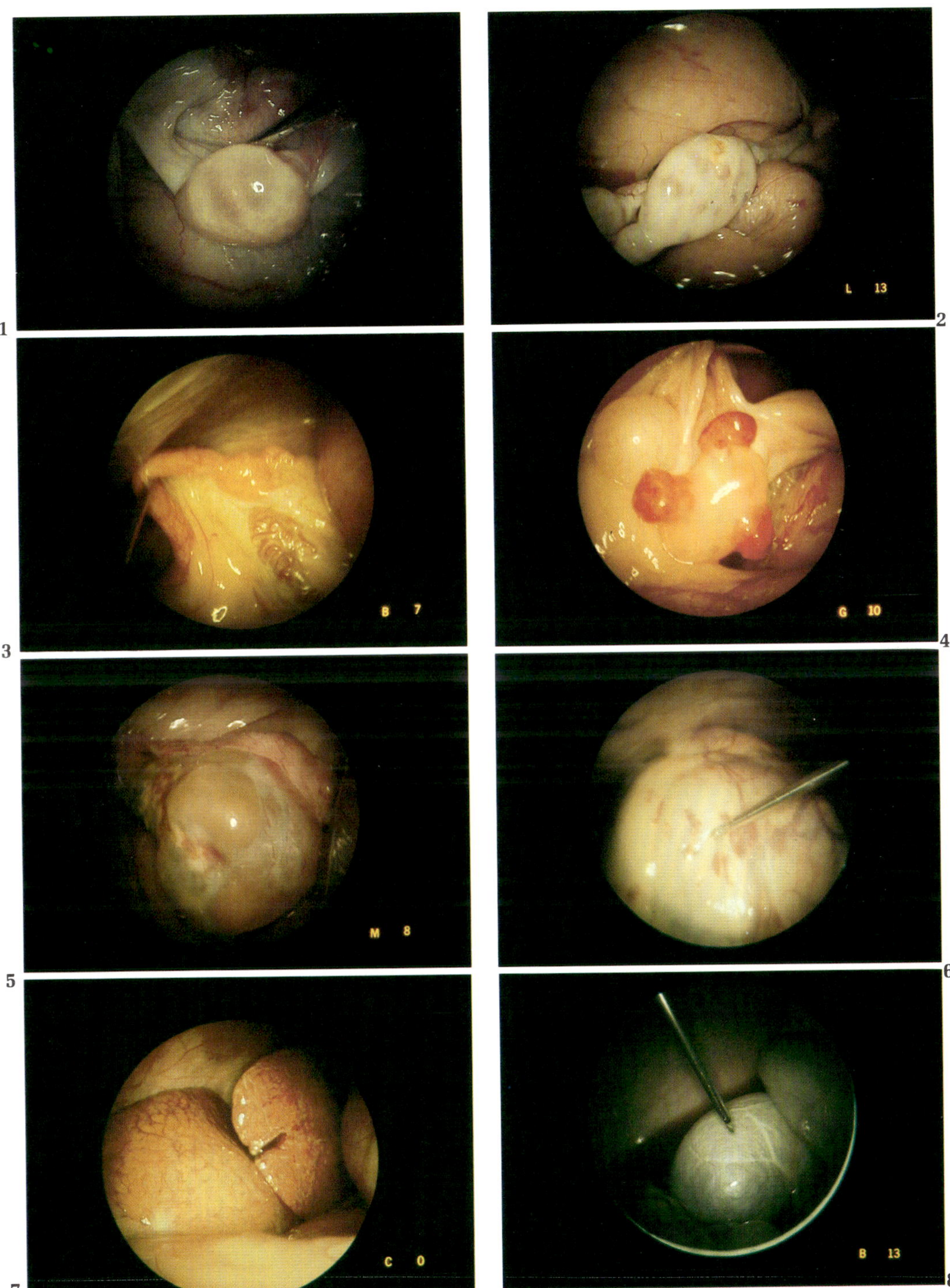

**COLOR PLATE 9. Figure 1.** Mature follicles on the ovary of a jaguar (Chapter 10). **Figure 2.** Ovary of an African lion (Chapter 10). **Figure 3.** Ovarian bursa of a spectacled bear (Chapter 10). **Figure 4.** Ovary of a cheetah following exogenous hormonal therapy; three corpora hemorrhagica (Chapter 10). **Figure 5.** Polycystic ovary of an aged Bengal tiger (Chapter 10). **Figure 6.** Enlarged abdominal tumor in a clouded leopard (Chapter 10). **Figure 7.** Liver of cheetah imediately following forceps biopsy (Chapter 10). **Figure 8.** Insertion of biopsy needle into cheetah kidney (Chapter 10).

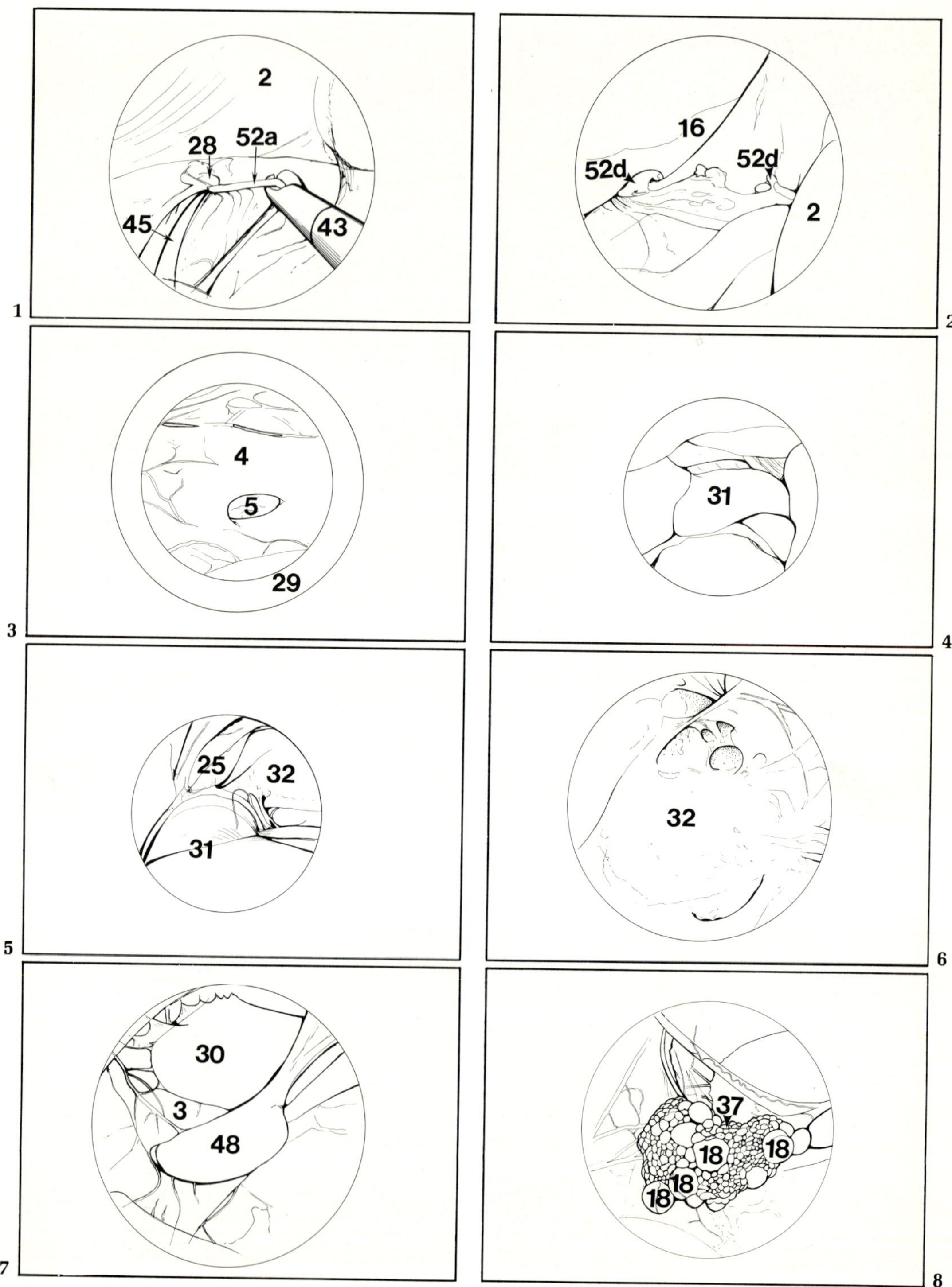

**DIAGRAMS FOR PLATE 10.** **2**—abdominal wall; **3**—adrenal; **4**—air sac membrane; **5**—air sac membrane opening; **16**—fat; **18**—follicle; **25**—heart; **28**—inguinal ring; **29**—inner rim of laparoscopic cannula; **30**—kidney; **31**—liver; **32**—lung; **37**—ovary; **43**—scissors; **45**—spermatic artery-vein; **48**—testicle; **52a**—vas deferens, left; **52d**—vas deferens, severed ends.

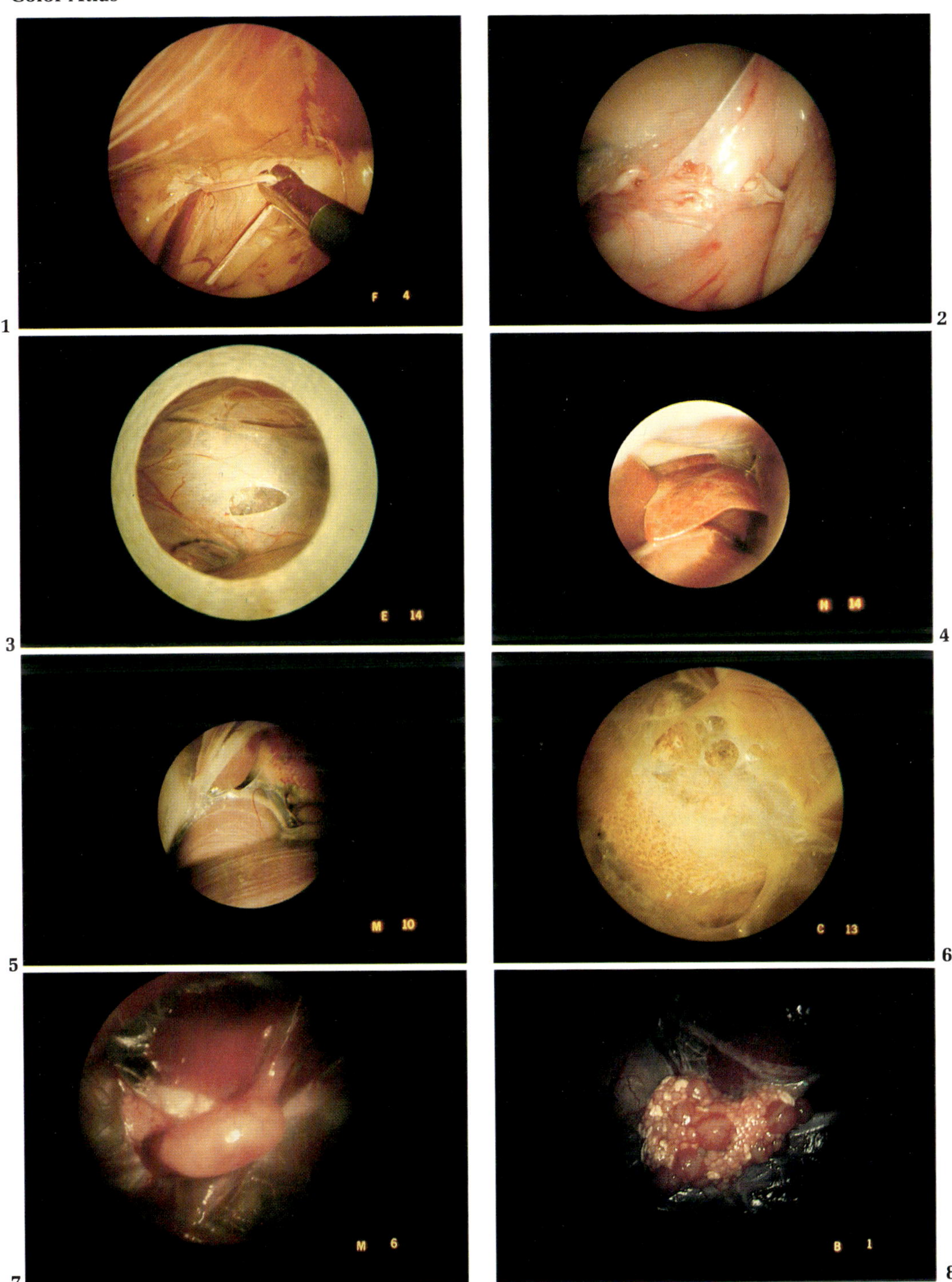

**COLOR PLATE 10. Figure 1.** Internal vasectomy in the crab-eating fox (Chapter 10). **Figure 2.** Separated vas deferens in the lion following laparoscopic vasectomy (Chapter 10). **Figure 3.** Air sac membrane opening in an emu. The laparoscope is passed through this opening to observe the adrenal, gonad, kidney, spleen, and intestines (Chapter 11). **Figure 4.** Liver of pigeon (Chapter 11). **Figure 5.** Heart, lung, and liver of pigeon (Chapter 11). **Figure 6.** Lung of a lesser sandhill crane (Chapter 11). **Figure 7.** Testicle, adrenal, and kidney of a vulturine guinea fowl (Chapter 11). **Figure 8.** Ovary of an adult blue peafowl (Chapter 11).

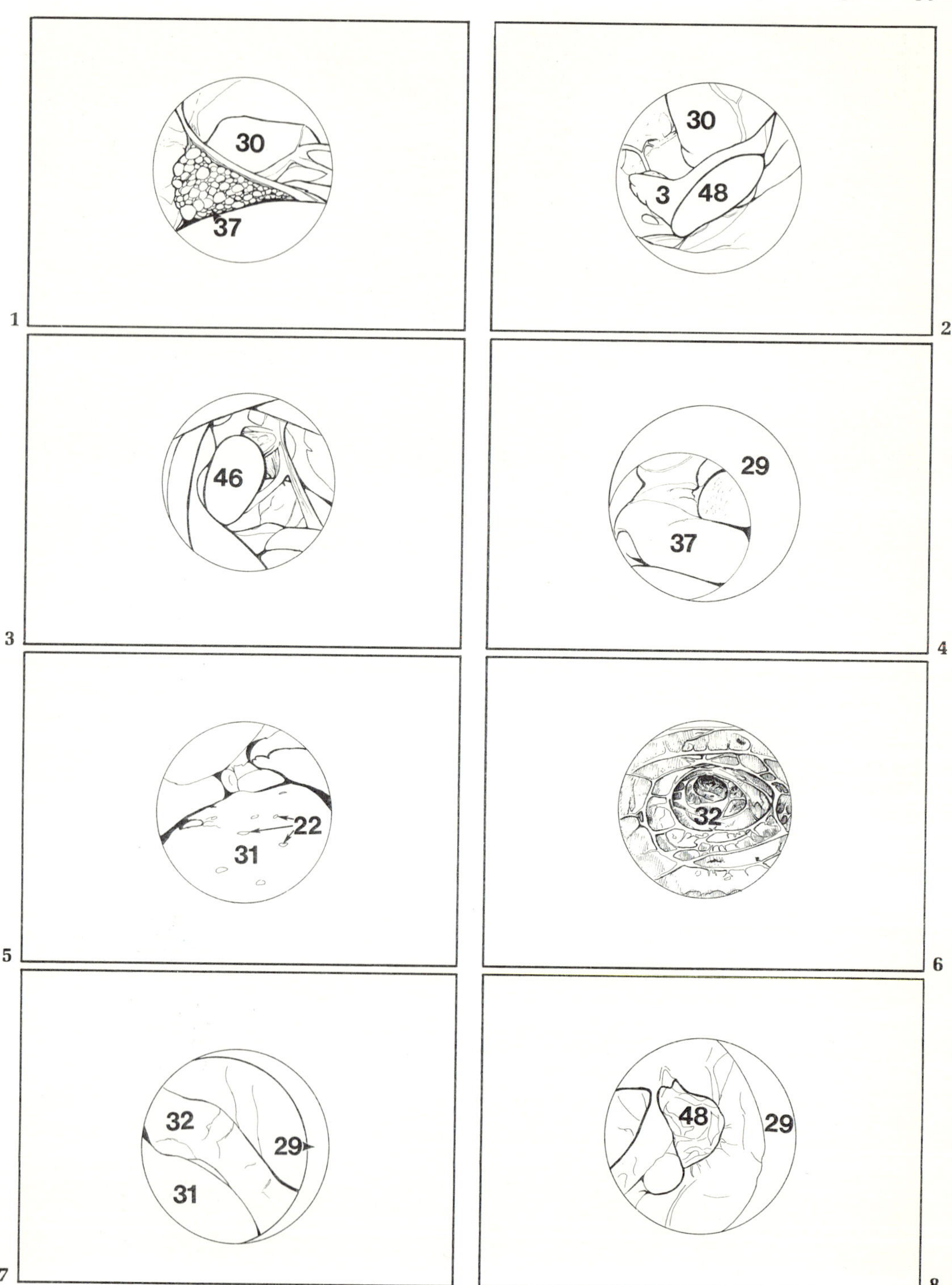


**DIAGRAMS FOR PLATE 11.** **3**—adrenal; **22**—granuloma; **29**—inner rim of laparoscopic cannula; **30**—kidney; **31**—liver; **32**—lung; **37**—ovary; **46**—spleen; **48**—testicle.

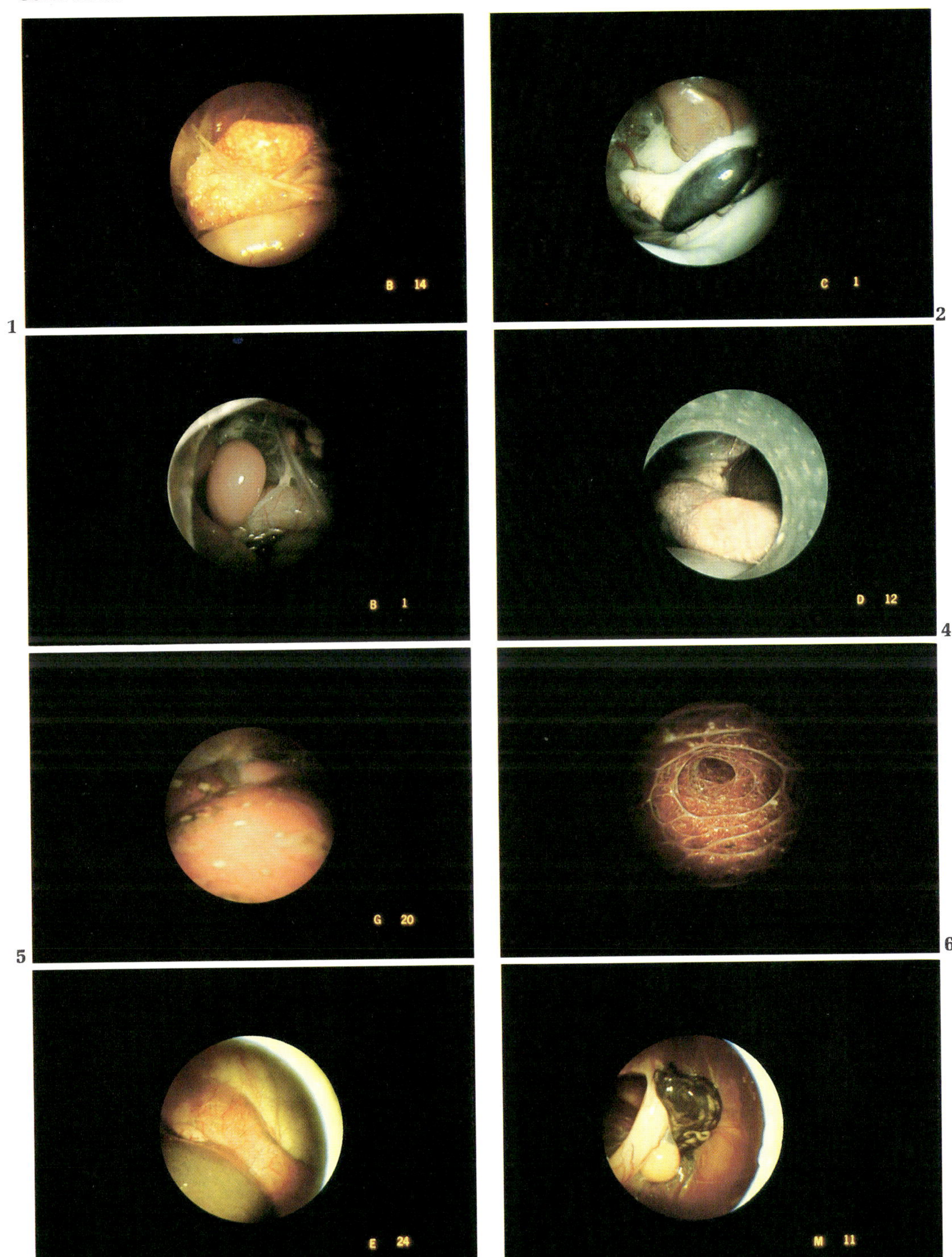

**COLOR PLATE 11. Figure 1.** The ovary and speckled kidney of a turaco (Chapter 11). **Figure 2.** Adrenal, testicle, and kidney of a salmon-crested cockatoo (Chapter 11). **Figure 3.** Spleen of a bare-throated tree partridge (Chapter 11). **Figure 4.** The flat granular surface of the immature ovary of a Patagonian crested duck (Chapter 11). **Figure 5.** Liver of a vulturine guinea fowl with avian tuberculosis; white granulomas on liver surface (Chapter 11). **Figure 6.** Lung of a leopard tortoise (Chapter 11). **Figure 7.** Lung and liver of an adult male box turtle (Chapter 11). **Figure 8.** Testicle of an adult male box turtle (Chapter 11).